# Nurturing Our Wholeness

## Perspectives on Spirituality in Education

Edited by
John (Jack) P. Miller
and
Yoshiharu Nakagawa

Volume Six of the Foundations of Holistic Education Series

Foundation for Educational Renewal

P.O. Box 328, Brandon, VT 05733-0328

# Table of Contents

## Practices

# Foreword

## John (Jack) P. Miller

Recently we have seen increased interest in spirituality in education. Several books have been published (Glazer, 1999; Kessler, 2000; Miller 2000) and *Educational Leadership*, one of the most widely circulated educational journals, devoted an entire issue to "Spirit in Education." Conferences are also being held on this theme around the world.

There are many reasons for this phenomenon. One obvious reason is the wider interest in spirituality in the culture at large. One need only look at the best seller list in nonfiction books. With regard to education the tragic shootings in schools in North America have made many of us look deeper into what really is the purpose of education. Is it merely to develop people to "compete in a global economy" and to achieve on "high stakes" tests? Is it too far fetched to see the link between an education system which stresses competition instead of compassion and the violence and fear in our schools? There is evidence (Peterson, 1998) that the students who committed the shootings were lacking in empathy or the ability to understand another person's feelings. Yet how often do we see compassion or empathy as a stated outcome? When our political leaders talk about education, the rhetoric is almost always about designing more tests rather than about how our schools can develop whole human beings who can think, act and feel.

This book is part of this growing movement which seeks to broaden the dialogue, aims and practices in our schools and other educational settings. Some would say, particularly in the U.S., that you cannot have spirituality in schools because it interferes with the separation of church and state. The Dalai Lama makes a useful distinction here between religion and what he calls secular spirituality. Secular spirituality is primarily concerned with fostering qualities such as wisdom and compassion in human beings. The development of wise and caring individuals should be at the center of our educational system. Unfortunately, we have tended to focus on the transmission of knowledge and the development of individuals who can "compete in a global economy." The student who can meet standards that are connected to competing in the global marketplace has become the primary focus of our educational efforts. The result of this focus is that schools become places where students grimly compete with one another rather than learning the deeper and more lasting values of wisdom and compassion.

## NURTURING WHOLENESS

The aim of education should include the development of the whole person: intellect, emotions, body and spirit. Instead schools now are focusing on a few skills that can be tested. The price we are paying for this narrow vision is huge. We treat our students like products whose only value seems to be their grades and test scores. Starting in Greece, the aim of education in the West was to develop human beings who became *citizens* in the complete sense of that term. Why we have turned back on this vision of our ancestors? What do you think Plato, Shakepeare and Emerson would think of our current obsession with testing? We need to reclaim this vision of wholeness that also can be found in the teachings of the East. To lead us out of our present confusion we need a synthesis of Eastern and Western visions of wholeness and spirituality. For that purpose this book offers a variety of perspectives on spirituality in education.

## TRADITIONS, TEACHERS, PRACTICES

*Traditions*. This book has three sections. The first section discusses various spiritual and religious traditions and their connection to education. Richard Brown, who teaches at Naropa University and is directing a new graduate program on Contemplative Education, has written a chapter on Tibetan Buddhism and how it can be a source for nurturing compassion and wisdom in teachers. Using personal narrative as a format, Sam Crowell has written a chapter on Taoism. Sam explores some basic principles of teaching from a Taoist perspective. Kathleen Kesson has written a piece about the spiritual science of Tantra which is connected to Hindu traditions. Kathleen wrote this chapter after returning from a recent trip to India.

Western spiritual traditions are discussed by Ron Miller and David Purpel. Ron Miller's chapter on the Quaker tradition explores how education can arise from recognizing the divinity within each person. Ron also links Quaker education to other movements and approaches within holistic education. David Purpel writes about the Hebrew prophets and how their approach is still relevant to dilemmas that we face today as educators.

*Teachers*. This is the largest section of the book as there are ten chapters on various spiritual teachers. Again both Eastern and Western teachers are discussed as well as the implications of their teachings for educational thought and practice. Some individuals like Rudolf Steiner specifically designed school curricula while others such as Huxley, Buber and Merton focused on ideas and principles that provide a basis for educational practices.

David Marshak and Karen Litfin have contributed a chapter on Aurobindo Ghose, a spiritual teacher from India, whose ideas have found actualization in the community of Auroville, India. There are several schools in Auroville based on Aurobindo's ideas and Litfin was able to visit these schools on a recent trip to India. Scott Forbes, who taught for many years at Brockwood Park, a school in England based on Krihsnamurti's ideas, has written a chapter on this well known spiritual teacher. Scott addresses the principal ideas that Krishnamurti brought to educational theory and practice. The third Eastern teacher discussed in this section is Tagore. Takuya Kaneda, a professor in Japan who has visited the school in India that Tagore founded, has given us an inspiring description of Tagore's contribution to education.

Two other Japanese professors have contributed chapters to this book. Interestingly they have written about two Western educators, Martin Buber and Aldous Huxley. Atsuhiko Yoshida from Osaka, Japan has explored the ideas of Buber and particularly the concept of "encounter." One of the coeditors of this book, Yoshiharu Nakagawa, has contributed a chapter on the work of Aldous Huxley. Huxley is not well known for his educational ideas but Professor Nakagawa has elucidated a broad spectrum of ideas that Huxley developed with respect to spirituality in education.

The other coeditor, Jack Miller, has written about three 19th century American Transcendentalists, Emerson, Thoreau and Alcott, and their contribution to education. All three of these individuals taught and had a life long interest in education. Thomas Del Prete, who has written a book on Thomas Merton and his educational theory, has contributed a chapter on the Catholic monk who was one of the most important contemplatives of the 20th century.

Finally three European educators are discussed in this chapter. Jeff Kane, editor of *Encounter*, has contributed a chapter on Rudolf Steiner and Waldorf Education. Ron Miller, who was trained as a Montessori teacher, has written a chapter on Maria Montessori from the perspective of her spiritual intentions as an educator. Montessori's work is often viewed from a much more limited perspective than the one that Miller has provided here. Bob London's chapter on J. G. Bennett, who was a student of the Russian mystic Gurdjieff, describes the key principles of his thought. Bob has been working with these principles for most of his adult life and has provided several examples from his own teaching experience of how these ideas can be applied.

*Practices*. Although almost all of the chapters in this book do discuss some aspect of practice, the three chapters in this section have educational practice as their principal focus. All three chapters draw heavily on the authors' experiences as teachers. Rachael Kessler has written a chapter on the erotic shadow in teaching, an unexamined subject to date. This chapter explores an aspect of teaching that has been ignored and even repressed. Rachael has brought her broad range of experience and understanding to this sensitive issue. Lourdes Arguelles' chapter could also have been in the traditions section but we have placed it in this section because she has brought so much of her experience as teacher to her writing. A practicing Tibetan Buddhist, Lourdes describes how she brings some of her spiritual practices into her teaching in a way that nourishes the spiritual lives of her students. Finally, John Donnelly, who has taught students with a variety of emotional, behavioral and physical disabilities at the secondary level for over twenty years, brings this broad experience to his chapter. John makes a powerful plea for compassion and engaged service in teaching.

This book does not include all spiritual traditions. We asked a colleague to contribute a chapter on Native American traditions but the person was unable to do so because of illness. Still we believe that this book provides a variety of perspectives, ideas and educational practices that should help educators who are committed to the education of whole human beings.

## References

Glazer, S. (1999). *The Heart of Learning: Spirituality in Education*. New York: Tarcher/Putnam

Kessler, R. (2000). *The Soul of Education: Helping Students Find Connection, Compassion, and Character at School*. Alexandria, VA: ASCD.

Miller, J. (2000). *Education and the Soul: Toward a Spiritual Curriculum*. Albany: SUNY Press.

Peterson, K. (1998). "Lack of empathy seen as key to spotting trouble." *USA Today*, June 1, p. 6D.

# Acknowledgments

We would first like to thank all of the contributors to this volume. Readers will sense the engagement of each author. Several of the contributors are part of the Spirituality in Education Network, including Lourdes Arguelles, Richard Brown, Sam Crowell, John Donnelly, Bob London, and Jack Miller. The members of this network played an important role in the development of this book not only in terms of their specific contributions, but also in their general support and encouragement.

We thank our two assistants, Constance Lien and Andrè Tremblay, at the Ontario Institute for Studies in Education at the University of Toronto who helped in formatting and proofing the text. Special thanks to Andrè who stepped in to finish the formatting.

We also appreciate very much the work that Charles Jakiela has put into guiding the manuscript through the publication process.

Finally we would like to express our gratitude to Ron Miller for his support for this project. His commitment to Holistic Education has been an inspiration to many of us.

—Jack Miller and Yoshi Nakagawa

# TRADITIONS

# CHAPTER 1

# Taming our Emotions

## Tibetan Meditation in Teacher Education

### Richard C. Brown

Tibetan Buddhist meditation offers a non-sectarian, spiritual practice for knowing and liberating our inner resources, so we can become more effective and compassionate teachers. Meditation, rather than being an escape from the stresses of teaching, is a method for relating more fully and honestly to the learning environment and ourselves. In the process the seemingly mundane and problematic aspects of ourselves and teaching relationships become transformed and sacred.

Over the last thirty years Tibetan Buddhist teachers have established many centers in North America and Europe. Chogyam Trungpa, Rinpoche, in particular, was interested in establishing non-sectarian cultural forms in North America, which could express the qualities of an "enlightened society." Because he was particularly interested in education, in the 1970's Rinpoche founded three non-sectarian schools in Boulder, Colorado: Alaya Preschool, The Vidya School (an elementary and middle school), and Naropa University. During the 1980's elementary and secondary schools were also founded in Halifax, Nova Scotia. With the exception of The Vidya School all of these schools still operate.

During this period I have been a teacher in the "Buddhist-inspired" schools in Boulder. For the past ten years I have been developing non-sectarian teacher education programs based on the principles and practices of Tibetan meditation. The first of these was an undergraduate degree at Naropa University in Early Childhood Education. Recently we

have begun a Masters in Contemplative Education for teachers at all instructional levels.

In this chapter I will use reports from Naropa University undergraduate student teachers' experiences to illustrate particular aspects of contemplative teacher development. I will briefly explore how a meditative
approach to knowing and accepting ourselves can lead to compassionate and effective teaching particularly in situations where "negative"
emotions are present.

Most of the students quoted in this chapter have been meditating for
only two years and are at the very beginning of their teaching careers.
Even so, we will see how the practice of meditation has begun to permeate their student teaching. The effects of meditation are cumulative and
the practice of contemplative teaching is a life-long journey. We are just
beginning to discover what it is to join Buddhist meditation with holistic
teaching.

## THE CONTEMPLATIVE TEACHER

According to Chogyam Trungpa, Rinpoche's view, Buddhism *per se*
was not to be taught in our "Buddhist-inspired" schools, except in
classes on comparative religion. Instead, Rinpoche suggested that we
should manifest the effects of our practice of meditation in our everyday
teaching. This he called "contemplative education," distinguishing it
from religious education, because it is applicable in many educational
settings. This integration of meditative principles and practice into everyday, non-sectarian education is, for me, one of the most intriguing
and personally rewarding contributions of Buddhism to holistic education.

In contemplative education the inner lives of teachers and students
are viewed as vital ingredients in teaching and learning. The primary
method for knowing ourselves in Buddhism is meditation. As Pema
Chodron, an American Buddhist nun and teacher, says: "The path of
meditation and the path of our lives altogether has to do with curiosity,
inquisitiveness. The ground is ourselves; we're here to study ourselves
and to get to know ourselves now, not later...So come as you are. The
magic is being willing to open to that, being willing to be fully awake to
that." (1991, p. 4)

Meditation practice develops precision regarding the elements of our
inner experience. Usually these sometimes-subtle states of mind go unnoticed during our active days. Thoughts, feelings and perceptions are

so intertwined that we are often consciously or unconsciously bewildered and anxious. Teachers may be aware of inner experiences while teaching, but often mask them because they seem tangential or problematic. The complexities and alienation, which result from maintaining a separate inner life, can be very stressful and compromise the quality of education for everyone. Meditation is a method of effectively integrating our inner experience into teaching; and the accumulated knowledge of Buddhist practitioners over the centuries offers a wealth of wisdom regarding the skillful transformation and integration of our inner selves into everyday activities.

Faced with meeting the many needs and demands of ourselves and our students, finding time to nurture inner experience may seem like an impossible luxury. However, by meditating regularly outside of our teaching schedule mindfulness of our inner life emerges and, over time, carries over into skillful and intuitive teaching.

An important aspect of this transformation and integration of inner experience for the contemplative teacher is the process of acceptance or "making friends" with ourselves. Through meditation we begin to notice and respect all that we are, including our foibles, gifts, and the experiences we can't even label. In this often-humbling encounter, we begin to see these elements of experience as inner resources. All of our emotional, intellectual, and physical experiences are relevant to the contemplative journey. When we experience ourselves directly and with compassion, we begin to relax and take our place in the classroom just as we are.

Teachers know that we all carry individual burdens that often hamper effective teaching. When we encounter these in ourselves during meditation, they may be experienced as complex habits that we have learned in the course of our lives. Under the gentleness of the mindful attention and non-attachment of meditation, needless patterns may naturally fall away or be transformed. In this non-judgmental practice we simply notice our momentary experience or habits and let them go with the breath. By mixing the objects of mindfulness with the breath, the elements of our direct experience are infused with spaciousness and, eventually, liberated from habituation. There are no other strategies for the elimination of harmful patterns during meditation. As Trungpa, Rinpoche writes:

> Generally, when the idea of ego is presented, the immediate reaction ... is to regard it as a villain, an enemy. You feel you must destroy this ego, this me, which is a masochistic and suicidal

approach....But true spirituality is not a battle; it is the ultimate
practice of non-violence. We are not regarding any part of us as
being a villain, an enemy, but we are trying to use everything as
part of the natural process of life. (p. 68)

Experiencing ourselves directly and thoroughly means not dismiss-
ing any of our base inner experiences because they don't meet our high
conceptual standards. Among the obstacles that holistic teachers may
encounter are preconceived ideas of what it is to be "holistic" or "spiritual." We can fall into the trap of thinking that spirituality in education is,
perhaps, only evidenced by an inspired, blissful state of mind or an en-
chanting classroom experience. However, Chogyam Trungpa suggests a
more earthy view: "The whole approach of Buddhism is to develop transcendental common sense, seeing things as they are, without magnify-
ing what is, or dreaming about what we would like to be" (p. 4). This
contemplative approach does not identify certain experiences as "spiritual," because the whole of existence is seen as sacred. The practice is to
synchronize with that. In the process of inner exploration, we may discover that our notions of the "spirituality in education" have become so
fixed that we are unconsciously restrictive or hurtful toward certain expressions of natural harmony.

## OPENING TO EMOTION

When we are too firmly attached to what we think education should
be, it is often experienced as aggression not only by our students, but also
within ourselves. Meditation with its practice of precise noticing and
then letting go has the effect of softening our sense of ownership and the
accompanying rigidity. Plans and inspirations that may arise for us as
teachers are transformed by this practice of acceptance and spaciousness. "My" plan, "my" feeling, "my" opinion, "my" theory, are experienced less as possessions of truth than as open, transitory, participatory
creations. Often this radical acceptance of and simultaneous non-attachment to our inner experience, can be a painful, disconcerting, and hum-
bling process, but it is the Buddhist path to compassion.

Because meditation invites our emotional lives to be included in our
practice, we gradually become familiar, relaxed and trusting of our feelings. By learning to experience emotions clearly, spaciously and without
attachment, meditation seems to enhance our natural compassionate,
empathetic and intuitive qualities. Here is an incident from a student

teacher's self-evaluation, which reflects a simple, basic experience of empathy:

> There is a child in my class who is not very verbal. He is often reluctant to speak, and when he does, he usually offers only enough words to get his point across. I watch his strong physical play and feel that he experiences the world this way, a way that is very different than mine. So, on this day, he was on the swings and he asked for a push. As I stood behind him, I watched as he would swing forward and then just as the swing was about to come back, he would arch his body back and close his eyes. His face smiled more than I had ever seen before. As I watched him, I could remember what that felt like, I could feel my stomach do that small flip flop it does, just after the swing stops in mid air to begin its way backwards. The feeling was so overwhelming it brought tears to my eyes... I was truly able to feel the experience this child had. This experience opened up a whole different approach to communication and a new dimension to my relationship with this child.

Teachers are usually expected to be objective, calm, mature mentors and leaders. When we begin, as contemplative teachers, to open to our emotional energies, they are usually experienced as the antitheses of these characteristics. As teachers we can feel guilty or unprofessional when we express, or even notice, strong emotions; we have little training or experience otherwise.

Tibetan Buddhism is unique among spiritual traditions in its depth of wisdom and skillful means related to working with emotion. When neither suppressed nor indulged, emotion is seen as the ground of compassion. Chogyam Trungpa Rinpoche describes this view of transforming emotional energy:

> The intelligent way of working with emotions is to try to relate to their basic substance, the abstract quality of the emotion, so to speak. The basic 'isness' quality of the emotions, the fundamental nature of the emotions is just energy. And if one is able to relate with energy, then the energies have no conflict with you. They become a natural process.... When there is no panic involved in dealing with the emotions, then you can deal with them completely, properly. Then you are like someone who is completely skilled in

his profession, who does not panic, but just does his work completely, thoroughly. (p. 67)

The synchronization that Rinpoche describes energizes our teaching by freeing us from resistance to our emerging emotions. The skill comes when we ride those energies for the benefit of our students.

A student teacher writes about her anxiety and expectations while preparing to teach. Her attention to her feelings and openness to her intuition seem to lead to an experience of effective teaching which is new to her:

> I was nervously preparing myself mentally to lead circle that day. At one point, I decided to let go of all my expectations of how it was supposed to turn out. Suddenly I got an inspiration... I noticed that I seemed more able to be calm and centered in the midst of activity; I was helping each child through their projects, remaining mindful of the environment, attending to a nearby conflict, and focusing on my project all at the same time. I felt coordinated, synchronized and clear! I felt more competent than ever – able to come up with the right words and solutions while thoroughly enjoying myself in the role of teacher. I had finally fallen in [a] smooth rapid groove and caught a glimpse of effective action.

Having the same attitude towards our emotions while teaching as while meditating can be very liberating. As Pema Chodron notes, "Feeling irritated, restless, afraid and hopeless is a reminder to listen more carefully. It's a reminder to stop talking; watch and listen" (1994, p. 115). In this way, 'negative' emotions can wake us up; we can be aware and effective teachers even while miserable. Ultimate generosity in teaching is the willingness to be thoroughly true to what we think and feel and to embody it skillfully and without attachment. This student teacher gives a vivid report of working directly with the energy of strong emotion in herself and a child:

> I have lots of difficulty allowing myself to feel irritated when with the children. I think there is an underlying feeling that it is wrong to feel irritation towards children and that I should be able to accept them fully and in a non-judgmental way. This sounds great but in reality is very difficult. To be able to come into the classroom fully and truthfully I need to be able to acknowledge anger and irritation in myself. There is a particular

child in our classroom who has taught me a lot about this energy and I have become much more able to work with it because of him. This child has an incredible temper and he is very intense in the way that he deals with things. As I worked with him I began to realize that my fear of becoming angry or irritated had a lot to do with being afraid of not being liked by the children if I wasn't always 'nice'. As I continued to work through situations with this child I began to be able to let go of that fear and count these emotions among the many other tools I work with. I found that if I acknowledged these feelings that I didn't even need to go to a place of anger or annoyance but was able to use them to cut through the situation in a much cleaner way than if I tried to be 'nice' about it.

## HARMONIZING WITH EMOTIONAL ENERGY

Experienced teachers are prepared for strong emotions in learning environments. Usually we notice emotions only when they are fully manifest in our students or ourselves. At that point we might forcefully plow ahead or abandon the situation altogether, causing confusion or anxiety. When we don't synchronize with emotional energies, we give mixed messages, become heartless or actually cause harm. In contemplative learning communities where ego-based agendas are naturally exposed, we make friends with emotions and are less likely to be reactive towards our students or ourselves when strong feelings emerge.

Through meditation practice we can begin to notice precisely when emotions begin to arise, feel their qualities, and notice their passing away. When we are present with our emotional experience, yet hold it very lightly, our ownership begins to loosen. There is a spaciousness and creativity when there is harmony with emotional energy. Rather than *having* an emotional experience we *participate* in an energetic experience.

> I remember one incident where a little boy was having a temper tantrum. There were two teachers slowly moving towards him and trying to talk to him. When they got close he would try to hit or kick them. I could see that he was lost in his own emotions and I remember knowing that he needed to be held. I was a little anxious to do anything because I didn't want the other teachers to feel I was stepping on their toes. He continued to cry until I finally decided to do something. At first, I sat down next to him for a few minutes, then slowly, I moved closer and picked him up. He was still crying really

loud so I carried him outside. I remember feeling his face nuzzle into my neck and his warm tears running down my shoulder. In that moment I could completely feel his sorrow. This situation really helped me to trust my own abilities and to trust that genuine action arises when I am really present with what is going on.

The Tibetan teacher Tarthang Tulku summarizes the Buddhist approach to transforming strong emotion, in this case anger:

> What we can do is concentrate on the anger, not allowing any other thoughts to enter. That means we sit with our angry thoughts, focusing our concentration on the anger — not on its objects — so that we make no discriminations, have no reactions.... Concentrate on the center of the feeling: penetrate into that space. There is a density of energy in that center that is clear and distinct. This energy has great power, and can transmit great clarity. To transform our negativities, we need only to learn to touch them skillfully and gently. (p. 52)

In this report a student examines her own negativity and its relationship to the negativity of a child. This insight changes her teaching approach with this child:

> There was one particular child that I had a difficult time with. The main and only way that it seemed he had to connect with people was to intimidate them. This was especially hard for me to deal with because I would be watching a group of children playing and he would come and try to purposely destroy the game that they had going. I felt that the teachers were constantly taking him aside, making him take a break, or losing patience with him. I also discovered that he definitely intimidated me. He was such a bright little boy that I felt useless as I tried to talk to him. Usually he would just laugh at me or roll his eyes. Insecurity and hopelessness would sometimes overcome me and I would be so shocked at how much this boy could affect the other children and myself.

> I decided to watch with 'curiosity' to see what I could do to change the interactions that we were having and how to end the negativity within myself... I was shocked to find that the only interactions I had had with him in the past were negative... I

started to engage with him and ask him about things that were of interest to him. He was so responsive and we ended up forming a friendship. I was able to witness my anger and frustration transform into curiosity and compassion.

## THE INTENTION OF COMPASSION

As the Dalai Lama points out, simply the intention of compassion itself can make a difference in relationships:

> If you approach others with the thought of compassion, then that will automatically reduce fear and allow openness with other people. It creates a positive, friendly atmosphere. With that attitude, you can approach a relationship in which you, yourself, initially create the possibility of receiving affection or a positive response from the other person. And with that attitude, even if the other person is unfriendly or doesn't respond to you in a positive way, then at least you've approached the person with a feeling of openness that gives you a certain flexibility and the freedom to change your approach as needed. (p. 69)

On the path of contemplative teaching we develop clarity and respect for what is happening in the moment, even when it is painful. Awareness through meditation not only leads to self-knowledge and acceptance, but also the integration of emotional energies into learning relationships. When we are open to the changing emotional energies of our students that usually produces an opening or directness on their part. In those moments there can be real connection, communication and discovery. When we honestly and compassionately manifest who we are, without attachment, we can experience ourselves and our students as ordinary *and* sacred. Such a genuine meeting of hearts and minds naturally gives rise to effective teaching and learning. This is education without aggression — education not based upon fear, rigidity or control, but upon uncovering, exploring and creating a sacred world.

## REFERENCES

Chodron, P. (1994). *Start Where You Are: A Guide to Compassionate Living*. Boston and London: Shambhala.

Chodron, P. (1991). *The Wisdom of No Escape and the Path of Loving-Kindness*. Boston and London: Shambhala.

Dalai Lama & Cutler, H. C. (1998). *The Art of Happiness: A Handbook for Living*. New York: Riverhead.

Thartang T. (1978). *Openness Mind*. Emeryville, CA: Dharma Press.

Trungpa, C. (1976). *The Myth of Freedom and the Way of Meditation*. Berkeley and London: Shambhala.

**CHAPTER 2**

# The Spiritual Journey of a Taoist Educator

## Sam Crowell

Ashley Montague once told me that ultimately "we teach who we are." Increasingly, I believe this to be true. Who I am and how I teach is woven together by the tapestry of my life's experiences and, I believe, by the ultimate quality of my commitments. We all journey through life trying to find our way. Sometimes it seems that all we do is coast along. Sometimes we feel the struggle of wondering which way to go. But whatever the nature of our wandering, this journey is ultimately a human struggle that has been present since the dawn of our history. Even if we are raised in a particular tradition, at some point it is likely that we will question its substance and application to our life. This process can't be done by anyone else. We stand alone as we measure the course of our lives.

Carlyle (Needleman, 1982) suggested that the paths we choose define us. "The thing a person does practically lay to heart . . . concerning one's vital relations to this mysterious universe, and one's duty and destiny there, that is in all cases the primary thing for him or her, and creatively determines all the rest" (p. 11). A path in this sense is not just a set of beliefs, rather it represents what we are willing to commit to as we live out the practical aspects of our lives. At least for me, the journey I've taken and the path I've chosen have had significant implications not only for my life but for my work as an educator. Our inner and outer worlds are constantly interacting to shape the person we become. As Jacob Needleman puts it, "We are meant to live in two infinities at once — one leading us outward toward action in the world around us; the other calling us to open ourselves to the world within us" (1996, p. 15). The "world within us" is not just a psychological profile but includes the spiritual essence of our lives.

"Spirit" literally means "breath." It refers to the source of life and to the source of all the tangible manifestations of life that we perceive. Spirituality in education is an awareness of the inner narratives of our lives and the inherent connectedness to the larger narratives of life. It is a recognition, or perhaps a remembrance, of the origins of our humanity, that special connection that we share with each other and with nature itself. It is a deep awareness of the questions that cannot be explained by material philosophies and that go beyond our neat answers and concise explanations.

Somehow we have chosen not to integrate these concerns into the fabric of our schools. But what are the consequences of not addressing the needs and questions of the human spirit? Both teaching and learning are part of our very humanity. They must somehow address who we are, not just what we know. Knowing cannot be isolated from a sense of self or from a sense of meaning and purpose. Thomas Moore (1992) said it well: "As long as we leave care of the soul out of our daily lives we will suffer the loneliness of living in a dead, cold, unrelated world. We can 'improve' ourselves to the maximum, and yet we will still feel the alienation inherent in a divided existence. We will continue to exploit nature and our capacity to invent new things, but both will continue to overpower us, if we do not approach them with enough depth and imagination" (p. 282). If teaching and learning are extricated from who we are as individuals, from our hopes and dreams, from our visions of a different kind of world for ourselves and our children, and from our belief that there is a special significance to each of our lives, then it will be doomed as a sterile activity with only short-term, instrumental purposes. I submit that all education should be "spiritual."

In sharing myself through this essay, I hope not to be self-indulgent or to set myself up in any way as an example of what anyone else should be. Each of us has a spiritual story that gives insight to our own journey through this life and that returns us to those things we perceive to be most significant — that which informs the very nature of who we hope to be. By taking this approach, I hope to reconnect each of us to the spiritual paths we have chosen and how these paths become manifested in our work. I also hope to provide some insight into Taoism and how it has influenced me as an educator. I do not claim to be a Taoist scholar or to be a master of any path. Nor do I claim that my path is right for anyone else. I only claim to be a traveler.

## MY JOURNEY

Early in life I felt deeply connected to the unseen, intangible qualities of life. This sense of connection has taken different twists and turns over the years but it has been the central theme of my life. As a youth and an adolescent, I was deeply committed to the Christian faith. The example of Jesus as an incarnation of love was the preeminent guide in my life. The Bible was a source of inspiration and understanding for me.

By the age of fourteen I was asked to give sermons at our church. Before I was twenty, I had preached in churches ranging in size from 50 to 2,000, I had spoken on radio and television, and I had gone outside the country to serve in various missions. By twenty-one, I was ordained and served as a church minister.

My thinking during this time was framed by a conservative understanding of the Bible, but as I look back over my sermons, they are surprisingly free of themes of fear, punishment and intolerance. The message that I preached was one of love and service, of inner peace and fulfillment, of purpose and meaning.

As I became more of a student of the Bible, I was able to see deeper messages, understand the historical contexts and perceive some of the symbolic and mythical aspects that expanded my thinking. As I translated parts of the New Testament from the original Greek, I was particularly drawn to the distinction between belief and commitment. It is the notion of "belief" that is so emphasized in most religions. The word "pisteos," however, which is usually translated as belief, more accurately means commitment. The verb form is often used, giving an active sense of the word "am committing." There is the idea that a life of the spirit is an on-going process of "becoming committed," of continuing to deepen the spiritual essence of our life, and how we manifest that in the world. This distinction had a great effect on me. I became less and less interested in the primacy of creed and dogma and more interested in the tangible ways that the loving example of Jesus could be manifested in the world.

Increasingly though, I could not accept the path I was on and the inevitable direction it would take me. Ironically, the God-language no longer spoke to my heart but rather, made it difficult for me to entertain ideas of a higher truth. First I rejected my denomination; later, I abandoned the

Christian faith as well. My decision to break from the Christian tradition was not just an intellectual exercise for me, it affected my entire identity and source of meaning.

Although I rejected the creed and dogma of Christianity, I did not reject its higher themes. I realized though that I would need to reconstruct a meaning system for myself that could articulate the truths I felt deeply in my heart and soul. I had no idea what new path to follow and delved into the classical writings of many spiritual traditions. Each filled me with uncertainty and doubt.

During this time I was introduced to systems theory. I resonated with its idea of an interconnected web of relationships. I could also see ethical overtones in its implications. The notion of purposeful systems that dynamically interact in an on-going process of development and change struck a chord with me that was deeper than just scientific observation. That our actions affect an entire ecology whether it be personal, social, organizational, or environmental made complete sense to me and stirred the spiritual inclinations within me. As I continued to read from and contemplate the perennial spiritual traditions of the world there seemed to be a great commonality of themes that reinforced my understanding.

My interest in open systems led me to explore the revolutionary ideas of quantum theory, holography, chaos theory, complexity sciences, and fractal geometry, collectively known as the "new sciences," that is, new scientific understandings of the world that represent a dramatically new way of understanding and perceiving the world. As physicist Paul Davies writes "It is, in short, nothing less than a brand new start in the description of nature" (1988, p. 23). Gabriel Garcia Marquez described this new world as "so recent that many things lacked names, and in order to indicate them it was necessary to point."

I felt as if my life mirrored this situation. These new ideas were like fingers pointing toward something significant in my life that I needed to pay attention to. My old world had died. Joseph Campbell's words captured my longing, "The old gods are dead or dying and people everywhere are searching, asking: What is the new mythology to be, the mythology of this unified earth as of one harmonious being?" (1986, p. 17). Although my questions were intellectual and philosophical, this was clearly a spiritual search for me. While the ideas described a particular scientific reality, my inner self was tuned in to the concepts that spoke to my soul.

The new sciences reintroduced my spirit to the great mystery and the awe of the cosmos. I could marvel at its complexity yet sense the simplicity of its patterns of order. I was able to open myself to a view of wholeness and interconnection without feeling threatened by conventional religious language. The new sciences debunked the "scientism" I had been so critical of and created the possibility of a radically transformed perception of the fundamental properties of matter and life.

As a philosopher, I explored the implications of the new sciences for a new conception of subject matter, curriculum, and teaching. I was an early voice for the need for a new paradigm that would create alternative visions of possibility. Yet as much as these ideas influenced my thinking, I yearned for the authenticity of lived experience. The core of my spirit recognized a need within me to not just articulate a set of ideas but to follow a path of commitment and cultivation of my inner self.

Science can only explore, describe and seek to explain. It cannot reach into the intangible qualities of soul and spirit that intertwine themselves into our existence. Science cannot tap the paradox of our lives that brings into question who we are and why we are here. It cannot satisfy the longing to be one with that which is not of the material world — with that quality of existence that is beyond and within the need to "be." At this time in my life I felt the need for a committed practice that would experientially ground my ideas and that would lead me to a greater realization of my place and purpose. Increasingly, I was drawn to contemplative Taoism.

## THE WAY OF TAO

My interest in Taoism began when I first read the *Tao Te Ching*. What attracted me was the beautiful simplicity of the language, the way Taoism is grounded in nature, the intuitive wisdom it communicates for real life, and the way it uses paradox and transcends our reliance on reason as an answer for all things. Even today, every time I read the *Tao Te Ching* and with every new translation, my heart opens to fresh and greater truths. As its mystical content is applied more experientially, I am slowly understanding its deeper meanings for my life.

The *Tao Te Ching*, purportedly written by Lao Tse, is the most notable text in Taoism. It is a tiny text organized in 81 chapters, written poetically, using numerous metaphors and analogies. It addresses virtually every aspect of life. In addition to the text by Lao Tse are the writings of Chuang Tse. Chuang Tse uses story and philosophy to effectively support the insights of the *Tao Te Ching*. Taken together these writings unify two complementary sides of human nature: 1) intuitive wisdom and practical knowledge and 2) contemplation and social action.

The term Contemplative Taoism has come to refer to the spirit of the original ideas of Lao Tse and Chuang Tse as well as the practice of "quiescence" or "quietism" as a contemplative approach to being one with Tao. Contemplative Taoism is to be distinguished from other forms of Taoism associated with organized religion, sects, and rituals. Taoism was never meant to be institutionalized as a formal authority. Taoism was meant to guide us to a self-exploration of our own truths. "If you want to worship the Tao, first discover it in your own heart" (p. 20). When we connect at the deepest level to the truth within us, then we open ourselves to inner transformation and possibility. Tao becomes, not a static truth, but a path to follow that reveals itself in the simplicity of nature and through our experience of inseparable unity.

Tao literally means the "Way" or "Path." It affirms that there is an essential nature within all things and the source of this essential nature is the ultimate mystery and undefinable presence of Tao.

> The Tao that can be expressed is not the eternal Tao;
> The name that can be defined is not the unchanging name.
> Non-existence is called the antecedent of heaven and earth;
> Existence is the mother of all things.

As a path, Taoism is not so much a prescriptive set of practices and beliefs so much as a perspective that is lived and realized in one's life.

Chang Chun-yuan (1948), in a wonderful and comprehensive treatment of Taoism, writes that "The understanding of Tao is an inner experience in which the distinction between subject and object vanishes. It is an intuitive, immediate awareness rather than a mediated, inferential, or intellectual process" (p. 19). This essential sense of oneness means that one is "living within the moving forces of the universe and is oneself a part of it" (p. 40). To realize this sense of oneness means to transcend our notions of a dualistic universe where things appear to be separate and unrelated. When we act in harmony with this essence, we act from a natural integration and wholeness that connects us with all things and makes our actions effortless and uncontrived.

Taoism is also about embracing paradox—the yes and no, the both/and, it is and it isn't. It is about cultivating the integration of body, heart/mind, and spirit. It is grounded in everyday action in the world and the experience of life. Yet, it brings forth the mystery of the universe as the intangible and essential aspect of all things and all action.

> From eternal non-existence, therefore, we serenely observe the mysterious beginning of the universe;
> From eternal existence we clearly see the apparent distinctions.
> These two are the same in source and become different when manifested.

It is the empty space from which all possibility arises. When we draw upon the power and possibility of emptiness, we can then act in harmony with Tao because we are, in fact, in harmony with ourselves.

> Thirty spokes meet in the hub,
> but the empty space between them is
> the essence of the wheel.
> Pots are formed from clay,
> but the empty space within it is
> the essence of the pot. (Tao 11)

An important concept common to Taoism and to many indigenous cultures as well is the law of opposites. This dynamic interplay of the opposing forces is present throughout all nature and is given the names *yin* and *yang*. *Yin* characterizes softness and receptivity, darkness, earth and the feminine. *Yang* is more reflective of the masculine, of hardness, activity, brightness and heaven. Within the law of opposing forces is the important understanding that each opposing force is part of the same unity and provides the transforming energy that the other needs. All of nature must respond to these conditions and it is when we are in harmony that we are most in balance. The Chinese symbol for "human" subtly conveys this thought. The symbol is similar to a vertical line connecting two horizontal lines, suggesting that we are meant to connect heaven and earth. It is in bringing together the yin and yang aspects of our lives that we can creatively participate in the transformative processes of life.

Many of the examples in Taoist literature are analogies from nature. The same forces that are at work in nature are at work within us as well. Living our lives in harmony with Nature also means to live life in harmony with our true nature. This has implications for our physical health, the ways we act in the world and for how we maintain a dynamic balance in our lives.

The Taoist concept of *Wu Wei* literally means non-action. "The Tao does not act but there is nothing it does not do." In our Western mindset, the term "non-action" is often misunderstood. *Wu Wei* does not mean passivity; rather it means uncontrived action. When we spontaneously act from our true nature there are no hidden agendas, manipulations, or self serving motivations. Rather we allow ourselves to act more intuitively and from the heart. If we are authentically true to ourselves and our hearts, there is no need for a strict moral code or standards; our actions will be what they need to be.

Taoism places great importance on self-cultivation and the development of "Te." *Te* has been defined as virtue/power. *Te* is developed through affirming a basic simplicity of life and becoming aware of one's inner self. Thus one encounters the real world through inner serenity and the strength of purpose that comes from the profound experience of oneness. It is a casting aside of negative energies and the ability to see things as they are. Through the process of self-cultivation, of becoming the "uncarved block," we are able to let go of our attachments and open ourselves to a higher potential.

The Way of Tao is not something one can outline easily for anyone else. It is not a dogmatic statement of beliefs but it does represent a perspective to be explored and experienced.

> A way can be a guide but not a fixed path;
> names can be given but not permanent labels (Tao 1)

My experience in Taoism has been full of mystery and intrigue, searching out its meanings, not really understanding but slowly achieving a new perspective and feeling it become a greater part of my life. One realization that has been important for me is that Tao is not so much to be articulated as it is to be lived. This moves Taoism from being simply a philosophy to being a "practice."

## THE PRACTICE OF TAO

It is through a commitment to practice that a spiritual path takes shape and becomes personal. Therefore its meanings can be applied more directly to lived experience and to the insights we may gain.

For me, the practice of Taoism began with meditation. "If you can cease all restless activity, your integral nature will appear" (Lao Tzu, 1992, p. 55). A very simple description of meditation is "To restore the mind to its unfragmented origin, sit quietly and meditate.... Just settle the spirit and breath, and trust nature" (Lu Yen, 1993, p. 159). Meditation is not an end in itself but is seen as a "temporary device," a means to greater realization of our oneness with Tao. Meditation is at the heart of contemplative practice.

My Taoist practice was greatly enhanced when I started a *tai chi* class. The gentle movements became more than just exercise. They became a tangible expression of words and ideas in the *Tao Te Ching*. The challenge to be balanced, not go too far, remain focused, and flow from a grounded source of energy were all physical embodiments of ideas I was trying to understand. The movements became a physical metaphor for other areas in my life. This has been equally true of other forms of physical meditation as I began to explore: *qigong* and *daoyin*.

Perhaps, though, the practice of Contemplative Taoism can best be described more directly through some of the words of the *Hua Hu Ching*.

> The first practice is the practice of undiscriminating virtue. (Lao Tzu, 1992, p. 4)

> To practice virtue is to selflessly offer assistance to others…. without prejudice concerning the identity of those in need. (p. 6)

> When you perceive that an act done to another is done to yourself, you have understood the great truth. (p. 50)

Undiscriminating virtue is that practice of selfless service to others. It is realizing that we truly are not separate and that when we act from the heart, for the benefit of others, we open ourselves to our true spiritual nature. Some teachings suggest that each day we seek to extend positive thoughts to others, and extend virtue through both words and deeds.

Service, however, is integrated with our own self-cultivation. As we perceive the world more and more in terms of its basic wholeness and interconnedness, we are able to also perceive ourselves differently. We are better able to let go of limiting concepts, attitudes, and actions. In an odd way we become the world and our thoughts and consciousness become real events that impact everything else.

> I confess that there is nothing to teach…. Simply be aware of the oneness of things. (Lao Tzu, 1992, p. 10)

> Serve others and cultivate yourself simultaneously. Understand that true growth comes from meeting and solving the problems of life in a way that is harmonizing to yourself and to others. (p. 52)

> Simply avoid becoming attached to what you see and think. Relinquish the notion that you are separated from the all-knowing mind of the universe. (p. 54)

> Live simply and virtuously, true to your nature, drawing no line between what is spiritual and what is not. (p. 62)

If the world is unfragmented and whole, then our being in the world affects everything else. Who we are, what we think, and what we do makes a difference. It is not an external morality that governs the person of Tao but rather the commitment to inner development and authentic action that comes from that process and the circumstances of one's life.

> If you want to awaken all of humanity, then awaken all of yourself. If you want to eliminate the suffering in the world, then eliminate all that is dark and negative in yourself. Truly the greatest gift you have to give is that of your own self-transformation. (p. 96)

The practice of Tao is a dual process of expanding and negating one's self. Through expanding our awareness and our virtue/power, we come to experience the mysterious unity of Tao and we experience the personal realization that non-existence is the very source of all existent possibility.

> Take time to listen to what is said without words.... The breath of the Tao speaks, and those who are in harmony with it hear quite clearly. (p. 106)

## TAOISM AND TEACHING

While Taoism has its roots in mysticism and contemplative practice, at its core it is eminently practical. When we are in harmony with any aspect of life, we are experiencing an aspect of Tao. Taoism is a path of self-cultivation and mastery as well as means for inner spiritual development.

For me, teaching has always been an applied philosophy. As Taoism came to have a greater impact on my life it was natural for me to see within it implications for my role as a teacher. Years ago I created a simple affirmation that said "I honor my work as part of my spiritual practice and my spiritual practice as part of my work." This has led to a greater exploration of the relationship between teaching and spirituality.

In conveying how I believe my Taoist practice has influenced my teaching, I have tried to consider the major questions and themes that I have developed in my work. These are (1) Depth and Substance, (2) Oneness, Interconnectedness, and Relationship, (3) Spontaneity and Naturalness, (4) Process and Transformation, (5) Simplicity and Harmony, and (6) Engaged Service. I will share how I have applied these understandings to my teaching.

1. My Taoist practice has broadened my understanding of what it means to teach with *depth and substance*. A central question from a Taoist perspective is "what is the essential nature of things?" Most often this is not what is most evident. What is most essential is usually related to the significance to our lives, to the underlying "truths," to the patterns of relationship and order that exist, to the unseen qualities that point to the mystery of Tao.

As I look at what is to be taught, I begin asking myself what is important — not in an academic sense but rather in regards to what is significant for our lives. I try to determine the larger story that connects what is to be learned to a deeper exploration of life. What themes does the content point toward that offer possibilities of deeper awareness, insight, and transformation? I confront myself with the question, "So What?" and ask if I am just going through the motions or whether there is something hidden that needs to be seen. Then I ask for the courage to go there and that I may learn its message for my own life as well.

For example, if I am going to be teaching about the nature of culture, I try to consider what is significant about this content that goes directly to the question of who we are. Can we explore through this information an understanding of ourselves as cultural beings? Can I create experiences that draw us into compassionate understanding of others and an appreciation of their stories? Can we begin to develop an ownership of others' stories and perceive ourselves as both unique and the same? Can we see ways that we can make a difference in the world?

Exploring the essential nature of things ultimately brings us back to exploring ourselves. This happens also to be a message of quantum theory, that whenever we investigate anything we inevitably are investigating ourselves. In this sense, all content becomes a vehicle for deeper insights rather than a goal in its own right. Content becomes a continuing mystery that holds possibility, awe, insight, and wonder. My teaching has been enlivened by posing these questions and has the potential for a more soulful quality.

2. Taoism emphasizes the concepts of *oneness, relationship, and inter-connectedness*. There is a sense of unity and wholeness that acknowledges that everything in the cosmos and the forces that operate within it are essentially unfragmented and whole. Dualism and separation are only illusions of our senses and our goal is to be one with the essential wholeness of Tao.

What it means to me as an educator is that part of what I search for are themes and experiences that illustrate the relational and interconnected qualities of life and our need to be whole and complete human beings. I can no longer be satisfied teaching in a fragmented, skills-based way. I am drawn naturally to integrated subject-matter and providing opportunities to explore connections. The themes of holistic education make sense to me as I try to give attention (even in college classes) to movement, art, music, and experiential activities. This includes involvement with nature and with one another. I want to tap the spiritual qualities of my students as well.

There is a Native American saying that "we cannot know anything until we understand how it relates to everything else." This is consistent with our understanding of systems sciences. My Taoist path helps me to explore these interconnections in my own experience and to be aware of the connected energy within me. It gives a greater authenticity to these ideas because as I explore them within myself, I am able to perceive them more clearly in the curriculum and instructional approaches I use.

Another important application of these ideas has been a greater emphasis on building community. The need for celebrations, interaction, and creating a unified and coherent sense of purpose are essential qualities I strive for. I create rituals and sometimes ceremonies whose only purpose is to emphasize our connectedness. I try to create an atmosphere of democratic participation where the class belongs to each of us, and each of us has unique and valuable contributions to make.

3. A significant concept in Taoism is the notion of *Wu Wei*. As explained earlier this means acting from our true nature — trusting the *spontaneous simplicity* of our intuition and *acting from the heart*. I try to understand what this means for my teaching. While much of what we do as teachers requires planning, preparation, and degrees of structure, often we depend so heavily on this that opportunities for spontaneity are lost. I have tried to develop a style of teaching that allows me to interact more naturally with students and their questions. I try to create what Donald Oliver calls "learning occasions" that make a significant point, but also

remain open to multiple interpretations, meanings, and understandings. I create time and space to revisit previous content and activities so we can find our place again in the story and give opportunities to explore tangents that are important to the students. I share my poetry, bring in harmonicas, drums, and activities that encourage personal expression and promote a creative response to knowing.

I have begun incorporating the techniques of "heartmath" in some classes, that open each of us to our intuitive knowing and provides a balance to reasoning and analysis.

*Wu Wei* contains the idea of "appropriate right action." It also can mean "acting with a true heart" or "acting true to your heart." Ray Griggs defines *Wu Wei* as virtue/power — the power that comes to us when we act from the heart. I can tell when I come from my mind rather than my heart and I continue to learn how acting from my heart impacts my teaching. As I become more involved in my practice, I am always amazed how contrived so many of my actions are and how easy it is to be afraid of our natural response to life. There are so many things we try to "force" and practicing *Wu Wei* makes me more aware that these moments are usually counterproductive to the situation.

4. As I observe the interaction of *yin* and *yang* in the processes of life, I am made more aware of how patterns of opposites work in the world. The dynamic movement of circumstances and events are filled with *process and transformation*. Increasingly, I am coming to understand the movement of time within all our activities and how content, objects, activities, methods, and ideas all emerge from one thing into something else. I find myself trying to be more and more open to what is needed. How long have my students been sitting or standing, listening or talking, interacting or reflecting? I am trying to understand more deeply the processes involved in any activity and also the processes embedded in information and content. I try to emphasize the "doing" of a subject rather than just learning "about" a subject. I try to provide time to consolidate and gather thoughts just as much as exploring and generating ideas.

Process and transformation are ideas I've believed in for many years but my Taoist practice helps me understand them more deeply through my experience. My perceptions are more accurate and it becomes easier to look at process and transformation in all aspects of my life. To help increase my perception of process and transformation, I sometimes try to avoid thinking in terms of nouns and try to understand nouns as verbs. For example, rather than seeing myself as a teacher or a professor, I am "teachering or professoring." Almost always I become more conscious of the negative traits of those roles that I take for granted and I also realize that my own actions in the moment define what "teachering" and "professoring" really are.

The concept of *yin* and *yang* is more than just an understanding of opposite forces, however. It is an understanding of dynamic unity in which each perceived action has embedded within it its own opposite. So wise actions must always consider the whole and perceive that any single action will always lead to others and must be considered in its entirety. Having recently served as an interim director of a charter school where many troubled youth attended, I realized that my actions always set in motion many responses. In many cases I began to see that the least action was the most effective. In other situations, it was necessary to act quite strongly.

The *Tao Te Ching* says "Know *yang* but act from *yin*." This wisdom suggest that force actions will often create the most forceful responses, whereas being receptive to others' feelings, confusions, and pain can often create the least resistance and an openness for future dialogue and relationship. Kids who had been discarded by the education system slowly let go of many of their resisting attitudes and opened themselves up to the possibility for change. Gentleness is not the same thing as weakness. Taoism uses the analogy of water being soft but nothing can match its power. Its gentleness is persistent yet hard rocks and mountains are eroded away.

Finally, for me a dynamic balance has curricular and instructional implications as well. I am a proponent of process approaches to instruction. But there has to be something to process. Content and process go together. They are embedded within each other. Skills and creativity are not mutually exclusive. Caring and participative decision-making are not antithetical with orderliness and self-discipline. I have seen so many wonderful instructional strategies fail because they were seen as all or nothing and teachers felt they could not incorporate natural elements of an "opposite" approach.

My Taoist practice continues to make me more aware of the dynamic balance of *yin* and *yang* and the powerful ideas of process and transformation. My reason for teaching is to tap the processes of inner transformation that enable one to be more fully human and to realize their own spiritual purposes. In my own experience, I find that this involves "unlearning" as much as it does learning. Awareness and insight cannot be taught but they can be valued and honored and given opportunity to flower within.

5. *Harmony and simplicity* are significant concepts in Taoism that speak to the quality of relationship we have with the world and how we act upon the world around us. The analogy of a musical harmony is the notion of separate sounds coming together to make a single complementary chord. There is an innate simplicity in the sound that comes through. The old Chinese symbol for wisdom means "to sweep away the clutter." Simplicity is such a powerful concept because in essence it is a process of uncluttering that allows us to get to the heart of things. As I try to apply harmony and simplicity to my teaching, I am learning to appreciate the small and ordinary events of a classroom. Teaching becomes a joyful experience if we unburden ourselves of all the external requirements and expectations it is so easy to become attached to.

Being in harmony with your own nature and with the needs of the situation create a feeling of dynamic unity and wholeness. There is a recognition that the energies within us must work together with everything else. As one works with an awareness of these energies, it becomes easier to notice when we are out of balance and why.

In creating a learning environment, I try to put together simple harmonies such as particular kinds of art and music, sometimes a plant or a candle, and occasionally fragrant oils that are gently noticeable. If I am having difficulty with my own stress, I will meditate for a while before class or during a break to achieve a more grounded feeling within myself. It is important to me to not just play the role of teacher but to be an authentic human being. I've noticed that when I am most into a role that there is a kind of sterility that accompanies it. Even if things go well, there is a lingering feeling that I missed the mark.

Harmony becomes important in the quality of relationships, the pacing of instruction, and the story of meaning that is created by students. It is an ineffable quality that can be felt if we are open to it. We can experience its power but we can't plan it or make it happen. It requires that we teach with a receptive attitude and cultivate an openness to respond to what is needed.

Ray Grigg (1990) writes "Begin therefore, with the mystery of the obvious, with the profoundly ordinary and the inexplicability of the simple. Understanding does not become wonder until the simplest and the lowest are amazing. Without wonder, understanding is not alive" (p. 77). This captures what I hope to create in my classes. I try to unclutter the curriculum by creating a story of the content. I try to find the "story" that needs to be told and then explore the various meanings of the story in a multitude of ways. But it is the simplicity of the story line and its significance that allow the complexities to be introduced meaningfully. I constantly revisit the content as if it were the characters and events of the story so the essential meanings and questions are not lost. What inevitably happens is that the students' stories become interwoven and indistinguishable from what we are studying. Ultimately we are learning about ourselves.

6. Finally, my Taoist practice leads me to cultivate myself for the benefit of others. It also leads me to cultivate myself through *service to others*. The *Hua Hu Ching* states that "True understanding in a person has two attributes: awareness and action. Together they form a natural *tai chi*. Who can enjoy enlightenment and remain indifferent to suffering in the world? This is not in keeping with the Way. Only those who increase their service along with their understanding can be called men and women of Tao" (p. 65). In my teaching I strive for what I call "*responsive learning....*" For me, this is a kind of learning that elicits a personal response to our knowing. It is when we transform our knowing into ontological action that true transformation begins. Service in this sense comes more authentically from the heart and is an outgrowth of our awareness and understanding. It is this movement into responsive learning that creates opportunities for spiritual growth and personal transformation. I still have a long way to go in understanding the subtleties of this process but it gives my teaching a depth of purpose that sustains me and, I hope, enriches my students.

## CONCLUSION

It is my hope that by sharing my spiritual journey, I have in some way connected you to your own. It is through the cultivation and commitment to our own paths that we can each make a difference in the world. From one traveler to another, I wish you joy and peace.

## REFERENCES

Bopp, B. J. M., Brown,L., & Lane, P. (1989). *The Sacred Tree: Reflections on Native American Spirituality*. Twin Lakes, WI: Bantam.

Campbell. (1986). *The Inner Reaches of Outer Space: Metaphor as Myth and as Religion*. New York: Harper & Row.

Chang, C. Y. (1963). *Creativity and Taoism: A Study of Chinese Philosophy, Art, and Poetry*. New York: Julian.

Davies, P. (1988). *The Cosmic Blueprint: New Discoveries in Nature's Ability to Order the Universe*. New York: Simon & Schuster.

Grigg, R. (1990). *The Tao of Being*. Atlanta: Humanics.

Lao Tse. (1948). *The Wisdom of Lao Tse* (Y. Lin, Trans.). New York: Random House.

Lao Tzu. (1992). *Hua Hu Ching: The Unknown Teaching of Lao Tzu* (B. Walker, Trans.). San Francisco: Harper.

Lu Yen. (1993). *The Spirit of Tao* (T. Cleary, Trans.). Boston: Shambhala.

Moore, T. (1992). *Care of the Soul*. New York: HarperCollins.

Needleman, J. (1996). *A Little Book on Love*. New York: Delta.

Needleman, J. (1982). *The Heart of Philosophy*. New York: Knopf.

# CHAPTER 3

# Tantra

## The Quest for the Ecstatic Mind

### Kathleen Kesson

In 1968, George Leonard, writer on education and the human potential movement, wrote a book entitled *Education and Ecstasy*. Capturing the spirit of the decade, it wove together ideas from the counterculture, brain research, new technologies, and psychedelic experimentation as well as the human potential movement, to attempt to seed new thinking about educational possibilities. Leonard's book was widely read by a mass audience. Like many of us at the time, Leonard was confident that the various revolutions taking place in consciousness, social patterns, and politics were about to usher in a new era of freedom, experimentation, and, well — ecstasy. We would, he hoped, soon take advantage of innovative new technologies to individualize instruction. We would take seriously the current brain research that insisted that pleasure — yes, pleasure! — was at the heart of meaningful learning, and we would affirm that the aim of human life was the fulfillment of latent human capacities, including the capacities for joy, freedom, inquiry, and relationship.

Well, it is the year 2001, over 30 years after the publication of this interesting book, and there is today little talk of pleasure or ecstasy, or even joy in the world of educational discourse. Now, the more familiar words are assessment, standards, zero tolerance, and accountability — the words of the corporate boardroom, not the human potential movement. In such a climate, it is perhaps absurd to attempt to resuscitate interest in the ecstatic possibilities of the human mind. But the quest for ecstasy — the search for meaning, pleasure, and lasting joy — is much older than the 60's cultural revolution. It is an important current in all of human history, and we can only hope that our contemporary obsession with the standardization and mechanization of learning may eventually give way to an engagement with more enduring human values, including that state of aesthetic fulfillment spoken of by sages throughout time, and widely misunderstood — the state of ecstasy, or bliss (*ananda*, in Sanskrit). It is this transformation to a state of blissful enlightenment that provides the foundation of Tantric spiritual practice. Understanding the mental model and the spiritual science underlying this practice may help orient us towards more expansive educational possibilities, should we ever tire of the corporate social engineering that characterizes the present era of education.

There are other reasons why it is vital for educators to understand various forms of spirituality and spiritual practice, even such esoteric traditions as Tantra. Let me share a personal story. I recently returned from a trip to India. On the leg of the flight between Kuwait and London, I sat between a woman from Mumbai, India and a woman from Karachi, Pakistan. The woman from Pakistan shared with us a handwritten piece of inspirational writing from her Muslim tradition, which we agreed had universal appeal. The woman from India, a Hindu, unpacked a gift she had received on her trip, and showed us the lovely, beaded statue of the legendary god Krishna that her nephew had given her for her birthday. An animated conversation ensued among us that covered the topics of idol worship, the names of God, deities, gender issues, and Pakistan/Indian hostilities. All of us were comfortable discussing our various beliefs and seeking the common threads in our understandings of these topics. The woman from India talked about her son who had become a computer programmer and wanted nothing more than to settle in America. I talked about my son, who is an aspiring Sanskrit scholar, married to a Parsi woman from Mumbai, and who wants nothing more than to stay in India. The woman from Pakistan, a geography teacher, was extremely interested in strategies to enliven her geography classes, which sparked a spirited discussion about the project method, experiential learning, John Dewey, and Howard Gardner's multiple intelligences theory. We chuckled at the ironies in all of this. And thus, global connections are made in this increasingly smaller world. In this era of globalization, easy international transportation, electronic communication, and immigration, it is crucial that we come to understand both our cultural differences and the similarities that promise to link us together in peaceful coexistence.

Religious difference is the one territory largely ignored by theorists of multicultural education. Perhaps this is because of great nervousness having to do with anything "spiritual" in the context of public education. And yet it is religious differences that lie at the root of many of the most devastating international conflicts, as well as those closer to home. In order to learn to live together in an increasingly pluralistic world, we must come to understand each other, and this understanding must begin with knowledge.

In addition to increasing our intercultural understanding, there are yet other reasons to study worldviews that are vastly different from our taken for granted ways of thinking. Tantra embodies a philosophy of mind and consciousness that challenges some of the most fundamental assumptions upon which we base our Western theories of teaching and learning. Its theories are derived from centuries of introspective practice, providing us with a wealth of historic, contemplative insight. Understanding such significant conceptual differences may help us think in fresh ways about our taken for granted assumptions, which could foster important new questions and insights about the aims and purposes, as well as the methods, of education. And finally, Tantra embodies a value system worth examining in this era of materialism, greed, and egocentricity *writ large*. Contemporary Tantrics are attempting to put their philosophical principles as well as their values into practice in education. I believe that we all have something to learn from this effort.

## THE SPIRITUAL SCIENCE OF TANTRA

What combination of cultural circumstance and internal psychological dynamic is it that causes some of us to be attracted to the "Other," that which is quite foreign to everything in our culture of birth? Why are some people content to carry on the cultural and spiritual traditions of their foremothers and fathers, and others only satisfied to forge less familiar paths? In my case, it was likely a convergence of factors. I was born in a neighborhood bordering the Golden Gate Park in San Francisco, a port city known for its liberality and cultural pluralism, to parents of mixed European heritage. One of my earliest memories, reinforced by family photographs and my mother's narratives, is of regular excursions in my stroller to the Japanese Tea Gardens in that park. Another vivid memory is of the Chinese New Year's Parade on Grant

Avenue — I recall being very small and very lost there, while above me a dragon's head dipped and swayed and firecrackers boomed. One might think such an early trauma would have left me terrified of all things "Oriental" (a common term signifying Asian back then), yet my fascination only grew. Mother and I went to Chinatown regularly, for lunch and shopping, and on one of these excursions I purchased a golden Buddha. Returning home, I set it up in my room, and proudly announced to my mother that I believed in reincarnation. I was a young adolescent at the time, so perhaps my announcement was designed for shock value. I think not however, for the attraction continued to grow and deepen. Fortunately I had parents who, rather than being shocked at my declaration, encouraged me to explore whatever interested me spiritually, which probably resulted in my later pursuing an undergraduate minor in comparative religion and philosophy.

When I left home to take up professional studies in dance and theater, one of the first books I bought myself was a handbook on Hatha Yoga. Laboring in the privacy of my own small Hollywood apartment, I worked to perfect the physical yoga postures. I approached them much as I approached my dance studies, with determination and the goal of technical perfection! In that book, there was some mention made of meditation, and this sounded like a good thing, so I tried to teach myself how to do it. There is some conventional wisdom in the world of spiritual practice that when the student is ready, the teacher, or the teachings, will appear. That did seem to be the operative principle in my case. In 1965, I was working as a dancer on a movie set at Allied Arts Studio in Hollywood. I can't even remember what movie it was now, 35 years later, but I distinctly remember the book that many of the leading actors were reading during the filming. It was *The Autobiography of a Yogi*, by Paramahansa Yogananda (1946). I was intrigued. The actors invited me out to lunch, and we went next door to the first vegetarian restaurant I had ever experienced, which happened to be associated with the Self-Realization Fellowship (the L.A. center of Yogananda's teachings). I was hooked — I bought the book, began to eat soybeans and yogurt and drink herbal tea, and immersed myself in what would become a lifetime of exploration of the various spiritual traditions of the "East."

At the core of many of these traditions is Tantra, perhaps the most ancient set of spiritual practices still in existence on the planet. There are scholarly debates about Tantra's origins as well as its relationship to the Vedic School of Indian philosophy, which is historically important in

Hinduism. The history of this tradition is hard to pin down due to the oral nature of transmission that has carried its teachings forth for centuries. Its Indian roots are in the indigenous nature worship that predated the Aryan invasions (approximately 1500 BCE) of that subcontinent. It both shaped and was shaped by the scriptures known as the Vedas, composed in India by the invading Aryans. Its many branches include "cults," such as Shaeva, Kaula, and Shakta cults, as well as profound influences upon major religious traditions, including Buddhism, Hinduism, and Jainism. It is at the heart of what we know in the west as "Yoga," due in large part to the work of Patanjali around 100 CE to systematize the beliefs and principles into a practice. The system articulated by Patanjali came to be called Astanga Yoga, the "Eight-Fold Path." Although Tantra is much larger, in both the historical and philosophical sense, than Yoga, the terms can be, to some extent, used interchangeably. According to Zimmer (1951), yoga means "the yoking of empirical consciousness to transcendental consciousness" (p. 580).

Tantra is a culturally specific spiritual practice, and thus connected with particular myths, legends, creation stories, deities, and forms of ritual and worship. Tantra and Yoga permeate Hindu mythology, such as in the epic poem, *The Mahabharata*, and one of its most important narratives, the *Bhagavad-Gita*. Despite its mythopoetic elements, Tantra is not itself a religion, but a "spiritual science," a set of practices that includes physical culture, mental development, and spiritual devotion. Although Tantra has a mystical and a philosophical dimension, virtually all writings about it stress the experiential nature of the practice, which requires no adherence to belief or dogma.

The most appropriate analog for this internal process in the modern world is probably psychoanalysis. Bharati (1965) uses the phrase "psycho-experimental-speculative" to convey the essentially exploratory nature of the practice. In this context, gods and goddesses, deities and demons have no ontological or existential status to the Tantric, rather they serve as archetypes — "necessary anthropomorphic ways of finding out 'what is inside the mind'" (p. 20). Axioms, principles and guidelines are tentatively held speculative constructs, to be amended on the basis of experimental data.

Below, I provide a necessarily abbreviated overview of the main concepts and assumptions underlying Tantra, then highlight one particular form of education — Neo-humanist education — that is making the effort to implement this philosophy.

## FUNDAMENTAL CONCEPTS

For ease of communication, what follows is an attempt to articulate some of the fundamental concepts of Tantra in the context of Western philosophical categories. I do this with some hesitation in this "post-ontological, post-epistemological" academic atmosphere. (For an exploration of the relationship between contemplative traditions and philosophical postmodernism, see Kesson, 2000.) For the purposes of this paper, however, rather than problematize the categories, I will lay out the ontological, epistemological, psychological, and axiological principles that seem most germane to my understanding of this very complex system.

## ONTOLOGY

When we study ontology, we study the nature of *being*. According to Tantra, human *being* is a multidimensional condition. At the level of the conscious mind, there is a sense of separation. But within every human resides the "*âtman*," variously defined as soul, mind, spirit, or self (Müller, 1962). Through contemplative practice, one realizes the essential unity of the *âtman* with the higher Self, variously called the Divine, the Supreme, the Absolute. In this tradition, this highest Self is the last point to be reached by philosophical speculation, and the goal is overcoming the limitations imposed by the individual ego. The working assumption here is that there is a "higher" form of existence, attained when the ego-bound mind is freed of illusion. This notion of a supreme state, variously called *nirvana* (Buddhism), *satori* (Zen), or *samadhi* (Tantra), represents humanity's longing for something larger and more significant than the limited self. Tantra supposes that the individual mind (or unit mind) can transcend its limitations to experience itself as part of the ocean of limitless consciousness. Tantric practice is a system of attunement in which the individual mind comes into resonance with the universal mind.

## PSYCHOLOGY

More properly phrased, in this context, *biopsychology*, Tantra proposes a model of the psyche that encompasses the entire human body, which is composed of both material and subtle energies as well as "energy fields" outside the body. Unlike Western models of the mind, which locate mental functions entirely in the brain, Tantra assumes a more interpenetrating bodymind system, a continuum of increasing subtlety as one moves conceptually from the dense material body to the more ethereal mental functions. To understand this comprehensive psychosomatic system, one must suspend deeply engrained, dualistic models of body and mind.

Perhaps the most elusive concept to people not practiced in this tradition is the notion of *kundalini* (*kula kundalini* literally means "coiled serpentine force"). The kundalini is a psycho/spiritual force that lies dormant at the base of the spine until "awakened" — most commonly by the invocation of a *mantra* (a special sound vibration that when repeated, either audibly or internally, fosters a resonance between the practitioner and the sought after state of cosmic consciousness), or through other psycho-somatic processes such as chanting, breath control (*pranayama*), visualization (either internally or on an external object) or concentration. The awakened kundalini moves upward through a system of seven *chakras* along the *shushuma nadi*, a psychic energy channel in the spine. Chakras are "the points of contact between the individual on the one hand, and non-physical energies and beings on the other ... psychic energy centres (sic) which are associated with particular areas of the body, but are not part of the body" (King, 1986, p. 55). Various Tantric texts allude to innumerable other energy centers in the body, "all of them interconnected by subtle energy channels, the psychic equivalents of nerves, arteries, and veins, which are called *nadis*" (p. 56). For our purposes, the main point of interest is that the various chakras are thought to control different aspects of human life (speech, digestion, emotions, mental activity, etc.) culminating with the seventh and highest chakra at the top of the head, which is the seat of pure blissful consciousness, *Sat Chit Ananda*. According to Tantra, physical, mental, and spiritual health depends on the proper balance and functioning of the energy of the chakras. The entire system, which includes physical exercises, meditation, vegetarian diet, and breathing techniques, is oriented towards creating such a balance, a state of well-being that is conducive to the realization of the higher, or limitless Self.

While the chakras may have no "objective" (physical) existence, they are a useful heuristic device. That they are "real" at some level of experience is suggested by the Tantric theory of the Sanskrit language, which is that the phonemes in that language are based upon the vibrational sound frequencies of the various "petals" of the chakras. Sanskrit is, according to this theory, a language of the body, and the many chants and mantras based upon these sounds do not merely correspond to arbitrarily assigned meanings, but have psychosomatic effects as well. Other traditional explanations of the origins of Sanskrit differ on this point.

While Tantra recognizes, with Western psychology, the conscious and the subconscious layers of the mind, it further elaborates the dimensionality of the mind by positing mental realms termed the "superconscious," where the capacities for intuition, discrimination (defined as the ability to transcend illusion), and union with the infinite abide. Western psychology pays little attention to these categories of the superconscious. One important exception to this neglect is the field of transpersonal psychology, which is perhaps best articulated in the work of the prolific interdisciplinary scholar, Ken Wilber.

## EPISTEMOLOGY

Epistemology is a philosophical category that encompasses efforts to understand how it is we can know anything at all. Ironically, in contemplative practice, it seems more important to explore the process of *unknowing* — that is, how we free ourselves of limited, conditioned responses. Some of the epistemological processes utilized to enable the mind to deconstruct its normal awareness are embodied in Tantric meditative techniques: *bhuta shuddi* (withdrawal of the mind from the external world); *asana shuddi* (process of withdrawing the mind from its conditioned identification with the body); *citta shuddi* (suspension of thoughts); *dharana* (focused concentration on a single point of awareness); and *dhyana* (unification of individual consciousness with cosmic consciousness, a blissful state of non-duality).

Many Eastern philosophies disavow all objective knowledge as illusory, which has in some historical cases led to cultural passivity. While Tantra is certainly an introspective practice, its essential dynamism is best represented by a *yantra* (image for contemplation) used by Ananda Marga, a contemporary Tantric group, which includes two interlocking triangles, one pointing upwards and one pointing downwards. These are said to symbolize the necessity for "objective" adjustment (action in the world) to complement the "subjective approach" of contemplative practice. Tantra's longevity may in part be due to its empirical method (it is an experiential, experimental approach to the development of consciousness). Unlike Western science, however, there is an emphasis on following all thought to its source, introspectively. This practice highlights the nature of all thought as dependent upon other thought. When the *jinána yogi* (one who seeks self realization through the path of knowledge) proceeds along this epistemological line, he or she inevitably reaches a point

> where both reflection and refraction end. That is, the mind of the inquirer reaches a point where it fails to comprehend that plate on which the processes of reflection and refraction operate. The point where the mind loses its capacity to analyse (sic) or compare further is the supreme point…. (Sarkar, 1998, p. 180)

Tantric practice thus embodies both a dynamic theory of knowledge and a keen sense of its limits, or the point where intellectuality gives way to intuition.

## AXIOLOGY

Morality is said to be the base of Tantric practice. In historical times, it is said that when disciples approached a *guru* (spiritual teacher) seeking enlightenment, they would often be instructed to develop a moral approach to life before given further teachings. Unlike the conventional morality in some religions, in which the precepts are rigid and connected to fixed structures of reward and punishment, the moral framework in Tantric Yoga is a set of guidelines oriented towards creating mental harmony. They include principles of relating to society *(Yama)* and principles for personal integration *(Niyama)*. The principles of *Yama* include: *Ahimsa* — action performed without the intention to harm anyone or anything by thought, word, or deed; *Satya* — a spirit of truthfulness, in which all thought, speech and action is guided by a feeling of benevolence; *Asteya* — trustworthiness, non-stealing, the spirit of not taking that which belongs to another; *Aparigraha* – an ecological and psychological principle that asks that we minimize our needs, and only use what is necessary for individual preservation; and *Bramacarya* — a state of mind in which one sees everyone as an expression of the Divine.

The principles of *Niyama* include *Shaoca* — the cultivation of a strong healthy body through proper exercise, diet and asanas (yoga postures), as well as attention to destructive mental habits such as greed, jealousy, fear, shame, etc.; *Santosa* — cultivation of a state of mental ease, contentment; *Tapah* — the practice of foregoing personal pleasures for the joy of serving others, an expression of our essential "oneness"; *Svadhyaya* — the effort to penetrate beyond dogma and ritualism to the truth in scriptures; and *Ishvara Pranidhana* — the mental effort, through meditation, towards union with cosmic consciousness.

All of these principles have been interpreted in various ways, and a more complex examination of the subtleties and differences of interpretation is well beyond the scope of this introductory paper. What is important is to understand that the pedagogical principles that emerge from these values play an important role in the educational design of Tantric schools.

## MISCONCEPTIONS AND DISTORTIONS OF TANTRA

In the Western mind, Tantra is most often associated with "spiritual sexuality," and sometimes with magical practices and the occult. It is not difficult to understand how these conceptions came about. Ideas in Tantric texts, according to Eliade (in Bharati, 1965), are frequently couched in secret, obscure language, with double meanings, sometimes expressed in erotic terminology. This has two intentions: first, to camouflage the teachings from non-initiates, and second, to "project the Yogi into the 'paradoxical situation' indispensable for his (sic) spiritual training" (p. 173). Many of the primal symbols of Tantra are overtly sexual in content. In India, one can still visit temples dedicated to Shiva and observe contemporary Shiva worshippers making offerings at an altar at which the primary symbol is a phallus (*lingam*) emerging from a vagina (*yoni*). In Tantric lore, the act of creation between people, as represented in the sexual act, parallels the cosmic act of creation, in which pure consciousness (often represented by Shiva) interfaces with active, dynamic forces in time and space (often represented by his consort, Shakti). Lama Yeshe (1987) suggests that the images of male and female deities in erotic embraces, rather than signifying degeneration (a charge that has been directed towards Tantra),

> is a symbolic portrayal of the inner unification of our own male and female energies. On a deeper level, their embrace symbolizes the aim of the very highest Tantric practices: generation of a most subtle and blissful state of mind that, by its very nature, is supremely suited to penetrate ultimate reality and free us from all delusion and suffering. (p. 31-32)

Ecstatic bliss, brought about by the "sense of freedom from the impoverishment brought about by ego-centeredness" is, according to Guenther (1972), a "peak experience of ... pure aesthetic perception and enjoyment" (p. 37). For most of us, sexuality is as close as we ever get to a peak experience (Maslow, the Western psychologist who developed the theory of the "peak experience" describes it as "the experience of awe, mystery, wonder, or of perfect completion" [1975, p. 312]). Is it any wonder that early Yogis used symbols derived from such fundamental human experience to describe what is, essentially, indescribable? In truth, while it is the erotocentric passages in Tantric texts that have made Tantra famous, these passages represent only a small fraction of the literature.

Because esoteric texts are widely available now, as opposed to a former time in which the teachings were transmitted orally by spiritual teachers who oversaw the moral and ethical development of their disciples, interpreters have made of the teachings what they will; thus a body of both sexual and occult practices has sprung up around Tantra, which according to some contemporary Tantrics, are but pale reflections of the genuine enlightenment tradition. The theme of ecstasy, says Bharati (1965), "has been victimized in recent times by fraudulent esotericism of the sort that is rampant in the Western world" (p. 285). While it is beyond the scope of this paper to develop an elaborate critique of these practices, let the reader be cautioned that especially in the West, practitioners have sometimes been guilty of appropriating those elements of the practice which suit their inclinations, without attention to the much broader and deeper spiritual tradition from which they have been extracted.

Herein, of course, lies one of the great dilemmas of this era of cultural pluralism, exchange, and synthesis: to what extent can we adopt aspects of "foreign" traditions to meet our own spiritual needs without being guilty of cultural appropriation? And, without neutralizing, trivializing, or distorting the original intent(s) of the tradition? It is an ethical dilemma with which I have personally wrestled. Lama Yeshe reminds us that it is "very important to be able to differentiate clearly between the essence of Tantra and the cultural forms in which it is currently (and historically) wrapped" (1987, p. 27). Tantra, he notes, is far deeper than language or custom might suggest. It is also important to remember that Tantra is nomadic, traveling as it has from India to China, Tibet, Japan (Zen) and more recently to the "Western" world. In transit, the essence remains, while forms change. And that essence, Lama Yeshe reminds us, is a teaching that embodies a way of breaking free from all the conditioning that limits our understanding of who we are and what we can become. In this sense, it is a truly universal spiritual practice.

## EDUCATING THE ECSTATIC MIND

Neo-humanist education has evolved from the teachings of Prabhat Ranjan Sarkar, a Tantric guru of the 20th century with a worldwide following. The fundamental principles were originally laid out in a little book entitled *The Liberation of Intellect: Neo-Humanism* (1982). Neo-humanism is defined as

> The love and respect for all people, extended to include all living beings, animate and inanimate. Neo-humanist education is the concerned effort to develop the highest human potential of every child. This translates into an emphasis on the whole child — physical, mental and spiritual — infusing children with love so that they grow into people who care to improve the world in which they live. (Nivedita & Bardwell, 1999, p. 147)

In contrast to a dominant Western view of education (increasingly adopted by "modernizing" nations the world over), which understands the individual as fundamentally alone in the universe and in competition with others for resources and status, this educational philosophy promotes a vision of humanity as "intimately linked with the fabric of the universe" (Bussey, 2000, p. 10). This fundamental concept of interconnectedness, derived directly from Tantric philosophy, is at the heart of their pedagogy. Also at the heart of the philosophy are concepts familiar to educators acquainted with the experiential, constructivist educational models of John Dewey and other "progressive" educators: continuity, interaction, engagement, and integration. Knowledge, in Tantra, is obtained through personal encounter, through concrete involvement with and through an understanding of the relationship of one thing to another as well as of the fundamental unity of things. This happens in an integrated way,

> through feeling, acting, thinking, which is the 'Way' as a process of unification. The result, the unity of knowledge, is then not a constructed intellectual scheme, but a personal acquisition, a living state of mind which can be recognized and known, but which defies all conceptual statements. (Guenther, 1972, p. 100-101)

Interestingly, according to Tantric scholar Guenther, in Buddhism, Tantra means both "integration" and "continuity." We can hear shades of Dewey in the words Guenther uses to describe the form of learning fundamental to Tantra:

> The world of man (sic) is not some solipsism (subjectivism at its peak) nor is it the sum total of all the objects that can be found in the world; the world of man is his horizon of meaning without which there can neither be a world nor an understanding of it so that man can live. This horizon of meaning is not something fixed once and forever, but it expands as man grows, and growth is the actuality of man's lived experience. (p. 3)

> …the human problem is one of knowledge and that knowledge is not merely a record of the past but a reshaping of the present directed toward fulfillments in the emerging future. (p. 3)

We can begin to glean from these descriptions an idea of the inherent dynamism of Tantra, and of its concerns with human growth and development and with lived experience. Its gaze is not otherworldly, but rather focused on concrete human experience, understood introspectively. This synthesis of the core ideas of Tantra raises a number of important questions for educators to consider: What sorts of educational experiences are *integrative*, involving body, emotions, mind — the full spectrum of human *being?* What sort of pedagogy might illuminate the ways in which the mind gets "stuck" in habitual thinking patterns, and how might we help students become reflective about those patterns? What sorts of educational experiences evoke shifts in perspective that lead to greater freedom, joy, sensitivity, compassion and purpose? What do we have to learn about the nature of deeply aesthetic experience, in which subject and object fuse in pure pleasure and appreciation?

Since I first wrote about Neo-humanist education for *Holistic Education Review* (Kesson, 1988), schools in this Tantric tradition have continued to proliferate all over the world (there are over 1000 schools in over 50 countries in both the "developed" and the "developing" world). Recently, practitioners in Neo-humanist schools contributed short narratives of their practice for a lovely, illustrated collection entitled *Neo-Humanist Education* (Ananda Rama, 2000). I was asked to review these papers and write a brief introduction, and was pleased to see that this tradition, from humble beginnings, is starting to make a significant contribution to the emerging literature on spiritual pedagogy.

The core values listed earlier in this paper under "Axiology" serve as a referent for educational decisions in this approach and further expand on the basic commitments noted above. Based on my study of this system, a few principles stand out as fundamental. First, Neo-humanist education confers a much needed sense of value on the profession of teaching. The work of teachers is thought to be one of the most important roles in society, and the work they do is thought to be far more than that of a technician. Morality, ethics, and the development of pro-social behavior are of great importance in this system, and it is believed that "adults' loving behavior and good role modeling are the most effective ways of helping children develop their morality" (Nivedita & Bardwell, 1999, p. 151). Therefore, the qualifications of a teacher must include "personal integrity, strength of character, righteousness, a feeling for social service, unselfishness, an inspiring personality, and leadership ability" (Jacobson, 2000, p. 20). It goes without saying that teachers should be deeply engaged with their own spiritual practice, for it is felt that working with children demands mindful self-analysis.

Teachers, above all else, must exemplify the notion of *bramacarya*, a state of mind in which everyone is perceived as an expression of the Divine. Teachers are encouraged to see the child in all of his or her potential fullness, as opposed to a "deficit model" in which students are perceived as incomplete, and in need of fixing. This fundamental shift in perception gives rise to a host of pedagogical commitments. Teachers act as facilitators, "encouraging and guiding the children to bring out what is within themselves" (Jacobson & Volpe, 2000, p. 21). Academic experiences encourage the creative self-expression of each child. And at the spiritual level, the validity of spiritual experience is affirmed through myth, story, play and the opportunity for reflection within the context of the overall life and rhythm of the class. Bussey (2000) reminds us that spirituality is not a doctrine, but a "living sense of one's connectedness within a greater whole" (p. 29).

This sense of interconnectedness finds concrete expression in the Neo-humanist commitment to fostering a "sense of place." On the material level, students practice *aparigraha* as they participate in organic agriculture, recycling, composting, land and water management, forestry, and wildlife care. At a more conceptual level, this move towards sustainability "must be created in local communities by people who have been stirred by a profound sense of wonder at the beauty and mystery of the world around them, who have experienced ecstasy in nature"

(Ananda Mitra, 2000, p. 53). The capacity for "wonder at the beauty and mystery of the world" is essentially an aesthetic capacity, and Neo-humanist schools understand art and the creative process as central to the full development of human *being*. Painting, music, dance, sculpture, and theater are at the core of the curriculum in these schools, not at the periphery, and these art forms are fully integrated into all subjects, for it is art that expands the inventive, intuitive, and imaginative powers of the superconscious mind.

A key element of the Neo-humanist vision is the belief that educational institutions are of great importance in the transformation of our world from its current conditions of war, poverty, environmental degradation, materialism, racism, and a host of other destructive "isms" to a world of mutual respect, peace, and justice that is free from dogma, superstition, and exploitation. To this end, Neo-humanist educators value the multitude of cultural expressions that make up the whole of humanity, fostering indigenous language, arts, and other cultural expressions in their schools. Multicultural education, in this context, is about "transcending the text of nationalism and creating a new type of globalism … (a) recognition of the differences that are part of the post-modern thrust but not its conclusion; a climax neither in capitalist homogeneity nor post-modern nihilism but in life-embracing unity" (Inayatullah, 2000, p. 72). One of the currents that Neo-humanist schools find themselves swimming against is what is termed "pseudo-culture," the homogenous (mostly American) music, films, and television shows that are designed not to uplift the human spirit, but to gain short term profits for their makers. These products are finding their way into every corner of the world, and eroding local cultural expressions and sentiments. This raging current of cultural products is countered in Neo-humanist schools by working to develop local art and craft forms, by media literacy and the development of a critical social/political awareness, and by fostering the creative transmission of cherished local values to future generations (through plays, murals, literature, and other forms of expression).

Neo-humanist schools are understood as communities in the broadest sense, with the welfare of all of the groups — parents, teachers, staff, and students — in mind. For example, schools in poverty-stricken areas of the world often have adult education, nutritional programs, and agricultural projects connected to them. Students in Neo-humanist schools are encouraged to direct their efforts outwards to the community in self-selected service projects, exemplifying the commitment to *tapah*. Service

— to people, plants, animals and the earth itself — helps to develop feelings of selflessness, and a sense that one is "involved in the web of life as a contributor and not only a taker" (Ananda Rama, 2000, p. 63).

Children in these schools are exposed to the basic Yoga practices embodied in Tantric philosophy. Students' all-around growth and development is fostered through eating wholesome vegetarian foods, the practice of asanas (physical postures that balance and strengthen the body), guided imagery, and ample opportunities for silent reflection and introspection. One powerful practice, sustained even into the higher grades, is the "morning circle," a collective activity in which the child has an opportunity to transcend one's own personal struggles to feel oneself an integral part of the whole. Morning circle may include singing, dancing, chanting, contemplation, or discussion, but whatever the content, the aim is that students "contribute to the collective intelligence and wisdom (and) at the same time they are supported by the powerful synergetic flow" (Merz, 2000, p. 30). Above all, joy and pleasure in learning are fostered in an atmosphere free from rewards and punishments, from externally mandated standards of learning, and from the unproductive stress of high stakes tests. Unlike state schools (in almost any modern, industrialized country), which increasingly are required to "cover the curriculum," whether or not the curriculum connects to anything of relevance to the students, Neo-humanist schools have the luxury of cultivating the more subtle human characteristics and interests: emotion, intuition, insight, imagination, aesthetics, reflection, service, and spiritual development. This educational philosophy and practice provides a stark contrast to the kind of education that dominates the planet right now, one geared toward high test scores, decontextualized knowledge, nationalism, and narrow vocationalism.

## CONCLUSION

George Leonard was convinced, back in the 1960's, that new global conditions such as the incredible destructive power of new technologies, population increases, and the compression of time and space called for entirely new responses, indeed for a new kind of human being. This sort of human would not be driven by "narrow competition, eager acquisition, and aggression" but would "spend his (or her) life in the joyful pursuit of learning." The chief ingredient in the form of education necessary to bring about this new human being would be "ecstasy — joy, *ananda*, the ultimate delight" (1968, p. 230). In the last chapter of his book, he acknowledged the fear that we have about this secret ingredient, and attempted to convince the skeptical reader that ecstasy is not necessarily opposed to reason, order, or morality. In fact, he suggests, "ecstasy is education's most powerful ally. It is reinforcer for and substance of the moment of learning" (p. 232). "To affirm, to follow ecstasy in learning…is to move more easily toward an education, a society that would free the enormous potential of man (sic)" (p. 234).

Although the Cold War, which was at its height in the 1960's, is over now, the times are, if anything, more complex, and every bit as treacherous. Population is steadily increasing, environmental destruction escalates, wars and rumors of war abound, consumerism and commercialism have seemingly conquered the hearts and minds of everyone, and the gap between the rich and poor persists. The need for a "new kind of human" is as compelling as ever. Perhaps we have something to learn from the planet's most ancient tradition about how to nurture the capacities that will help us develop a peaceful, healthy, and happy society, a society in which learning is engaged in for sheer and utter pleasure, and for the genuine welfare of humanity. This is truly a revolutionary idea — perhaps one whose time has come.

## REFERENCES

Ananda Mitra. (2000). "Environmental education." In *Neo-humanist Education*. Germany: Ananda Marga Gurukula Publications, pp. 52-53.

Ananda Rama. (2000). *Neo-Humanist Education*. Germany: Ananda Marga Gurukula Publications.

Bharati, A. (1965). *The Tantric Tradition*. London: Rider.

Bussey, M. (2000). " Sa' visya' ya' vimuktaye: 'Education is that which liberates' " In *Neo-Humanist Education*, edited by Ananda Rama. Germany: Ananda Marga Gurukula Publications, pp. 10-11.

Guenther, H. V. (1972). *The Tantric View of Life*. Berkeley: Shambala.

Inayatullah, S. (2000). "The Multicultural Challenge to the Future of Education. In *Neo-Humanist Education*, edited by Ananda Rama. Germany: Ananda Marga Gurukula Publications, pp. 72-73.

Jacobson, E., & Volpe, K.( 2000). "The role of the teacher." In *Neo-Humanist Education*, edited by Ananda Rama. Germany: Ananda Marga Gurukula Publications, pp. 20-21.

Kesson, K. (2000). "Contemplative spirituality, social transformation, and currere: Finding our 'way'." In *Educational Yearning: The Journey of the Spirit and Democratic Education, edited by* D. Carlson and T. Oldenski. New York: SUNY Press.

Kesson, K. (1988). A neo-humanist model of education. *Holistic Education Review, 1*(3), 12-18.

King, F. (1986). *Tantra For Westerners: A Practical Guide to the Way of Action.* New York: Destiny.

Leonard, G. (1968). *Education and Ecstasy.* New York: Dell.

Maslow, A. H. (1975). "Some educational implications of the humanistic psychologies." In *Four Psychologies Applied to Education*, edited by T. Roberts. New York: Schenkman.

Merz, A. (2000). "Morning circle." In *Neo-Humanist Education*, edited by Ananda Rama. Germany: Ananda Marga Gurukula Publications, p. 30.

Müller, M. (Trans.). (1962). *The Upanisads.* New York: Dover.

Nivedita, A. A., & Bardwell, K. (1999). "Expanding the child's mind: Sarkar's theories on early childhood education." In *Transcending Boundaries*, edited by Inayatullah and Fitzgerald. Australia: Gurukula.

Sarkar, P. R. (1998). *Discourses on Neo-Humanist Education.* Thailand: Ananda Marga Publications.

Sarkar, P. R. (1982). *The Liberation of Intellect: Neo-Humanism.*

Yeshe, L. (1987). *Introduction to Tantra: A Vision of Totality.* Boston: Wisdom Publications.

Yogananda, P. (1946). *Autobiography of a Yogi.* Los Angeles: Self-Realization Fellowship.

Zimmer, H. (1951). *Philosophies of India*, edited by J. Campbell. New York: Pantheon.

# CHAPTER 4

# "That of God in Everyone"

## The Spiritual Basis of Quaker Education

### Ron Miller

The Religious Society of Friends has represented a distinctive dissenting voice in Western religious and cultural life since the mid-seventeenth century. Responding, in part, to the turmoil surrounding the English Civil War, George Fox and his followers turned away from established Church practices and dogmas to seek an authentic *experience* of the Divine. Because many of the early Friends were so deeply, literally moved by this experience, they were called "Quakers," a name by which they are most commonly known today. By turning inward in contemplative silence, these dedicated seekers encountered what they called "the Light" of Christ — the actual presence of the spiritual force that nourishes the created world. They believed that this Inner Light is universally present within all human souls, that "the sacred is always within us as potentiality, waiting to be addressed, answered, called into fuller being" (Lacey, 1998, p. 3). Fox claimed that this Light represented no less than "that of God in everyone."

This turn from exterior ritual to interior awareness, from a theological emphasis on the transcendent (otherworldly) nature of God to an insistence that divinity is immanent within the human soul, represented a significant step in the evolution of Western religious consciousness. In recognizing that spiritual reality could be encountered directly by silencing the ego and allowing a deeper dimension of knowledge to appear, Quaker practice seems to confirm the pattern of spiritual development that Ken Wilber (1983) has identified in the history of consciousness: Over the course of many centuries and throughout diverse civilizations, he explains, religious understanding has evolved from magical practices to archetypal mythologies to intellectual models to direct apprehension of transpersonal reality. Fox and other Quaker seekers recognized the need to go beyond institutionalized ritual and theological dogma in order to truly experience the Light. In so doing, they began to break free of cultural (mythological and ideological) identities that differentiate human beings and make them adversaries; they saw instead that a more fully realized spirituality reveals the universal source of human identity. As the Bible puts it, in Christ (that is, in true spiritual consciousness) there is neither "Jew nor Greek," male nor female, slave nor free; there is instead that of God in every one. The Quakers took this to heart.

## A SPIRITUALITY OF SOCIAL JUSTICE

This religious viewpoint leads to potentially radical social and educational ideals, as the Society of Friends has amply demonstrated. To Quakers, the Light within represents nothing less than a "bond linking all human beings" in spiritual equality and brotherhood, and Quakers' "unyielding devotion to the Inner Light, as well as their belief in the universal nature of that Light, formed the basis of the Friends' humanitarian impulse" (Kashatus, 1997, p. 17). Consequently, Quakers have been led to proclaim "testimonies" against slavery, war, and exploitation, and their moral passion has supplied potent leadership and ideals to movements for social justice and peace. Numerous Friends have been moved by their spiritual awakening to "speak truth to power" — to confront injustices perpetrated by governments, armies and others with authority despite personal risk. At many times in the past three and a half centuries, Quaker activists in both England and the United States (and increasingly elsewhere) have sought to arouse a greater public commitment to values such as community, equality, simplicity, and nonviolence or "harmony." Friends have been involved in movements for prison reform, improved medical and psychiatric care, gender equality, human rights for Native Americans and other marginalized populations, conscientious objection to military service, environmentalism and other forms of political and humanitarian action.

Indeed, Quaker spirituality has had a profound influence on modern social movements, though it is not explicitly recognized very often. Recently, however, sociologist Paul Ray, who has studied so-called "cultural creatives" and the social vision they have carried forward from the 1960s, was asked about the "earlier struggles" that influenced the rise of social activism in that decade. "Well," he replied, "you could argue that the Quakers started the whole thing...." centuries earlier, along with a handful of other groups. "Those people did the first versions of [cultural] reframing — it's just that the rest of the culture didn't pick up on it at the time" (van Gelder, Ray and Anderson, 2001, p. 17).

This pervasive concern for justice, equality and peace has also informed Friends' educational endeavors. Since William Penn founded the Friends Public School in Philadelphia in 1689, American Quakers have applied their religious and social ideals to a distinctive tradition of holistic, spiritually rooted educational thought and practice. In a recent study of the origins of Quaker education in Philadelphia, William C. Kashatus (1997) described the cultural and political forces that have shaped educational practices within the Quaker community. He found that, while Friends schools, like other denominational schools, were to one degree or another established to preserve the sect's integrity by providing religious instruction "guarded" from the corruption of secular society, Quakers' guiding testimonies and social conscience have clearly informed many of their educational efforts. Friends' education aims for far more than religious indoctrination. According to Paul A. Lacey, it seeks

> to encourage people to make the world better, to become informed, skilled agents of positive social, political, economic, and educational change, devoted to the fullest possible expression of the particular world image and style of fellowship represented by the Quaker testimonies.... (Lacey, 1998, p. 80)

For example, Quaker educators take seriously the teaching that a divine "seed" animates *every* human soul, and they understand their primary mission to be nourishing this seed so that all people may reach their intellectual, social, moral and spiritual potential. Penn himself argued that "education was an essential form of outreach to children from a variety of socio-economic backgrounds" — a civic responsibility to build an inclusive and mutually supportive community (Kashatus, 1997, p. 29). Consequently, Quaker educators such as Anthony Benezet in the mid-eighteenth century were among the first to insist that African American youths be provided equal educational opportunities. Diversity has become a central goal, if not a hallmark, of Friends schools, and a major concern of Quakers who work for public school reform. For them, practicing respect for all human beings regardless of racial, ethnic, cultural, class or gender identity is not a politically correct act but a spiritual imperative. Such identities are partial and incidental, and the task of building harmonious communities depends upon recognizing our common humanity.

## RESPONDING TO THE INNER TEACHER

The Quaker "world image" affects other dimensions of educational practice as well, beginning with a fundamental respect for young people's autonomy and integrity as learners. Friends have placed a great emphasis on reason over the authority of tradition. Reflecting on their own experience of persecution at the hands of an established Church, they maintain that first-hand, experiential knowledge, refined by the exercise of judgment and reason, enables people to discern deeper truths than those they passively receive through dogmatic instruction. Like other Quakers, "Penn believed that human nature could only be improved if society respected the liberty of one's conscience," wrote Kashatus. "Only in this way could the individual exercise reason, pursue the search for inward truth and become a constructive member of the larger society" (p. 21).

Significantly, this trust in the individual's ability to discern truth does not arise from some romantic, libertarian belief in personal freedom, but from a profound faith in the power of the Inner Light. Friends often speak of Christ as the Inner Teacher — a voice that contains the wisdom and insight that people need to achieve moral and spiritual maturity. Paul A. Lacey comments that "perhaps in no tradition is this metaphor — God is a Teacher — more central than in Quakerism, where the very core of the liberating message is, in George Fox's words, that 'Christ has come to teach his people himself.' George Fox invariably describes his ministry as turning people toward the Teacher within them, the Light which has enlightened every person who has ever come into the world" (Lacey, 1988, p. 4).

This divine voice is not heard through the words of others but inwardly through one's own receptive conscience, yet a certain self-discipline is essential to cultivating this receptivity. The Inner Light, according to respected Quaker author Howard Brinton, "can be reached only by 'centering down,' to use an old Quaker phrase: that is, by concentrating our attention on the inward side of life where the soul's windows open toward the Divine...." (Brinton, 1953). "Centering down" means turning away from ego-driven pursuits, from selfish individual concerns, and allowing oneself to be moved by a spiritual intelligence greater than one's everyday consciousness. And, though truth cannot be obtained from others, neither is it a "personal possession"; as Lacey and other Friends writers point out, Quaker spirituality involves the gathering of community to "practice *discernment*" — that is, to test the authenticity of what one believes to be a divine leading. "We turn to the Christ within us, but what we find there, if it is true, will be found within others who also turn inward with a willingness to be taught" (Lacey, 1988, pp. 8, 9, 11). Or, as the well known educator and author Parker Palmer has said, "It is part of the genius of Quakerism, I think, that the movement of the spirit is not enclosed as a private matter, but is made manifest in public ways and put to public test. The most important consequence of any meeting is the nurture of community, of recentered and reconnected selves" (Palmer, 1976, p. 6).

Liberty of conscience, then, means freedom *for* thoughtful, selfless pursuit of truth within a fellowship of seekers, not freedom *from* all influences outside the individual. This is an important distinction, not only in Quaker practice, but in holistic educational thought generally. Quaker education, like all carefully considered holistic approaches, views the individual within a social and communal context, as well as a transpersonal (spiritual or divine) context, not as an isolated psychological atom. This does not diminish the integrity and even sacredness of the individual's inner life, but it holds the individual accountable to larger realms of meaning (Miller, 2000).

A disciplined conscience comes through the experience of *silence*. As practiced in Quaker worship, silence is an active effort aimed at "greeting the sacred" and "centering outside the self" (Lacey, 1998, p. 9). The individual strives to put personal wants and preconceptions aside, and to listen carefully for guidance from a deeper source. Silence, as a spiritual and educational practice, is a means of opening one's heart and mind to dimensions of truth and wisdom that lie beyond our current understanding. We need to cultivate the humility and sense of receptivity to acknowledge that Truth is not contained by our presently held ideas, assumptions and understandings; rather, it is continually being revealed in ever greater fullness throughout our lives. "Every moment bears in it the dynamic of new truth, a life-changing insight, a hitherto unexplored perspective often coming through unexpected and unlikely channels," as one Quaker educator has commented (Brown, 1982). This is a truly radical conception of knowledge! It demands of each person that we continually re-examine our beliefs and attitudes in light of new experience. This notion is very similar to John Dewey's attack on the "quest for certainty" that underlies so much of modern Western knowledge, though with a more spiritual conception of the source of experience.

Even further, Friends' insistence on spiritual equality erodes social ranks and distinctions, claiming that the Light will appear through any soul that is open to it. This challenges our common assumption, based on vestiges of a long history of authoritarian social control, that teachers, textbooks, and government standards contain the only important elements of learning. Everyone's voice is valuable, because every person's experience represents some measure of Truth, and until we listen, until we afford compassion and respect to dimensions of human experience outside accepted norms, we cannot know what measure this might be. All people, even students and youths, have access to knowing that is deeper than common knowledge if they are prepared to receive it. And we become prepared through silence and the caring support of spiritual fellowship, not professional rank or academic training.

## COMPASSIONATE KNOWLEDGE

An education grounded in this practice has been described by some Quakers as "worship across the curriculum." In this spirit, academic disciplines no longer hold total authority over self-awareness and personal conscience, but become vehicles for cultivating an ethical and spiritual relationship between person and world. All fields of study are attempts to engage the world in a deep way, to know the mystery of things as well as established facts, to respect the wholeness and integrity of the world as it is. Parker Palmer captured the essence of this Quaker understanding in his wonderful book *To Know as We Are Known*. He contrasted modern scientific knowledge, motivated by a desire to control the world for our own material benefit, with a knowledge arising from love and compassion — that is, a sincere effort to know the world on its own terms, in all its subtlety, complexity and unfathomable depth.

A knowledge born of compassion aims not at exploiting and manipulating creation but at reconciling the world to itself.... A knowledge that springs from love will implicate us in the web of life; it will wrap the knower and the known in compassion, in a bond of awesome responsibility as well as transforming joy; it will call us to involvement, mutuality, accountability. (Palmer, 1983, pp. 8, 9)

Palmer had been dean of studies at the Quaker retreat center Pendle Hill before he wrote this book, and his conception of knowledge reflects core values expressed in Friends' testimonies and teachings. In this light (or, we could say, in this Light), education is not viewed as training for a competitive job market but as the cultivation of a respectful, receptive, compassionate, connected and accountable attitude toward the human community and the world as a whole. This is an education for peace, for acceptance and celebration of diversity, for collaboration and partnership, and for ecological wisdom.

It is important to note, however, that Friends education has generally been eminently practical as well, recognizing the importance of academic and vocational accomplishment and nourishing these very successfully. Most of the authors on Friends education emphasize this element, and it is reflected very clearly in the high quality and stellar reputations of many Quaker high schools and colleges. Still, academic success is viewed within a larger social and moral context. Intellectual attainment is expected to be put into the service of making a better world, in collaboration with others in the community. Personal success is an important goal, but without a moral conscience making one accountable to larger contexts, the essence of Friends education is lost.

Reviewing various publications for and about Quaker educators (Miller, 1989), I concluded that they "tend not to emphasize techniques so much as distinctive attitudes or an atmosphere as being essential to a Friends school." There is general agreement that the school environment should cherish and nurture every member of the school community despite differences in ability or background, that educators should encourage imagination, self-awareness, and self-expression, that cooperation is essential, and that decisions should be made democratically, even by consensus if possible. Quaker congregations have traditionally run their affairs by a spiritually grounded form of consensus they call the "sense of the meeting" — an open-minded acknowledgement of "the gathered wisdom" of the community. These meetings for business maintain the same respect for silent attentiveness to deeper truth as do meetings for worship. In a pamphlet written for Pendle Hill that previewed the ideas he expressed in *To Know as We Are Known*, Parker Palmer saw a natural extension of this core Quaker process to education.

> Where else should the search for truth have greater prominence than in the process of education? Of course, for many of us, "education" has come to mean a scramble for information, which leads to grades, which lead to a diploma, which leads to a job. There are too many educational institutions where truth is not the point! Perhaps the image of a "meeting for learning" will remind us of forgotten depths in the educational process, just as the silent meeting for worship once stood as a rebuke to ways of worship which put the human before the divine.

> A meeting for learning is, in the first place, a genuine encounter between persons, a "meeting" in the literal sense.... In a meeting for learning the individual is always in relationship, and knowledge emerges through dialogue. (Palmer, 1976, p. 2)

Friends schools have, indeed, emphasized this communal nature in the search for knowledge. Douglas H. Heath observed that "Friends believe that growth occurs most fully when an 'individual-is-in-Community'.... To create a school, a class, that corporately searches for truth means some radical changes in the way we typically teach and learn...." (Heath, 1969; Heath, 1979). In place of individual competition for grades, status and personal success, Friends schools encourage activities such as reflection, listening and collaboration and values such as compassion and service.

## EDUCATION FOR TRANSFORMATION

Given all these elements of Friends pedagogy, it is not surprising to find more student-centered, experiential forms of teaching in their schools than in many traditional private and denominational schools. Methods such as cooperative learning, project-based instruction, whole language, and multiage groupings are familiar to many Quaker educators. During the twentieth century, a number of Quaker schools became associated with the progressive education movement in its various forms (for example, they were prominent in the Network of Progressive

Educators that was active in the 1980s and early 1990s). Lacey (1998) explicitly recognized an affinity between Quaker educational ideas and the work of holistic education pioneers such as Pestalozzi, Froebel, and Montessori. Although there is little evidence of cross-fertilization between their ideas and Friends education,[1] they hold similar views about the nature of the human being. Starting with a basic trust in the process of human development (whether this is seen in a biological/social context, as in progressive education, or in a more spiritual sense), all these holistic educators insist that true education is an encounter between an active, aspiring, evolving being and the larger world with which we are co-evolving. This encounter requires respect for, and dialogue with, the learner. In yet another essay, Parker Palmer (1978) expressed this point very clearly:

> Adults will always have the power to coerce children. But caring rests on the power of hope and trust, not the power of containment. If we try to keep our children within safe boundaries, we prevent them from undertaking any great experiment with Truth. (pp. 9-10)

Palmer went on to state that the primary responsibility of mature, authentic adults is *caring for new life* — a phrase that impressed me so deeply that I recently used it as the title for a collection of my writings about holistic education.

Palmer, along with other Quaker educators and the larger holistic education tradition, is essentially concerned with honoring, protecting and nourishing the creative vital forces that give rise to life and to our human identity. It should be the function of education to cultivate these energies, to see where their evolution will lead us, and not to impose the existing culture's prejudices on each new generation to keep young people's consciousness within "safe boundaries." Thomas S. Brown (1982) maintained that "our Quaker experience of education is different from education understood as the transmission of the group's inherited wisdom..."(p. 9). Using this term, transmission, precisely recalls Jack Miller's (1996) distinction between "transmission" and "transformation" orientations in education, and brings us to the very essence of Friends education as I understand it. In the Quaker tradition, education is not primarily about transmitting authorized knowledge to passive learners, but achieving personal and social *transformation* by unleashing and nourishing the creative power of the Inner Light. Again, it is Paul Lacey (1988, p. 26) who summarizes this point so well; indeed, his words provide a fitting close to this chapter:

> When it is faithful to its foundations, Quaker education is neither student-centered, nor discipline-centered; it is inward-centered. Quaker education operates from the conviction that there is always one other in the classroom — the Inward Teacher, who waits to be found in every human being.

## NOTE

1. One example of contact between these traditions is the interesting case of Amos Bronson Alcott, the romantic Transcendentalist who attempted to practice holistic teaching in New England in the 1820s and 1830s. As a young man he had left home to become a traveling peddler, and it was immediately after visiting a Quaker community in North Carolina that he returned to New England to teach and to begin a life-long spiritual journey. He was further inspired by his studies of Platonic and romantic philosophy while teaching in the Philadelphia area (where he was probably further exposed to Quaker influence) between 1830 and 1834. He did not join the Society of Friends but it does seem that his exposure to Quaker spirituality left a lasting impact. As further evidence of the connections among diverse holistic perspectives, Alcott did explicitly call his educational method "Pestalozzian," and over 150 years later his work was published and promoted in anthroposophic (Waldorf education) circles.

## REFERENCES

Brinton, H. H. (1953). "Education." In *The Quaker Approach to Contemporary Problems*, edited by J. Kavanaugh, (pp. 78-80). New York: Putnam.

Brown, T. S. (1982). *Reflections from a Friends Education* (C. A. Dorrance, Ed.). pp. 9-10. Philadelphia: Friends Council on Education.

Heath, D. H. (1969). *Why a Friends School?* Wallingford, PA: Pendle Hill.

Heath, D. H. (1979). *The Peculiar Mission of a Quaker School*. Wallingford, PA: Pendle Hill.

Kashatus, W. C. (1997). *A Virtuous Education: Penn's Vision for Philadelphia Schools*. Wallingford, PA: Pendle Hill.

Lacey, P. A. (1988). *Education and the Inward Teacher* (pamphlet). Wallingford, PA: Pendle Hill.

Lacey, P. A. (1998). *Growing into Goodness: Essays on Quaker Education.* Wallingford, PA: Pendle Hill.

Miller, J. P. (1996). *The Holistic Curriculum* (Rev. ed.). Toronto: OISE Press.

Miller, R. (1989). Quaker education: Nurturing the divine seed within. *Holistic Education Review* 2(2): 37-40.

Miller, R. (2000). "A holistic philosophy of educational freedom." In *Caring for New Life: Essays on Holistic Education* (pp. 90-105). Brandon, VT: Foundation for Educational Renewal.

Palmer, P. J. (1976, May). *Meeting for Learning: Education in a Quaker Context.* Wallingford, PA: Pendle Hill Bulletin

Palmer, P. J. (1978). *And a Little Child Shall Lead Them* (pamphlet). Philadelphia: Friends Journal.

Palmer, P. J. (1983). *To Know as We are Known: A Spirituality of Education.* San Francisco: Harper & Row.

Van Gelder, S., Ray, P., & Anderson, S. (2001). A culture gets creative. *Yes! A Journal of Positive Futures.* Winter 16: 15-20.

Wilber, K. (1983). *Up from Eden: A Transpersonal View of Human Evolution.* Boulder, CO: Shambhala.

**CHAPTER 5**

# The Prophetic Tradition and Education

## David E. Purpel

### WHO WERE THE PROPHETS?

Let me begin this essay with some historical and definitional considerations before moving on to the larger meaning and significance of prophetic spirituality. The capitalized form of the term "Prophet" derives from its prominent place and particular usage in the Hebrew Bible. The Hebrew word is *navi*, usually defined as a "seer," but although they talked a great deal of what the future held, the Hebrew Prophets are not to be regarded as soothsayers or fortunetellers. Their notion of what the future would be was more of an extrapolation of present trends within a framework of a strong belief in a particular course of human destiny. The Prophets predicted that unless the community renounced its present evil ways it would inevitably bring upon itself the wrath of God; but if it returned to the righteous path, it would surely receive God's blessings.

It is quite clear that the Biblical Prophets claimed to have directly experienced the presence of God and to have had quite specific communications with the Divine. Prototypically, these communications dealt with the relationship between divine intentions and the particular and current policies and practices of the society. Prophets served as divine messengers but they did not act, in Abraham Heschel's phrase, as merely "God's microphones." Rather, they engaged in direct and contentious dialogue with the community, interpreting the meaning and long-term consequences of God's concerns over persisting serious violations of the Covenant. In general, the message was one of severe condemnation of hypocritical piety attendant to these violations combined with both the threat of harsh punishment as well as the promise of shining redemption if the people were to alter their wicked ways. The following passage is a good example of the rhetoric and content of prophetic writing in which Isaiah quotes God as saying to the people of Israel:

> Though you pray at length,
> I will not listen,
> Your hands are stained with crime —
> Wash yourselves clean;
> Put your evil doings
> Away from my sight.
> Cease to do evil;
> Learn to do good.
> Devote yourself to justice;
> Aid the wronged.
> Uphold the rights of the orphan;
> Defend the cause of the widow.
>
> (Isaiah, 15-17)

Michael Walzer, in commenting on the political role of prophets in the Biblical era, has this to say:

> Prophets are not agitators in the modern sense. They don't aim to create a political or social movement; they make no effort to organize their audience.... On the other hand, they are also unlike modern social critics, who sit in their studies writing books and magazine articles and can hardly be imagined speaking in the streets. The prophets are religious preachers, something like contemporary revivalists, and although they criticize the whole of society and hope for its moral transformation, their precise demand is for individual *teshuvah*—"repentance"; the literal meaning is a "turning back" to the law of the covenant. (Walzer, p. 217)

Although such generalizations about the Biblical Prophets as a group are reasonable enough, their individual writing styles and sayings vary and are specific to particular historical times and situations. What they have in common is their piety and intensity in the context of their direct experience of God and their anguish over the moral state of the nation. They present themselves as God's agents willing to sacrifice their own well being in order to be true messengers of God's expression of severe displeasure even in the face of the inevitably sharp hostility of the now severely chastised community leaders.

Apparently, prophets were often, if not usually, part of the official order serving to offer advice to the rulers as to the spiritual propriety and likely consequences of particular policies and decisions. In this sense, they were called upon (or gratuitously volunteered) to serve as a kind of sounding board to the religious validity of political activities. It is clear that the ruling class was not always pleased with what the prophets had to say and, indeed, frequently sought out the prophets who would offer more pleasing pronouncements. Hence, prophets were certainly not of one voice, and indeed one of the most debated issues in Jewish writings is the basic question of how true prophets are to be distinguished from false ones, a problem that was to plague centuries of Jewish history.

When the Second Temple was destroyed in the first century, C.E., the traditional Jewish religious practices rooted in Temple ritual and sacrifice came to an end and were ultimately replaced by what has come to be called rabbinic Judaism. This tradition puts far greater reliance on human interpretation of sacred texts than on divine revelation for guidance and direction. Indeed, the sages of the early phase of this new era proclaimed the end of prophecy and ruled that insight into God's will was thereafter to be derived by serious and devoted study of the sacred texts.

The disputes regarding the distinction between 'true and false prophecy' is a crucial one in that it crystallizes the problematics of the validity of prophecy itself. First of all, it brings into question the credibility of the various accounts of personal encounters of God. Moreover, the question reveals the dilemma involved in predicating the truth of such claims on personal testimony, i.e., if I am to say that God has chosen me to reveal his word, who are you to doubt me in the face of such an extraordinary event? Secondly, the question suggests, at worst, the possibility of deception and fraud by the erstwhile prophet or, perhaps more charitably, the possibility of self-delusion and misperception. More ominously, it raises the question of the ambiguity and complexity of God's will and the human capacity to fully know it.

In spite of this skepticism and doubt, it is clear that many people have claimed the mantle of divinely appointed prophet and with it the right to speak with divine authority. What complicates the issue, of course, is that often the messages from these self-appointed prophets either confound prior understandings and/or contradict other prophetic messages. Absent clear and unambiguous signs, how then can we separate truth from falsity, genuineness from deceit, revelation from belief, and epiphany from madness? Even if we accept the possibility of divine revelation we are still left with the problem of sifting and judging the validity of individual claims of the reports of such events as well as the interpretations of them. The issue of the meaning of these divine communications becomes an even more difficult task in the face of those prophets who saw themselves much more as messengers than as interpreters.

In this regard, Michael Walzer, in his book on Jewish political thought, makes an important distinction between prophecy and wisdom:

> Kings are *challenged* by prophets … and *counseled* by wise men. Wisdom is prudent, politic, worldly, and human; prophecy is radical, impolitic, utopian, and divine. Wisdom is at home in the royal court, prophecy in the desert and then in the streets and gates of the city and the temple courtyards. Rabbinic Judaism in some sense escapes this tension with its claim to be the joint heir of the wise and the prophets. (Walzer, p. 202)

## PROPHECY AS METAPHOR

Obviously, there continue to be deep and significant differences about how and what ways our religious and spiritual traditions and texts are to be interpreted, particularly in the split between those who believe that these texts should be taken literally and those whose take on them is largely metaphorical. In using the term "metaphor," I have in mind the formulation of a figure of speech that seeks to describes one thing with another. The assumption for the value of such a process is that what is being described has an elusive, ambiguous, and multi-textured meaning which can only be evoked rather than defined. The result is that the metaphor being used 'is and is not' the same as what is being described (McFague, 1987).

A literal view of the prophets is that they are, in fact, people who have, miraculously enough, had a conversation with the actual persona of God regarding divine intentions. The difficulties with a literal interpretation include issues of plausibility and dogmatism, i.e., it strains credulity and invites intolerance of the skeptical. How can we reconcile these accounts of divine revelation with rational thought and how can we discern the Truth when we have such a wide variety of differing, if not conflicting testimonies? By what criteria do we judge the wisdom of these testimonies? Yet, at the same time we cannot logically entirely dismiss the possibility that some of these accounts can be literally true and still be valid.

A metaphoric view might regard prophets as people who have startling and powerful insights whose origins remain unclear, if not mysterious, *as if* they were divinely derived. It can also be a metaphor for the very real human and yet mysterious impulse to connect with the divine through the relentless pursuit of justice and mercy. There are a number of advantages to a metaphoric approach in grappling with the spiritual realm. For one thing, it allows and, indeed, encourages both humility and awe since we can affirm the existence of a spiritual realm without the arrogance and rigidity of certainty and literalness. Furthermore, metaphorical thinking provides the opportunity for the celebration of diverse interpretations and expressions of spiritual phenomena as well as for continuous good faith dialogue. Such open-ended dialogue also allows for an expanding and developing understanding of this realm as our historical contexts change and our experiences deepen.

Our notions of prophecy have certainly changed over the centuries while the question of who are the true prophets remains as crucial and controversial as ever. The literal minded approach is one that bemoans this reality and assumes that there is a correct answer to the questions of authenticity while a metaphoric one sees the ambiguity and uncertainty as inherent and irresolvable. Accepting a metaphorical approach is not without its difficulties, however. The problematics of a permanent absence of basic clarity offers anguish, doubt, and uncertainty as well as the opportunity for excessive poetic license. Nor does such an approach provide a barrier to divisiveness since there are those who totally reject the basic assumptions of interpreting spiritual matters metaphorically.

Furthermore, there are probably as many differences among those who take a metaphorical approach to understanding to matters spiritual as there is between the two camps. Although it is possible to argue, for example, that Jesse Jackson, Jerry Falwell, the Ayatollah Khomeini and Nelson Mandela are all exemplars of the prophetic tradition, it would be ludicrous to view them as embodying the same point of view. If we were to accept a metaphoric notion of prophecy it would also mean that we would have to cast considerable doubt on the prophets' claim to be primarily agents and messengers of God's will. The question then becomes not so much whether or not we want to adopt prophetic spirituality, but rather *which* particular prophetic spirituality. Such a view requires that the prophets' audience not only attend to the prophet's message but that it also has the further responsibility to critically examine and evaluate the significance and meaning of the message. Indeed, Michael Walzer, in his discussion of the distinction between prophecy and wisdom, points out that when

> The king's counselors, known by their worldly wisdom rather than their divine calling, give their advice about this or that policy matter, they no doubt raise ... questions about trustworthiness ... but what they explicitly invite is a debate about the advice itself: Is this really what prudence requires in our present circumstances? The prophet, by contrast, does not invite a debate of that sort. Indeed, if they have actually been sent by God, there is no room for any debate at all. The only way to challenge them is to call their credentials into question, not the content of their prophecies.... But the sages [the early highly esteemed founders of Rabbinic Judaism] call themselves wise and make room for arguments about both prudence and principle. And they do everything they can to neutralize the disruptive force of prophecy. They are as bound as the prophets were to God's word, but they are its interpreters now, not its messengers. (Walzer, pp. 204-205)

Employing a metaphorical approach, therefore, allows us to choose from among the many dimensions of the Biblical prophetic traditions as well as providing us with the opportunity to enrich and extend it with the properties of other traditions. In doing so we also give up the claim of certainty and divine authority and, thereby, take on the human responsibility for examining the possibilities and limitations of our views.

## PROPHECY AND SPIRITUALITY

For the true believer, the nature of the spiritual dimension of prophecy is self-evident and obvious, namely that the experiences of the prophets are but an additional revelation of a living and present God who actively participates in history. It is, of course, possible to attribute such experiences to psychological phenomena such as madness, delusion, and hysteria, or even to outright fraud and deceit. To do so, however, would be to deny the validity of the fundamental beliefs and feelings of an enormous number of people across time and space who, as a matter of faith, have accepted the possibility of such extraordinary encounters. Indeed, for those with religious faith, the pre-existence of a larger reality provides the ultimate and requisite context of understanding human experience. As Mircea Eliade puts it:

> Whatever the historical context in which he is placed, *homo religious* always believes that there is an absolute reality, the sacred, which transcends this world but manifests itself in this world, thereby sanctifying it, making it real. He [sic] further believes that life has a sacred origin and that human existence realizes all of its potentialities in proportion as it is religious — that is, participates in reality. (Eliade, p. 202)

However, the relatively narrow religious aspects of prophecy do not exhaust its spiritual possibilities. The experiences of the prophets raise basic questions about the origins of the human impulse to seek and sense meaning and purpose in life, to question the validity of the material and the visible, and to delve into the mysteries of existence. Moreover, one does not have to be a person of a particular religious faith to register one's wonder and awe at the magnificence and grandeur of creation and to yearn for (as well as acknowledge the possibility of) genuinely connecting to that immensity in ways suggested by the Prophets.

## PROPHECY AND MORAL VISION

Prophecy represents a spirituality of meaning, hope, and possibility guided by an energy directed at creating a world of social justice, human compassion, and personal joy within a universe radiant with transcendent love. Within this framework, the original Prophets experienced the failure to create such a society with intense disappointment and anguish but always held on to their faith in the human possibility to transcend human limitations. Abraham Heschel, in his magisterial work on the Prophets, has this to say:

> Almost every Prophet brings consolation, promise, and hope of reconciliation along with censure and castigation. He begins with a *message of doom*; he concludes with a message of *hope*.... [H]is essential task is to declare the word of God to the here and now; to disclose the future in order to illustrate what is involved in the present. (Heschel, p. 12)

Prophetic spirituality focuses very sharply on the moral attitudes and conduct of society with the determination that the social and cultural aspects are in accordance with divine commandment. The Biblical

Prophets measured social and cultural policies and practices by the strict and demanding criteria set down in the Covenant received at Sinai and further elaborated in later revelations. This insistence on examining both the general and the specific is a very clear manifestation of the concept of *praxis*, the process by which the full meaning of principles and theories enfold in the context of practice and application. The Biblical Prophets expected and demanded that the people be not only fully aware of the divine commandments, but also that they fully and genuinely integrate them into communal life so that there would be a seamless web of the temporal and the spiritual.

It is in this sense that the Prophets must be seen not only as mystical and spiritual seers but as astute and critical observers of the social and cultural milieu in which they live. Prophets use their intellectual and analytical powers to thoroughly examine and interrogate the degree to which particular policies and practices of the time match the fundamental social and cultural aspirations and commitments of the historic community. Indeed, they probably do not make hard and fast distinctions between theory and practice and between what is spiritual and what is secular in the way that much of modern culture does. What is important to note is that Prophets are people who see it as their responsibility to integrate criticality with faith and empiricism with belief.

Michael Walzer interprets the Prophets, however, as people without a particular political program but who, instead, angrily demanded that the rich and powerful repent their failure to achieve justice and to revere God. However, Walzer is not uncritical of the Prophets. He also points out that in their outrage at gross violations of the Covenant, they invoke a God who is destined to inflict terrible indiscriminate collective punishment on the community unless the rich and powerful reaffirm their obligations to God and the powerless:

> None of the prophets takes aim at the political or social hierarchy, only at the individual men and women who occupy its high places; there is no prophetic program for a democratic program and politics, or a classless society. All that the prophets demand — but how radical they make it sound! — is that the rich stop trampling the poor and that the powerful ... act forcefully to protect the weak. (p. 218)

> Even if idolatry could be the sin of the whole people, great and small alike, oppression can't be — there are always guiltless vic-

tims, oppressed men and women … the prophets speak with enormous courage on behalf of the oppressed against the powers-that-be. But they don't speak, as Abraham did, against the Power-That-Is: "Will You sweep away the innocent along with the guilty?" (Gen. 18: 23) (Walzer, p. 219)

## PROPHECY IN MODERN TIMES

Walzer's citation of Genesis is in reference to the episode in which Abraham courageously objects on moral grounds to God's threat to totally destroy the wicked towns of Sodom and Gomorrah. This criticism of the Biblical Prophets is an instance of a tradition that maintains that it is a continuing human responsibility to interpret the divine commandments in the light of historical events as well as the responsibility to maintain a critical stance toward our most influential texts. Walzer's criticism reflects an era when we have come to affirm and celebrate democracy and when we have come to challenge any rationale for privilege. Furthermore, we inhabit an era that remains anguished about the nature of God's relationship with humanity in the light of the devastating horrors of the 20th century. This is not to say that historical differences of such magnitude in any way undermine the basic thrust of prophetic thought — the utter incompatibility of God's vision of human society with injustice and oppression. It underscores, though, the necessity for understanding that this message is both eternal and contemporary, as we struggle to find the proper balance between individual responsibility and social expectations and between what is morally non-negotiable and what is historically contingent. Abraham Heschel has articulated this perspective with characteristic eloquence and power:

> Modern thought tends to extenuate personal responsibility. Understanding the complexities of human nature, the interrelationships of the individual and society, of consciousness and the subconscious, we find it difficult to isolate the deed from those circumstances in which it was done. But new insight may obscure essential vision, and man's conscience grows scales, pretense, self-pity … Above all, the prophets remind us of the moral state of the people: Few are guilty, but all are responsible. If we admit that the individual is in some measure conditioned or affected by the spirit of the society, an individual's crime discloses society's corruption. (Heschel, pp. 14, 16)

Walter Brueggemann is a distinguished theologian who has written extensively and brilliantly about the persistence across time and space of the tensions between those who are wont to preserve the privileges that attend to the preservation of the status quo and those who would re-create a more just and loving order. In his book *The Prophetic Imagination*, Brueggemann refers to these two positions as the "royal and prophetic consciousnesses." A royal consciousness permeates a society that is locked into a sense of "static triumphalism" made more secure by co-opting God to legitimate a society of affluence and exploitation. Such a society, very much like contemporary America, swaggers and gloats in a sea of smugness even as it is dimly aware that something of fundamental importance is amiss. But it cannot confront this nagging worry because

> Now and in every time, it is grossly uncritical, cannot tolerate serious and fundamental criticism, and will go to great length to stop it. [It is a] wearied culture, nearly unable to be seriously energized by new promises from God. (p. 14)

In sharp and direct contrast with this 'royal' sensibility is a way of being called the 'prophetic consciousness' that Brueggemann describes as a mode in which the major emphasis is justice and compassion in a community where basic equality is the goal. In this consciousness, humanity is free to create a life of meaning for all and has a cosmology in which God is also free from entanglements with the establishment. This consciousness is energized by its devotion to its principles and openness to transcendence (i.e., to the possibilities of a re-created world).

The prophetic moral view recognizes that humans can be expected to be greedy, oppressive, and cruel but which, at the same time, affirms the hope and possibility of becoming fully human, i.e., by creating a just and loving community. The very strong emphasis on justice for the weak is not merely an abstract principle about spirituality and the equality of souls, for it also demands material social equality, i.e., that we see to it that "the poor, the orphaned, and the widowed" are to be clothed, sheltered, and fed. Neither is the thrust of this commandment for social justice merely a pragmatic and shrewd process designed to provide for social and commercial stability for it is also to be regarded as an expression of God's vision of what constitutes a "good" (i.e., Godly) community. Furthermore, the injunction to respond to the needs of the powerless is not to be seen only as charity for the poor but as an essential and non-negotiable responsibility that is also required for the spiritual well being of the rich and powerful.

## EDUCATION AS PROPHECY

There are strong historical connections between the prophetic tradition and American education, as most strikingly reflected in the educational policies and practices of the New England colonies. In more recent times echoes of the prophetic consciousness have been reflected in the ideas of the Progressive and Reconstructionist educators. For example, Lawrence Cremin, quoting John Dewey's *My Pedagogic Creed* has this to say:

> What is apparent here is the ancient prophetic role which Dewey himself had in mind when he wrote in 1897 that the teacher is always 'the prophet of the true God' and the 'usherer in of the true kingdom of God.' The millennialist tone of these phrases has always left me a bit uncomfortable, but the insight is nonetheless profound. Prophesy [sic]; in its root meaning, the calling of a people, via criticism and affirmation, to their noblest traditions and aspirations. Prophesy, I would submit, is the essential public function of the educator in a democratic society. (Cremin, 1976, pp. 76-77)

In this selection, Cremin not only provides us with some historical perspective and an elegant definition of prophecy but also gives us some insight into the metaphoric usage of the concept of prophecy. Dewey's use of the term in this selection is clear even though Dewey's overall attitudes toward the religious and spiritual were ambiguous, if not unfriendly. Cremin himself, even as he affirms prophecy, distances himself from part of its theological overtones. Yet in an essay titled *Schools of the Prophets*, his social vision is strongly resonant with the moral imperatives of the Bible:

> — a truly humane society — a democratic society, committed to the dignity of all human beings and the worth of their individual lives; a free society, wherein each and every person is afforded a rich and varied opportunity to develop his or her potential to the fullest; a transnational society, which conceives its public life as extending to every man, woman, and child on ... "spaceship earth." (Cremin, p. 89-90)

I strongly believe that the prophetic tradition can provide us with the sharp insight and powerful wisdom that we need as we grapple with our now distinctly different educational situation. The teachings of the Biblical Prophets seem especially appropriate in an era when education has been largely permeated with a very strong technological, functional, and instrumental orientation.

## AFFIRMATION

It is now my task to attempt to speak to our current educational situation in a prophetic voice; a voice that, I hope and trust, in some important ways resonates with the Biblical Prophets yet is in harmony with the historical moment. I certainly do not want to claim that this is my own unique and original voice but rather one that I hope is in unison with particular spiritual traditions of criticism and affirmation. These are traditions that focus on issues of social justice, cultural diversity, personal meaning, and political democracy that witness our moral failings with outrage and that confess our highest aspirations with faith. It is a tradition that speaks in many dialects and accents but whose energies are grounded in a spirit that impels us to not only witness and confess but to act; not only to feel but to think; and not only to blame and rage but to be responsible and compassionate. I count among those in this tradition such people as Martin Luther King, Mohandas Gandhi, Nelson Mandela, Abraham Heschel, and their countless adherents and supporters who have struggled to create a world of loving-kindness and justice in the context of particular historical challenges and crises.

What then of our own time and context? What challenges and crises do we face today and what might constitute a prophetic response to them?

First, I believe that we must acknowledge the powerful historical forces that may have faded from our active memories but which still loom over our horizons. We have just ended a tumultuous century filled with promise and despair, horror and redemption, and the full range of human expression from generosity and compassion to cruelty and bestiality. In one century the world has witnessed the development of both life-saving medicines and of weapons of mass destruction; the hell of the Holocaust and the redemption of Israel; the end of European colonization and the start of the global economy. Powerful events and people still significantly influence our consciousness: the Great Depression; the incredibly bloody World Wars; Auschwitz; Hiroshima; the Cold War;

Chernobyl; Hitler, Churchill, FDR, Stalin, Freud, Einstein, Anne Frank, Martin Luther King, Mohandas Gandhi....

In the very first moments of the 21st century many of us tend to consider these events as ancient history and to see our era as a time of permanent peace and prosperity as we revel in the destruction of the Evil Empire and the triumph of the free market. Some have proclaimed that the market economy will end the boom and bust cycles and that we have entered an age of centrist politics that (except for some relatively harmless partisan bickering) will ensure lasting social harmony and stability.

However, there are those who are not without serious misgivings and nagging doubts. Many of us believe that we also live in a culture that seems primarily driven by ambition and greed directed at increasing material wealth, political power, and personal liberty. It is a culture where many people confuse indulgence with freedom, intellectual mastery with wisdom, who see technology as liberating, and who blur personal achievement with spiritual worth. We live in an era when we are urged to grasp for advantage and privilege by working hard with cunning and ferocious competitiveness instead of striving to develop closer communal ties and greater social harmony. Our popular culture increasingly reflects a society consumed in a relentless, if not joyless, pursuit of mindless pleasure. There are large and enthusiastic audiences for violent and pornographic films; for racist, homophobic, and sexist music; and for sports played by arrogant and brutal millionaires intent on humiliating and maiming each other.

We live in a society focused on the maniacal drive for ever more consumer consumption, industrial productivity, and global domination. What has been sharply eroded in this process is our tradition for caring and compassion, particularly for those who do not share in the recent prosperity, the current equivalent of the failure to respond to the plight of the 'widows and orphaned.' We have failed in our covenantal commitments to end unnecessary human suffering, in spite of the fact that we have the capacity and resources to do so. We have come to view the homeless as unworthy of pity, to regard those on welfare as malingerers, and to interpret social protest as the actions of a few twisted fanatics. For a nation as rich as ours, we have a shamefully high infant mortality rate and for a culture as enlightened and pious as we claim to be, we have an obscene rate of incarceration. It should be added that in both these examples, people of color suffer a disproportionate burden of the pain — a powerful indication of the continuing ugly persistence of racism in America.

Politicians talk endlessly of tax relief for the middle-class and the desirability of capital punishment but manage to avoid serious discussion of profound poverty and of the chasm between have and have-not nations. We have rhetoric that embraces human dignity and the right to clean air and water but enact policies that cruelly exploit people as well as nature in order to feed the insatiable demands of capital. Meanwhile, the beat goes on — the rich have gotten a lot richer, the middle-class are under even more stress, the working poor are getting more desperate, and the indigent have become entirely invisible.

Educational institutions are more and more seen as important instruments in the legitimation, support, and development of the politics and economics of the free market as they are expected to provide a technologically sophisticated, compliant, and highly motivated workforce to compete, achieve and consume. Parents increasingly see schools and universities as primary modes for providing advantage and privilege for their children, or at least to offer an antidote to the possibility of economic and social failure. Politicians have seized on these concerns and fears and have succeeded in turning complex questions of educational policy into simple-minded partisan campaign issues. The public has come to embrace a mantra that the "nation is at risk" because of the failures of organized education and hence there must be drastic educational "reform." Educators, in their haste to respond to public pressures and to do their masters' bidding, have reacted to these demands for reform with alacrity and energy.

Much of this so-called reform movement has been regressive both in its style and substance relying for the most part on punitive, oppressive, and vulgar measures. Primary attention has been on what is now called 'high-stakes' testing in which students (and in many instances, teachers) are required to take frequent standardized tests designed to evaluate not only the test-takers but the efficacy and efficiency of the schools. The results of these tests have had significant consequences for such matters as school graduation, college admissions, school funding, personnel assignments, and teachers' salaries. This emphasis on "accountability" has served to create frenzied efforts to get "good numbers" ranging from the allocation of considerable class time focused on specifically preparing students (teaching to the test) all the way down to actual fraud and collusion. Furthermore, it has served to vulgarly transform something as complex and variegated as the learning process into the acquisition of bits of isolated information and to reduce the art of teaching to the techniques of cramming. Teachers have less and less autonomy and have more to fear from being imaginative and creative in the classroom as they are heavily pressured to produce higher and higher scores while the definition of what constitutes a proper education becomes increasingly narrow and pedestrian.

The K-12 curriculum has gradually shifted to one that is heavy on computer technology and applied sciences with significant losses to such important realms as drama, dance, art, music, and physical education and recreation. There is much more homework required and it is being assigned at younger and younger ages, so much so that the attendant stresses for families have become a major topic for advice columnists. Many schools have adopted specific learning requirements for kindergarten graduation and the practice of so-called "social promotion" has been abolished in many states. At the university level, the number of MBAs, business, and computer technology majors continue to zoom while the numbers of those majoring in the traditional liberal arts continue to decline. All of this in the name of reform!

These reforms serve mainly to buttress social and cultural policies directed at American economic and political domination, continued corporate growth, and access to personal privilege. It represents a deadly amalgam of Social Darwinism and meritocracy, a harsh and unforgiving system that provides handsome rewards to the competitive and/or to those with selective talents while affording scorn and ignominy for the rest. It is not an educational policy that holds as central a concern for the enrichment of democratic traditions and institutions nor is it a program designed to deepen intellectual curiosity and stimulate the imagination. This is an education that is materialistic in all senses of the term, one that does not allow for, or even recognize, the opportunity for students to reflect on their quest for meaning and wholeness. Most tragically, it undermines our profound and ancient commitment to affording dignity to all through the creation of a just and loving community. Our current educational policies and practices do not urge us to love unconditionally but to reward conditionally; they do not urge us to seek justice but to chase success; and they do not validate our struggle to be as one with our sisters and brothers but rather they serve to legitimate our instincts for division and conquest.

Perhaps the most disheartening aspect of our times is the rise in cynicism and despair about the possibility of resisting such disturbing policies. It is clear that although there are many people who are profoundly disturbed by our social, economic, cultural, and political circumstances, a great many of them feel overwhelmed by the enormity of the barriers to genuine transformation. The "system" seems too powerful; the struggle to "fight city hall" seems more quixotic than ever; and in today's moral climate, the concept of idealism is much more likely to evoke ridicule than celebration.

I believe, alas, that these are indeed times when optimism about the creation of a loving and just society is unfounded, if not misplaced. From a rational and empirical perspective, the battle appears to be lost and to continue believing that we can overcome the forces of greed and selfishness would seem to be a case of denial and delusion.

However, to entertain the idea of surrendering to the struggle only adds to the crisis and, therefore, giving up becomes unthinkable. In such a despairing time we must, instead, go beyond the rational boundaries of expectation and optimism and instead, rely on the hope and energy that are so powerfully manifested in many of our religious and spiritual traditions. We have, miraculously enough, an especially rich resource that has the power to energize and give hope to us at precisely such moments of doubt and despair, i.e., the miracle that is prophetic spirituality. This is a spiritual tradition that has sustained us in other deeply troubled times from Babylonian exile to American slavery and from the destruction of the Temple to the construction of the gas chambers. Its origins are mysterious but familiar; its powers are ineffable but real; and its meaning is awesome but knowable.

Prophetic spirituality is about acknowledging and acting upon the deep connection between the divine and the material, between the promise and the reality; between criticism and affirmation; and between despair and hope. It does not seek to challenge the technical and organizational dimensions of society nor even its material ambitions but rather to denounce its moral aspirations and social conscience. When we, therefore, examine educational issues we ought to be more concerned with such issues as the poverty rate rather than with SAT scores and we ought to grieve for the pain of those who are labeled school failures rather than exult in those who win scholastic high honors. We must also remember in such times that there is a readily available tradition of highly imaginative educational ideas and practices directed at the enhancement of personal fulfillment and social justice. Moreover, we need to celebrate the untold number of people who courageously continue to fight for humane and meaningful education for all students. There are great ideas and great people out there; what is needed to help us to move from despair to possibility is the will and determination that emerges from profound faith in human possibility.

This is not to say that such a path is not without its difficulties and pains. There are aspects of the prophetic tradition that remain troubling. For example, I personally find it difficult to accept the idea that some people have had direct experiences with the divine and with the notion of a harshly vengeful God. Nor do I share the degree of anguish about the idolatrous violations of religious observance that many of the Biblical Prophets often railed against. Moreover, there is always the deeply troubling matter of sorting out which prophetic utterances are more compelling than others, i.e., of being able to discern the true from the false prophets.

In spite of these difficulties, however, I continue to maintain my commitment to the compelling truths that emerge from my understanding of the prophetic tradition. In part, I am able to do so by supplementing this faith with other human resources. We can and should rely on the power of critical thought both in personal reflection and rigorous dialogue to increase our insight into what is knowable. In addition, we have no choice but to deal with the ambiguities and complexities with courage and faith by accepting the wisdom that comes from humility and reverence in the face of mystery. We must as citizens and educators also take the risk of making moral affirmations in the full knowledge of the dangers of certainty as well as flaccidity:

> I affirm traditions that not only recognize that humans are fated to create our world but believe above all we are called upon to create a world resonant with divine intention — a world of peace, justice, love, community, and joy for all. These are traditions that accept as givens the potentials of human abilities as well as the limits of human fallibilities; they posit our capacity to be generous as well as to be selfish; to be angelic as well as demonic, compassionate as well as cruel; wise as well as foolish. Such traditions revere knowledge but only as it is tempered with wisdom that advances justice and mercy; a perspective that acknowledges the enormity of the task but dismisses human despair as sinful; and one that represents a

consciousness of outrage in the wake of cruelty and injustice but always in the faith that witness, confession, and healing offer the possibilities of transcendence and redemption. What is absolutely crucial to redemption is human responsibility and human agency since these traditions require that we act as God's agents, dedicated to constructing and sustaining communities based on joy, love, peace, and justice. (Purpel, 1999, p. 196)

I mention my own views as testimony to the enduring and compelling power of prophetic spirituality to inspire us to pursue the good, to guide us to know what is good, and to give us the hope and energy to sustain the struggle. Their words continue to bristle with scornful indignation at human folly yet mercifully they also show us the path to redemption through the healing that attends justice and love.

... Behold on the day of your fast, you pursue business as usual, and oppress your workers. Behold you fast only to quarrel and fight, to deal wicked blows. Is this the fast I have chosen?

... This is My chosen fast: to loosen all the bonds that bind men unfairly, to let the oppressed go free, to break every yoke. Share your bread with the hungry, take the homeless into your home. Clothe the naked when you see them, do not turn away from people in need. Then cleansing light shall break forth like the dawn, and your wounds shall be healed. Your triumph shall go before you and the Lord's glory shall be your rearguard. Then you shall call and the Lord will answer, you shall cry out and He will say, here I am. (Isaiah, 57:14–58:14)

## REFERENCES

Brueggemann, W. (1978). *The prophetic Imagination*. Philadelphia: Fortress.

Cremin, L. (1976). *Public Education*. New York: Basic Books.

Eliade, M. (1959). *The Sacred and the Orofane*. New York: Harcourt Brace.

Heschel, A. (1962). *The Prophets*. New York: Harper & Row.

McFague, S. (1987). *Models of God*. Philadelphia: Fortress.

Purpel, D. (1999). *Moral Outrage in Education*. New York: Peter Lang.

Walzer, M., Menachem, L., & Zohar, N. (Eds.). (2000). *The Jewish Political Tradition*. New Haven: Yale University Press.

# TEACHERS

## CHAPTER 6

# Aurobindo Ghose

## David Marshak and Karen Litfin

Aurobindo Ghose (called Sri, a title of respect for his saintliness, by his devotees) was born in Calcutta, India, in 1872. His father, an upper-caste member, sent Aurobindo to England at the age of seven for his schooling. Aurobindo completed his studies at Cambridge University in 1893 and returned to India. When he first stepped onto Indian soil, he discovered within himself a deep, unshakable feeling of inner peace. He later described this experience as the first step in his spiritual awakening.

In the decade after his return to India, Aurobindo devoted himself to studying Indian languages and cultures as a teacher at Baroda College. He also began a secret involvement in the movement for Indian independence. In 1906 Aurobindo moved to Calcutta to become principal of the Bengal National College. Here his previously secret commitment to political work became public, as Aurobindo wrote and spoke about the need for passive resistance to British rule and participated in the organization of a secret revolutionary group.

In 1908 the British colonial authorities charged Aurobindo with treason and imprisoned him for a year. In 1909 he was tried and acquitted. Immediately after his release, Aurobindo returned to his political work. Within a few months, however, Aurobindo received what he felt to be a divine command to abandon this work and take up an entirely spiritual life. He left Calcutta and traveled first to Chandernagore, then on to Pondicherry in French India, a hundred miles south of Madras, where he remained for the last forty years of his life.

Aurobindo had begun his practice of yoga in 1904. In 1907 Aurobindo experienced his first of four major spiritual openings. While in prison, Aurobindo devoted most of his time to spiritual practice and study, and his sense of mission broadened from India's liberation to that of the entire planet when he experienced his second spiritual opening.

When Aurobindo received his message to abandon political work, he realized his own profound work would be teaching humanity about the next step in its evolution. He discovered the evolutionary need not to reject any part of reality, as many previous Hindu mystics had done, but to understand all of reality as divine and worthy of liberation.

In his first decade in Pondicherry, Aurobindo published most of what would constitute his major writings, including *The Life Divine*, *The Human Cycle*, *The Ideal of Human Unity*, and *Bases of Yoga*. In 1920 Mirra Alfassa (Richard), a French woman, joined Aurobindo as his student. Soon afterward he recognized her as The Mother, his own spiritual partner and successor.

In the 1920s a community of devotees grew around Aurobindo and became the Sri Aurobindo Ashram, a spiritually based community very much in the world. In 1926 Aurobindo experienced his final illumination when he felt the Overmind, a higher spiritual level of being than mind, descend into the physical plane of this planet. Immediately after this experience, Aurobindo turned over the responsibilities for administering this community to Mirra Alfassa. He retired into seclusion for the rest of his life, although he stayed very much in touch with the world through periodicals and letters and did appear in public on four occasions each year.

Aurobindo Ghose died in 1950. The Mother, who had started the Ashram school in the early 1940s. lived on until 1973. For twenty-three years after Aurobindo's death she guided the Ashram and its attempt to embody his teachings. In 1968 the Mother and Ashram residents founded Auroville, a spiritually based "city of the future" near the Ashram, which has been recognized by the Indian government as an international city-state. The final section in this chapter explores education in Auroville.

## Aurobindo's Vision of Human Nature

Aurobindo Ghose's understanding of human nature is informed by his conception of the universe as consisting essentially of consciousness that is expressed on many different planes of being. Consciousness is "the fundamental thing in existence . . . not only the macrocosm but the microcosm is nothing but consciousness arranging itself" (Ghose, 1957, p. 257). The planes of being are "linked in graded continuity from the lowest matter to the highest spirit" (Bruteau, 1971, p. 438). These planes include the material plane, the vital plane, the mental plane, the transitional spiritual planes of higher mind, illumined mind, intuitive mind, and Overmind, the Supramental plane, and the divine consciousness.

Aurobindo's vision of human nature describes us as "divine being(s) in an animal and egoistic consciousness" (Ghose, 1960, p. 2). Each person is a unique individual, a self-developing soul. We are partially divine beings who are evolving toward greater divinity. Human beings are dynamic systems that consist of five major sub-systems:

- the material or physical being — the body of matter, of flesh and blood, and the physical consciousness;
- the life-force or vital being — "the life-force acting in its own nature (through) impulses, emotions, feelings, desires, longings, ambitions, and so on" (Ghose, 1957, p. 349); the vital being is also the seat of the instincts;
- the mental being—"a faculty for seeking knowledge ... (yet) mind is only a preparatory form of consciousness. It is an instrument of analysis and synthesis, but not of essential knowledge" (Purani, 1966, p. 144). The mind often perceives a part of some knowing that it cannot apprehend as a whole;
- the ego—the ego is not a being, yet it plays an important role in unfoldment. Its function is to protect the person by giving her a clearly felt though ultimately illusory sense of a center within herself until she learns about her true center within the psychic being;
- the psychic being or soul—a spark of the divine that has individual identity and is immanent within us; and
- the spirit—the spirit is transcendent to us, yet we have access to its expression through the psychic being. It is the infinite divine.

Each of the five sub-systems includes several or many elements within it. Each exists primarily on its own plane of being. Yet because the various planes of being are integral, not isolated from each other, these sub-systems interpenetrate each other and are profoundly interrelated. Whenever one sub-system changes or is affected by some force, every other sub-system is affected in some way.

Aurobindo's description of human nature is profoundly rooted in his conception of the evolution of consciousness as the central process in the existence of the universe. This evolution is a dual process: the emergence of consciousness from its involved state in matter into higher planes of being, and the simultaneous descent of spirit into the material, vital, and mental planes to aid the evolution of consciousness. "Evolutionary ascent is not by the negation of that which is lower, but by its complete appropriation and integration into a higher-level experience" (Langley, 1949, p. 73).

Central to Aurobindo's vision of human nature is the understanding that evolution does not stop with humans. We are transitional beings, as were all that have preceded us. We openly embody the mental plane as well as the vital and material, yet latent, involved within us, is the Supramental. In the next step in evolution, the Supramental will appropriate mind and transform it. At this stage in the process, the mechanism of evolution is the individual soul, each person's connection to the Supramental and her potential for bringing forth that plane of being within herself.

Aurobindo teaches that evolution has itself reached a radically new stage in its unfoldment. During the past century for the very first time, the beings that evolve—ourselves—have become conscious of the process of their evolving. With this awareness as guidance, humans can consciously choose to participate in evolution, to bring the energy of their will to organize their consciousness and, through spiritual discipline, learn to manifest the Supramental in this world. For in the movement from the mental to the Supramental, the primary medium of change will be consciousness, not matter.

## AUROBINDO'S VISION OF HUMAN BECOMING

Aurobindo describes human becoming between birth and age twenty-one as a process of unfoldment in which the person's innate potential seeks to emerge and grow. Each newborn child is an organismic whole that contains within it a developmental urge toward growth and self-mastery. This urge originates within the person's psychic being and is the manifestation of the divine consciousness seeking to propel the evolution of the individual and, through the individual, the evolution of the species.

Aurobindo discusses the nature of the developmental urge and the person's innate wisdom for seeking growth tasks that are appropriate for her particular stage of unfoldment. The Mother describes three distinct eras or ages of unfoldment: birth through six or seven years; six or seven years through twelve or thirteen years; and twelve or thirteen years through twenty years. The *first age* is a time marked prominently by the child's need to direct her own activity. During the first three years, the child belongs to the family. In the next three, she needs to reach out into larger social contexts. What is consistent through most of this age is that the child knows her experience as play, that is, self-directed activity that is purposive and more rewarding in its process than in whatever it achieves.

Around the age of seven years, the *second age* unfolds as a new quality of concrete, operationally-focused thinking becomes important to the child's consciousness. Her locus of interest shifts increasingly away from the family and toward the school and peer group. Also at the beginning of the second age the psychic being awakens for many children which opens their capacities for love, compassion, giving to others, and higher aspiration.

At seven through nine years the child is engaged in the task of grounding herself, of gaining a sense of her place in her family, school, and peer group. At eight through nine years she experiences a new intensity of social needs that continues into the teens. She wants to be with her peers more, to be engaged in activity with them and accepted by them. At ten through twelve years the child begins to take on the patterns of individuality that will be hers throughout the rest of her life. This is also a time in which she has the potential for beginning to discover her calling on this planet.

At twelve or thirteen years the child unfolds into the *third age*. This growth is marked by the youth's development of a more complete reason, including the capacity to work with abstraction, and by her new awareness of her own inner life. In this age the youth seeks freedom to explore both within — her feelings and passions, thoughts and intuitions and questions — and without — ideas, people, and experiences. She seeks freedom and adventure. It is a time when she wishes to explore the world beyond the family and school and to establish new relationships with it. This age is also a time when the youth brings energy and passion to her investigation of the meaning of life.

Sri Aurobindo and the Mother detail a number of developmental needs that must be met for a child to grow toward health and wholeness. The first need of the child, particularly in the first age, is the experience of an interwoven trust and happiness. This kind of trustful happiness plays a significant role in the child's life, for it is both her primary need and a sign that no other important needs are being neglected.

Among these other needs are the ones listed below. Each is important in all three ages though in different ways in each age:

- The child needs to grow in all of her beings as is appropriate to her stage of unfoldment.

- The child needs to grow in freedom and independence according to her own inner calling, the expression of her soul or psychic being. This need does not require adults to accede to the child's every wish, for every child expresses desires, whims, greed, and so on that are not needs. What it does demand of adults is a profound respect for the child's expression of herself and a willingness to accept that expression as it manifests itself, not to try to mold or shape it to meet the expectations or desires of the adults.

- The child needs the security of knowing that her growth will not be hampered by or interfered with by adults. She needs to know that she will not be compelled to do things for which she is not ready.

- The child needs support, affection, sympathy, and love, particularly on the soul level.

- The child needs to be given the opportunity to complete that which she begins. Her behavior is purposive. When she becomes engaged in an activity and gives attention to it, she wants to experience a sense of completion in relation to that activity before she moves on to something else.

- The child needs to experience beauty in people and in her environment. She also needs to experience gratitude, awe, and reverence.

- The child needs to learn how to satisfy her needs herself. She needs to learn how to take responsibility for her expression of a need, accept the consequences from her attempts to meet her needs, and learn from these experiences.

## AUROBINDO'S VISION OF EDUCATION

The process of education that Aurobindo and the Mother described and that their students sought to implement at the Ashram school is called *integral education*. The integrality refers both to the understanding of reality as a series of integral planes of being and to the nature of humans as immensely complex systems composed of various interrelated and interpenetrated sub-systems or beings. The term integral education also speaks to the purpose of education: helping the various beings and their faculties unfold according to their potential and learn to work together for a common purpose, a purpose that is conveyed from the spirit through the psychic being. The focus of integral education is first on the inner unfoldment of the child and then on the relationship between the child's inner life and her actions.

Aurobindo explains that the development and harmonization of the child's various beings is best nurtured by helping her psychic being to unfold as well as supporting the growth of her other, lower beings. The child's psychic being can be apprehended by the teacher through the teacher's own psychic being. It can also be known through the expression of the child's developmental urge, for this urge is the direct manifestation of the psychic being.

The psychic being, then, is a powerful *inner teacher*. In a profound sense,

> ... the child, with the tremendous motivating potential within, is his own teacher. The nurture of the child means this actualization of the inner motivating potential through the careful nurture of the developmental urge. (Joshi, 1975, p. 52)

The *inner teacher* is manifested as the child's curiosity, urge for exploration, aspiration for achievement, and pursuit of excellence.

> It is never by external compulsion that a child acquires interest, the key of all learning, but by finding within herself a security, a sanction, an authority from her own nature and the law of her own being. (Dowsett, 1977, p. 155)

Aurobindo summarizes the purposes of education by explaining that young people need to learn to think for themselves, change their consciousness, evolve their true personality in an integral way, and live the truth which they discover. Yet education must focus not only on the individual but also on one's relationship to opportunities and responsibilities as a member of one's community, nation, and species.

The guidelines that Aurobindo offers for education include the following:

- Invite the child to begin academic studies when she is seven years of age. Before that time she should be in an environment that is designed for play. Beginning the learning of academic subjects too early can interfere with the child's unfoldment.

- Treat girls and boys equally in all activities.
- Know that the focus of education is the actualization of the child's inner potential, the manifestation of her personal capacity for evolution. Education is not the acquiring of mental information. Such information is useful when it relates directly to the accomplishment of another appropriate goal. It is not a goal in itself.
- Understand and respect the child's unfoldment, and invite her to participate in environments and activities that are appropriate to her stage of unfoldment. For example, for children who think in concrete terms, offer stories, images, and parables rather than abstract concepts.
- Organize the learning environment and activities to suit the present needs of the child, not some set of projected future needs. At the same time, understand that education is for the unfolding and evolving soul of the child and the future in which she will live, not for the past or even present society.
- Organize the learning environment to function as "a student activated classroom ecology" (Dowsett, 1977, p. 19). Invite the spirit of freedom to permeate the entire atmosphere of integral education. "Activate a climate of curiosity, discovery and free progress — through living situations of self discovery rather than the acquisition of knowledge" (Dowsett, 1977, p. 20). Interact with the child so that you suggest and invite, never command or impose. The Mother called this kind of approach to education *the free progress system*. Within a free progress system of education, the child can and must learn about freedom and discipline: not one or the other but both in relation to each other.
- Invite the child to set the pace for her own learning.
- Give responsibility, power, and meaningful roles to the child as is appropriate to her level of unfoldment. For example: tutoring younger children; cooking, cleaning and maintenance; leading games and sports.
- Invite the child to discover and experience reverence and gratitude, so that she can experience moving beyond the narrow identity of her ego consciousness.

- Help the child "to develop his instruments of knowledge with the utmost thoroughness…" (Ghose, 1924, p. 27) and help her to gain a mastery of her native language, which will be the medium for much that she learns. Once she has developed her instruments of knowing, she can learn and grow in whatever directions her *inner teacher* carries her.
- Invite the child to learn about one subject at a time in depth, both as a whole in itself and in the ways it relates to other subjects.

Aurobindo emphasizes that ultimately the aim of education is to put all of the parts of the child's being in contact with the influence of the psychic being. So education must focus first on the whole child and, given that holistic frame, must simultaneously address the needs of her sub-systems, which Aurobindo describes as follows:

*The physical being*—a sound and fundamentally healthy body; the education of the senses; the awakening of the body consciousness; discipline and self-mastery; strength and fitness, with dexterity and control; grace, beauty, and harmony; and relaxation.

*The vital being*—"to become conscious and gradually master of one's character" (Ghose and Richard [Alfassa], 1956, p. 109) through the training of the vital energies for the building of character and will, that is, moral education; and the education of the aesthetic sensibilities of the child.

*The mental being*—to train its various faculties to unfold to their potential and learn to work together harmoniously. These faculties include the following: expression; memory; observation; discrimination; concentration; inner silence; imagination; intuition; will; judgment; and reason and logic.

*The psychic being*—The teacher is the key to the process of psychic education. She must be aware of the psychic being within the child and know its inherent goodness, light, and love. To gain this awareness and knowledge, the teacher must be engaged in her own spiritual practice and thus in nurturing her own psychic being. The most powerful teaching she can give to the child is through her influence and her example as these relate to her own psychic and spiritual life. Empowered by her own spirituality, the teacher can invoke soul qualities in the child's consciousness and behavior.

It is the teacher's responsibility to encourage and validate the child's expression of psychic qualities. She must also teach the child about the psychic plane. From the very earliest age the child must be taught that there is a reality within—within herself, within the earth, within the universe. From an early age, the child needs to learn and practice a spiritual discipline through which she can learn to quiet the mind, experience the inner silence and the witness consciousness, and grow more and more open to her psychic being.

Finally the arts are another way of opening to a consciousness of universal harmony and unity, to a perception of the divine. Experiencing beauty and harmony through artistic expression and experience can also help the child to know and explore her psychic being.

## EDUCATION IN AUROVILLE

In 1954, four years after Sri Aurobindo's passing, the Mother first articulated her vision of what was to become Auroville, "City of the Dawn."

> There should be somewhere on earth a place which no nation could claim as it own, where all human beings of goodwill who have a sincere aspiration could live freely as citizens of the world and obey one single authority, that of the supreme truth.… In this place, children would be able to grow and develop integrally without losing contact with their souls; education would be given not for passing examinations or obtaining certificates and posts but to enrich existing faculties and bring forth new ones. (*Mother's Birth Centenary Library* XII, 1985, pp. 91-92)

Auroville, an international township born on February 28, 1968 in South India, aims to realize a deep-felt human unity. After over three decades of hard work, including a good deal of turmoil during the early days, Auroville is now home to about 1500 people from forty different countries. There are about 50 different settlements in Auroville spread out over a 20-square mile circle. Most of the settlements' names represent spiritual values: Verité (Truth), Sincerity, Discipline, Revelation, to name a few. While most Aurovillians are westerners, India is the single largest nationality represented. Located in rural Tamil Nadu, about 15 kilometers from Pondicherry, Auroville established itself in the midst of several Tamil villages, where perhaps 50,000 people live at subsistence levels. As such, the community represents a living experiment in cross-cultural communication, both within itself and with the surrounding area. These enormous socioeconomic, cultural and linguistic differences make Auroville a sort of microcosm of humanity's problems. This perspective is further dramatized by the extremely degraded condition of the land upon which Auroville was founded. Ecological restoration, especially reforestation, and the establishment of sound living practices have been a major part of Auroville's work. Thus, Auroville itself is a place of education; international cooperation and sustainability are learned through the practical circumstances of life.

Education is not understood as a separate realm of activity in Auroville, as it is in modern schooling systems. Rather, according to The Charter of Auroville, issued by the Mother upon Auroville's founding, Auroville will be the place of an unending education, of constant progress, and a youth that never ages. Auroville wants to be the bridge between the past and the future. Taking advantage of all discoveries from without and from within, Auroville will boldly spring towards future realizations. Auroville will be a site of material and spiritual researches for a living embodiment of an actual Human Unity.

Thus, to be an Aurovillian is to be deeply and fundamentally committed to learning, both in an inner sense and in practical terms. While there are schools for the children, the real "school" is understood to be the community itself, for *both* adults and children, and the objective of this school is the inward sense and outward expression of human unity.

Unlike the Sri Aurobindo Ashram in Pondicherry, Auroville is mostly comprised of families, so the question of formal education for children emerged in the community's early days. A wide range of experiments in schooling has emerged in Auroville since the early 1970s. Like the Ashram school, these schools have sought to model themselves on the Mother's *free progress* conception of education, according to which each individual should be encouraged to progress at her own pace and on the lines of her own inner development. Progress should be guided by the soul, not by habits, conventions, or the quest for diplomas and degrees; teachers should be yogis contacting and inspiring the souls of their students. The Mother articulated the main stages for education in Auroville as proceeding from "Last School," before the community would be ready to abandon all formal education, to "No School," when Auroville will have transcended the need for structured schooling.

Because Auroville considers itself to be a "living laboratory of human evolution," its schools may be aptly understood as experiments. Some of the major experiments include the following:

1. Aspiration School. Founded in 1970 within the largest of Auroville's settlements, this was the first serious attempt to organize formal schooling. By 1976, some 80 children were attending school there on a daily basis. In that year, the teachers, with support from members of other settlements, decided to decentralize the school in order to more effectively integrate formal schooling into the larger community. Beginning in 1977, a host of diverse educational environments sprang up throughout Auroville for the younger children. This began a volatile period during which "formal" education essentially ceased, partly in reaction to the perception that the first experiment, Aspiration School, had become too conventional.

2. Last School. Originally named "High School," Last School was initiated in 1985 by older students who wanted a more consistent study program. Today, about fifty students attend the school, with about half of these coming from the local Tamil villages. The campus includes a computer center, a science laboratory, a library and an art center.

3. Transition School is the main school for most of Auroville's children between the ages of 7 and 12. Because one third of the students are Tamil and dozens of other nationalities are represented, there is a strong emphasis on language skills. English is the primary language of instruction. The classrooms are open, spacious, and orderly.

4. New Creation School. The largest of Auroville's schools, New Creation offers a dynamic and innovative learning environment for about 200 Tamil children from local villages. Apart from the usual academic subjects, there is a strong emphasis on the arts.

5. Isai Ambalam School began in the late 1970s as a Waldorf School and was later more consciously organized along the principles of the Mother's *free progress* model developed at the Sri Aurobindo Ashram. The students are village children between the ages of 6 and 14, many of whom would not otherwise attend school at all. Instruction is in Tamil, English, and, to a lesser extent, French. The school also has an innovative program to train local village women to be teachers in the school.

6. Fertile. While this is not formally a school, children may decide to come to this Auroville settlement when they are not satisfied with more formal learning environments. Here, the emphasis is on practical living skills, such as building a house, raising farm animals, and installing plumbing. According to the coordinator, "Learning in the West has become detached from physical life; what you learn here is a form of survival."

The Sri Aurobindo International Institute of Educational Research (SAIIER) was set up in 1984 to serve as an umbrella under which all the educational activities of Auroville could be coordinated and supported. SAIIER is in close communication with the Sri Aurobindo Ashram and its International Centre for Education.

As with the Ashram School, Auroville's schools are modeled upon the teachings of Sri Aurobindo and the Mother. While the degree of structure varies widely among Auroville's schools, each school is committed to integral education (i.e., promoting the inner unfoldment of the student and the expression of that inner life through body, heart, and mind). Physical education, aesthetic expression, moral learning, and mental challenge are all part of an integral education. According to Sri Aurobindo, "nothing can be taught." The teacher can only serve to awaken the knowledge within the student, encouraging her to grow according to her own nature and to follow the promptings of her own soul. Thus, the development of concentration and the cultivation of mental silence are part of formal schooling in Auroville. The Mother and Sri Aurobindo offered no clear guidelines or any standard curriculum for integral education. Rather, the teacher is challenged to go deeply within in order to contact her own soul and, in so doing, to be able to work from that level with the students. Thus, there is enormous room for freedom and innovation. Indeed, "the more organized forms of education have always been a fertile mixture of inspiration, improvisation, and, at times, despair; of responding creatively to particular needs as they arose" (*Auroville Today*, 1998, p. 69).

While there have been many disappointments over the years, teachers from all of Auroville's schools seem to concur that most students are exceptionally engaged in the learning process. It is not unusual, for instance, for students with virtually no exposure to English to become fluent within a year. In the words of one teacher from New Creation School, "It is just amazing. It is like planting a seed and watching it burst forth into blossom. What more can a teacher ask for?" (*Auroville Today*, 1998, p. 76). Because children have a choice about attending school, because they are not exposed to the punitive and competitive dynamics of more conventional approaches, and because the teachers at least aspire to relate to their students at a soul level, the educational environment in Auroville is quite positive.

Despite considerable disagreement about the degree to which education should be formalized and structured in Auroville, the community has embraced Sri Aurobindo's fundamental principle of education: "the mind should be consulted in its own growth." Thus, formal schooling in Auroville is optional for all children. If a child finds no joy in her schooling, she can simply leave. This radical approach means that teachers have a special responsibility to seriously engage the students at all levels: physically, emotionally, mentally, and spiritually. They must generate a sense of excitement and tap into the students' native desire for growth. Not surprisingly, the result is that virtually all children in Auroville genuinely enjoy going to school. According to one student, who had attended schools in India and the U.S. before coming to Auroville, "Outside it is either for the teacher that you're studying or for your parents, but in Auroville going to school is always your own choice, so you learn a lot more from within." Not surprisingly, the children exhibit an unusual honesty and frankness in their relations with adults. According to Deepti, one of the core teachers at Last School for many years, "Of course, these children have their outer crusts, but if you just scratch the surface you find this sweetness and soul quality, which is much more disguised in more sophisticated children" (*Auroville Today*, 1998, pp. 75-76).

Despite these high ideals, no school in Auroville has escaped the need for often painful introspection, dealing with internal issues such as discipline and the support, or lack thereof, from parents and the community at large. A persistent problem, and one that stems from the disparate educational and cultural backgrounds of the children, is that it is almost impossible to find a group of children that has the same level of comprehension in any given subject (Sullivan, 1994, p. 185). A more vexing issue is whether the curriculum at Auroville's schools should enable the children to take exams in order to study elsewhere in India or abroad, or whether the entire examination process is contrary to the "free progress" of the soul. Aurovillians recognize that the high ideals of the Mother are often beyond the abilities of both students and teachers. Ironically, the desire to remain faithful to these ideals has sometimes been an obstacle to the development of more pragmatic solutions (*Auroville Today*, 1998, p. 71).

While the freedom and openness of education in Auroville seem to work well for the younger children, a fair number of high school students have been frustrated with the lack of rigor and structure (although that situation does seem to be changing in recent years). During the 1980s and early 1990s, many students dropped out of Last School. Most went either to the *Lycee Francais* in nearby Pondicherry or the far more distant International School in Kodaikanal; others, sometimes referred to as "the lost generation," simply drifted (*Auroville Today*, 1998, p. 78).

The sense of dissatisfaction that many adolescent Aurovillians experience, however, should not be solely attributed to the schools. They find themselves in the paradoxical situation of living in a community that aspires towards human unity, while at the same time being aware that Auroville is something of an enclave. Thus, most teenagers in Auroville experience a strong yearning to study or travel abroad, to see "the real world." The fact that many, if not most, of those who follow that yearning eventually do choose to return to Auroville suggests that their experience has been a strongly positive one. Within recent years, an increasing number of babies have been born in Auroville; most of the parents of these children were themselves raised in Auroville. The community is growing organically and becoming increasingly multi-generational.

## REFERENCES

*Auroville Today*. (1998). *The Auroville Adventure: Selections from Ten years of Auroville Today*. Auroville: Auroville Today.

Bruteau, B. (1971). *Worthy is the World: The Hindu Philosophy of Sri Aurobindo*. Rutherford, NJ: Fairleigh Dickenson University Press.

Dowsett, N. C. (1977). *Psychology for Future Education*. Pondicherry: Sri Aurobindo Society.

Dowsett, N. C., & and Jayaswal, S. R. (Eds.). (1975). *The True Teacher*. Pondicherry: Sri Aurobindo Society.

Dowsett, N. C., & Jayaswal, S. R. (1976). *Education of the Future*. Pondicherry: Sri Aurobindo Society.

Ghose, A. (1921). *The Ideal of the Karmayogin*. Chandernagore: Prabartak Publishing House.

Ghose, A. (1923). *Evolution*. Calcutta: Arya Publishing House.

Ghose, A. (1924). *A System of National Education*. Calcutta: Arya Publishing House.

Ghose, A. (1936). *Bases of Yoga*. Calcutta: Arya Publishing House.

Ghose, A. (1949). *The Human Cycle*. Pondicherry: Sri Aurobindo Ashram.

Ghose, A. (1950). *The Ideal of Human Unity*. Pondicherry: Sri Aurobindo Ashram.

Ghose, A. (1952). *The Supramental Manifestation*. Pondicherry: Sri Aurobindo Ashram.

Ghose, A. (1957/1958). *The Synthesis of Yoga*. Pondicherry: Sri Aurobindo Ashram.

Ghose, A. (1953). *The Mind of Light*. New York: Dutton.

Ghose, A. (1953). *Sri Aurobindo on Himself and the Mother*. Pondicherry: Sri Aurobindo Ashram.

Ghose, A. (1957). *On Yoga I*. Pondicherry: Sri Aurobindo Ashram.

Ghose, A. (1958). *On Yoga II*. Pondicherry: Sri Aurobindo Ashram.

Ghose, A. (1960). *The Life Divine*. Pondicherry: Sri Aurobindo Ashram.

Ghose, A., & Mirra, R. (Alfassa) (the Mother). (1956). *On Education*. Pondicherry: Sri Aurobindo Ashram.

Joshi, R. K. (1974). Sri Aurobindo on education during childhood. *The Advent* 31(2).

Joshi, R. K. (1975, February 1). On education. *The Advent* 32(1).

Joshi, K., & Artaud, Y. (1974). *Exploration in Education*. Pondicherry: Sri Aurobindo Ashram.

Langley, G. H. (1949). *Sri Aurobindo: Indian Poet, Philosopher, and Mystic*. London: David Marlowe.

The Mother. (1952). *On Education*. Pondicherry: Sri Aurobindo Ashram.

The Mother. (1985). *Mother's Birth Centenary Library*. 16 vols. Pondicherry, India: Sri Aurobindo Ashram Press.

Purani, A. B. (1966). *Sri Aurobindo: Some Aspects of his Vision*. Bombay: Bharatiya Vidya Bhavan.

Sullivan, W. M. (1994). *The Dawning of Auroville*. Auroville: Auroville Press.

## NOTE

Parts of this chapter are adapted from *The Common Vision: Parenting and Educating for Wholeness* (Peter Lang Publishing, 1997) and reprinted with the permission of the publisher.

# CHAPTER 7

# Krishnamurti's Approach to Education

## Scott H. Forbes

For 74 years Krishnamurti wrote and spoke about education. His observations about religion, tradition, nationalism, relationships and the psychological state of humanity were considered radical and controversial when he first made them, but many have now found their way into modern Western culture. However, Krishnamurti's insights on education are still radical and frequently ignored. This is possibly due to Krishnamurti's presentation of education as a religious activity in an age when most people predominantly see it as preparation for succeeding in a material world — a dissonance shared with holistic education in general. Yet it is this very emphasis on the religious nature of education that has attracted so many parents and teachers to holistic education in general and Krishnamurti's approach to education in particular. Modern education has so obviously failed to educate people to solve the world's problems, has fallen so short of societies' aspirations, and has ignored the learning required to meet the challenges we all have in life (e.g., loneliness, fear, death, etc.). Krishnamurti's insights into education involve learning about the most fundamental aspects of living with the necessary but mundane; they marry the religious with the secular.

It has been argued elsewhere that a reasonable framework for examining any approach to education lies with answering three questions about that approach: 1) What is the goal or intention of an approach? This is not the goal towards which lip service is paid, but the goal towards which the majority of its resources of time, energy, space, and money are directed. The authentic goal of an educational approach is also visible in the forms of knowledge that preoccupy daily life in the school. 2) What needs to be learned to achieve or approach the stated goal? One might substitute "acquired" or "developed" for "learned" as the word learning often has restricted meanings in academic circles, and many educational approaches would want to include skills, attitudes, characteristics and even more subtle attributes to what they feel needs to be learned in order to achieve or approach the stated goal. 3) What does the educational approach contend facilitates the needed learning? "Facilitates" is used deliberately instead of "cause" as many educational approaches hold that important learning is not causal. For example, one can not "cause" another to develop courage, yet there may be many things one can do to facilitate it being developed.

This chapter will briefly answer these three questions for Krishnamurti's approach to education. This is not intended as a summary of his work on education, but rather a presentation of one perspective of his approach which, it is hoped, will act as an invitation to explore this rich and complex body of work.

For those readers unfamiliar with Krishnamurti, a brief description of his work may be useful. Krishnamurti explored the nature and state of humanity, investigating the most universal and troubling aspects of human living: fear, egotism, violence, cultural and personal conditioning, religion, and death. He felt that if people engaged in a detailed examination of the nature of thought and mind in general, and of their own in particular, eschewing all authority and dogma and negating all that was false; they could have insights into their own nature, that of the world, and into the deepest religious and psychological truths. He encouraged questioning, doubting, dialogue amongst equals and silent perception as tools for this discovery. With such insight people could come upon real psychological freedom, compassion, and a contact with what is sacred beyond anything made by humans.

Krishnamurti is thought of in many ways (a philosopher, a sage, an icon, etc.) but he is rarely thought of as an educator. This seems remarkable if for no other reason than the number of years he publicly addressed questions of education. His first book on education was published in 1912 and he kept writing and speaking on education until his death in 1986 — a seventy-four year span of publicly addressing questions of education which is, to my knowledge, unparalleled. His not being thought of as an educator is even more remarkable in view of his having started ten schools in his lifetime (Rudolf Steiner started five) all but one of which have survived. Educators credit him with inspiring the beginning of untold other schools through his many talks and books on education, especially *Education and the Significance of Life*, *The Beginnings of Learning*, and *Letters to the Schools*.

One of the reasons Krishnamurti is not thought of as an educator might be because his approach to education is so radically different from what commonly exists by that name. A person could understandably think, "Two such very different things can't be the same thing, therefore one must be something else" — if what goes on in their local school is education, then what Krishnamurti proposes can't be. This same logic might lead someone to presume that Krishnamurti didn't care about leading a religious life — he was not involved in any religion, he had no dogma, he did not believe in any "spiritual practices," and his whole approach to what he termed "religious," "spiritual" or "sacred" is so contrary to the norm that many people would find it difficult to use those words for him. Yet, he was an educator — a most extraordinary one. He was a proponent of leading a religious life — a most profound one. And he claimed that the principal reason for education was to lead a religious life.

Krishnamurti was a man of profound religiosity, yet he eschewed all religions. He felt that religions are human creations — cultural and social institutions which might aspire to the "other-worldly" and what transcends humans but which, by their very nature, must be culturally conditioned, time bound, and image generated — all things which the sacred, according to Krishnamurti, necessarily cannot be. Krishnamurti held that to confuse what is not sacred with that which is sacred is to conflate the profane with the sacred; and such conflation has led humans to kill each other in the name of God and commit every other possible obscenity and atrocity "in good faith." Having delusional ideas, images, and projections about what is sacred is worse than having none.

The question naturally follows: what ideas, images, or projections (if any) are not delusional? Krishnamurti felt that none are because all ideas, images and projections (like religions) are human creations, and all are, therefore, necessarily, destructive to a genuine religiosity.

This generates some severe dilemmas for many who would like to introduce spirituality into education. A supposition in most attempts to bring about or generate something in any social institution (like education) is that one knows what that thing is and that it is subject to human agency. Otherwise, how can one bring it about or generate it? If, on the other hand, one cannot have knowledge (ideas, images, or projections) of what is truly religious (and a great many religious exemplars have claimed that the sacred is unknowable), does that leave us with nothing to do to aid, foster or support spirituality or religiosity in education?

Krishnamurti coherently presented the case that there is a great deal that we can do without presumptions of knowing things we can't know; without conflating the profane with the sacred. He sometimes called it a "negative approach" because he felt that we might be able to approach that which is sacred by knowing and avoiding what it *is not*. He, therefore, encouraged people to see the falsely religious projections of our thoughts and images, the delusions of cultural conditioning, and the easy convictions of convention. Krishnamurti eschewed all notions of spirituality in education that involve attempts at learning to be "spiritual" or feeling "spiritual" or acting "spiritual;" he decried all attempts to change activities, practices or behavior so they conform more closely to some notion of "spiritual." In fact, all positive approaches towards the "spiritual" have such traps of delusion imbedded in them. Krishnamurti proposed instead that in investigating life's challenges as fully, deeply and honestly as possible, in discovering and living relationships of integrity and goodness, and in knowing oneself profoundly, that something genuinely religious may be touched and experienced without the destructive mediation of ideas, images or projections.

Krishnamurti questioned the desire to be "spiritual" or "religious," contending that "the urge to be successful in the material or in the so-called spiritual sphere" was often just a search for security (Krishnamurti, 1953b, p. 9). When that is the case, such urges are just more self-serving, and could never lead to the transcendence of the self, an aspect of what is truly religious.

## THE GOAL OR INTENTION OF KRISHNAMURTI'S APPROACH TO EDUCATION

The goals or intentions of different forms of education are not as similar as one may initially suspect. It is fashionable to declare lofty goals in the mission statements of schools. Declarations concerning character, morals, health, values, citizenship, and even spirituality are common. However, an examination of the allocation of resources (e.g. teacher time, student time, school space, finances, etc.) will generally reveal that very little is allocated to these loftier goals. There is generally an implicit understanding that schools are aimed at preparing children for the next level of schooling which a child should pursue as far as one can as this impacts worldly success. It is success in the material world (as fame, fortune, or simply a rewarding career) that is the goal towards which much education is directed. It is not my intention to denigrate this as a goal, simply to make it explicit.

Other schools have society as their focus and the making of good citizens as their principal goal. This was John Dewey's principal aim in education. In this view a good society is a general good, and a good society needs people to act in capable, socially responsible and informed ways. It is the job of society's educational system to ensure that children become such capable, responsible and informed adults. Again, it is not my intention to denigrate this goal of education.

For more than two hundred years holistic educators have argued that what education should have as its aim is the fullest possible human development, and Krishnamurti concurred. This fullest possible human development (called Ultimacy by some authors, and hereafter in this chapter) is a religious apotheosis for some holistic educators, in which a religious state (e.g., enlightenment, salvation, etc.) is reached. For other authors the apotheosis is more psychological as in Carl Rogers' "becoming fully human" or Abraham Maslow's "self-actualization." For still others, like Carl Jung, the locus of the religious is the psyche so that the psychological and the religious fold into each other, and Ultimacy (as in Jung's "Unus Mundus" — being one with existence) is both a psychological and spiritual accomplishment.

One claim that is common amongst all proponents of Ultimacy is that it necessarily encompasses all other aims. A person who approaches or achieves Ultimacy (and whether one achieves it or only approaches it varies with different authors) is said to be well suited for worldly success (as long as it is not in conflict with more substantive issues — e.g., becoming rich at the expense of morality) and is also seen as the best possible citizen since they can contradict the mores of a society for a higher good (e.g., conscientious objectors, or civil disobedience) thereby altering society for the better. The greater is seen as encompassing the lesser, so that a person who cares about Ultimacy will also care about other things such as their health and their aesthetic appearance, but these only ever assume a relative importance.

Krishnamurti held that the sacred was separate and distinct from the psychological, but that the psychological had to be in order for the sacred to be perceived. This is perhaps most clear in his many discussions about the brain and the mind. The brain is seen as the center of the nervous system and the organ of cognition. It is therefore responsible for co-ordination of the senses, memory, rationality, knowledge, etc. Krishnamurti claimed that the mind, however, is not material and is not located in the skull. The mind is related to insight (non-visual perception of "what is"), compassion (an objectless love that is not an emotional state), and profound intelligence which Krishnamurti claimed had nothing to do with cognition or IQ. The mind does have a great deal to do with Ultimacy and, therefore, with the meaning of life and the goal of education. Krishnamurti held that education of the brain alone is not only a partial education, it is also dangerous as it gives enormous capacity to effect things without the depth of understanding such capacity requires. He frequently stated that such distorted development was the cause of the awful destruction humans have perpetrated on other humans and nature.

Another key to understanding the relationship that Krishnamurti felt existed between the psyche and Ultimacy is to be found in his notions of "conditioning." This single notion has probably caused more misreading of Krishnamurti than any other, as he does not use the term in any of the conventional ways. Krishnamurti held conditioning to be an acquired set of beliefs, ideas, understandings, etc. that influence or distort a person's objective perception of reality. For a person to objectively see *what is* they need to eliminate the effects of conditioning. This, however, does not mean that we forget our conditioning, in the sense of our culture, language, etc. As such, conditioning, as Krishnamurti used the term, is like a false memory planted in subjects of psychological experiments: when the subject has been shown proof that the memory is false, the false-memory remains, but as the subject knows it is false, it no longer has the effect on the subject that it did when the subject thought the memory was true. Krishnamurti felt that what he called conditioning is like a lens that distorts what is seen through it. Once the person sees that the lens is distorting what they are seeing, they can compensate for it and perceive without the effects of that distortion.

This view of conditioning has implications not only for the relationship between the psyche and the sacred, it also has tremendous implications for Krishnamurti's approach to education:

> The real issue is the quality of our mind: not its knowledge but the depth of the mind that meets knowledge. Mind is infinite, is

the nature of the universe which has its own order, has its own im-
mense energy. It is everlastingly free. The brain, as it is now, is the
slave of knowledge and so is limited, finite, fragmentary. When the
brain frees itself from its conditioning, then the brain is infinite,
then only there is no division between the mind and the brain. Education then is freedom from conditioning, from its vast accumulated knowledge as tradition. This does not deny the academic
disciplines which have their own proper place in life.
(Krishnamurti, 1985, pp. 22-23)

Krishnamurti used many expressions to denote the Ultimacy he felt is
the goal of education. He sometimes spoke of "Intelligence" and the full
development of the mind which he distinguished from mere development of intellect, speaking of education as being about the "awakening
of intelligence." At other times he referred to the "flowering of goodness" which required the full development of all of a person's capacities
as well as contact with "an immensity" that lay beyond the individual. In
some of his writings and speeches in the 1940s and 1950s he claimed that
the true task of education was "integration" of the heart and the mind —
integration of what was finest within the individual with what is most
sublime outside of the individual. At still other times he expressed that
the purpose of education was "the enlightenment of man"
(Krishnamurti, 1981b, p. 106). These should not be seen as conflicting
contentions, but simply different attempts to put the ineffable into
words. The important point for our present purposes is that, for
Krishnamurti, the goal of education is Ultimacy. The task of communicating to the teachers and students in his schools something of the nature
of Ultimacy occupied a large part of his talks to them.

While it is beyond the purpose of this chapter to discuss in detail the
nature of the Ultimacy that Krishnamurti spent so much time expressing, several important characteristics of this view of Ultimacy do need to
be presented as a great deal of his work in education only makes sense if
these are understood.

One of these characteristics is that Ultimacy is not seen as existing in
the future. Unlike some versions of salvation (which might occur after
death) or some versions of enlightenment (which might occur after several reincarnations), Ultimacy, for Krishnamurti, could only be spoken
of as existing (or not existing) in the present tense. This is important as it
means that the principal concern in his approach to education lies not in

the child's future but in the child's present. In much of education there is an emphasis on shaping the child into something other than what the child is, with the emphasis on what the child *might be*. When the time reference shifts from the future to the present, the task is discovering *what is*; education changes from being preparation for what *might be* to engagement with *what is*. When the time reference is in the future, the educator engages in X to produce Y, whereas with the time reference in the present, the educator engages in X because X is intrinsically worth engaging in. The religious literature of the world frequently refers to this distinction; e.g., one should be charitable and compassionate for their own sakes and not for something that may come from them. That such engagement may be the best way of facilitating someone else's learning about the intrinsic value of such engagement seems strangely missing from most modern forms of education, but it is a mainstay of Krishnamurti's approach.

## WHAT NEEDS TO BE LEARNED, ACQUIRED, OR DEVELOPED

If "the awakening of Intelligence" or "the flowering of goodness" or "integration" (or any of the other expressions for Ultimacy that Krishnamurti used) is the goal of education, the question naturally follows: what must a person learn, or what skill must one acquire, or what capacity must one develop in order to accomplish or approach that goal? Again, Krishnamurti employed a great many expressions over the years to convey his perspectives on this question, but this does not denote contradiction. A careful reading of what he said he meant by the different expressions he used over the years shows remarkable consistency.

In keeping with Krishnamurti's approach to what is religious by describing what it isn't, he frequently began discussions of what needs to be learned for Ultimacy by describing what doesn't. He was a strong advocate of conventional academic learning, but felt that this had only secondary importance. It is like his advocating a healthy diet — eating healthy food is important but it is not what gives life meaning or what determines a person's relationship to Ultimacy. Unlike giving undue importance to a healthy diet, giving undue importance to merely cultivating technical or intellectual capacity "leads to destruction, to greater wars; and that is actually what is happening in the world" (Krishnamurti, 1953a). Greater capacity without greater wisdom to direct that capacity is dangerous. Krishnamurti also stated what his approach to education wasn't by making such statements as "Merely to stuff the child with a lot of information, making him pass examinations, is the most unintelligent form of education" (Krishnamurti, 1948).

When Krishnamurti stated in more positive terms what needs to be learned, perhaps most prominent as well as most consistently expressed, is self-knowledge. Krishnamurti felt that knowing the self in general (its nature, which is common to us all) as well as knowing the particular self of an individual is of paramount importance. He would frequently say such things as "To understand life is to understand ourselves, and that is both the beginning and the end of education" (Krishnamurti, 1953b, p.14), or, "When there is self-knowledge, the power of creating illusions ceases, and only then is it possible for reality or God to be" (Krishnamurti, 1953b, p. 47).

An important aspect of Krishnamurti's perspective on acquiring self-knowledge is that it involves a process of discovery. The self is not something to be deliberately created or shaped by the individual or others (like teachers or parents). Rather, the self is to be discovered or uncovered, and this can only be done by the individual with teachers and parents only supporting this process. This does not mean that the individual is unchangeable in one's attitudes, perspectives, behavior or ideas. These superficial aspects do necessarily alter with real learning as in the discussion above about going beyond one's conditioning, but they are seen as altering automatically in response to a deeper or larger understanding rather than being altered for their own sake (e.g., to have attitudes, perspectives, behavior or ideas more in keeping with some view of what these *should be*).

Krishnamurti frequently encouraged students to find their "vocation" which he described as "what you love to do" (Krishnamurti, 1974, p. 75). To spend one's life *not* doing what one loves to do, but doing something only for money, fame, prestige, etc. is not only a waste of life, it is also a denial of who one is. Consequently, Krishnamurti felt that "Right education is to help you to find out for yourself what you really, with all your heart, love to do" (Krishnamurti, 1974, p. 76).

Krishnamurti's statements about self-knowledge or understanding life, however, beg the question as to what he meant by "knowledge" or "understanding," and it is in looking at what he meant by these terms that the complexity and depth of Krishnamurti's work on education becomes evident. "Knowledge" and "understanding" for Krishnamurti were never only an acquisition of information or even a simple meaning

construction. It is beyond the scope of this chapter to provide a full expo-
sition of Krishnamurti's very complex and subtle epistemology, and it
must suffice to say that Krishnamurti emphasized the differences between various forms of knowledge. One might understand this by seeing that the kind of knowledge involved in knowing how to ride a
bicycle is different from the form of knowledge involved in knowing the
distance from the earth to the sun. One is experiential and the other is
conceptual. Still, while these forms of knowledge are different in many
ways, they share the fact that both involve the accumulation of information. Controversially, Krishnamurti proposed that "there is a learning in
which there is no accumulation, a constant movement of learning which
is non-mechanical" (Krishnamurti, 1975). This is a form of knowing acquired through direct contact with that which is known — a contact unmediated by mental constructions (ideas, images, prejudices, etc.) which
reflects "*what is*" (Krishnamurti, 1953b, p. 22) in a way that at least
broaches the unconditional. This form of knowing does not have any
ideation as a prerequisite so that it is essentially universally accessible; it
is not restricted to those with certain learning, conditioning or experiences. A person with no formal learning is not disadvantaged in knowing the *what is* of anything significant to Ultimacy even if that person
doesn't know the *what is* of intellectual things.

One of the characteristics of the knowledge or understanding that
Krishnamurti promoted as important is that it had an inevitable impact
on action. Krishnamurti would insist that if a person "thinks" they know
that something is bad or wrong for them, and yet still does that thing,
that proves that one doesn't really *know* or *understand* that thing, but only
*thinks* one knows it. This distinction between what we might call "false
knowing" and "real knowing" has been noted by many other educators,
philosophers and psychologists over centuries. It is often related to questions of knowing through abstraction or representation, as in a person
knowing about love through abstraction or concept (e.g., as it appears in
literature, philosophy or art) while having no direct experience of actually loving. Krishnamurti insisted that one simply can't know what love
is without engaging in the act of loving; no description, depiction, conception or representation can be a substitute.

Another characteristic of the knowledge or understanding that
Krishnamurti valued is that it is never static to the extent that it is never
the same thing. Some things are never static (e.g., electrons) but they remain constant in their essential nature. However, the knowledge or un-

derstanding that Krishnamurti promoted seems not even to have that concreteness. In many ways, he uses the terms "knowledge" and "understanding" as verbs in that they can only be said to exist when they are being engaged in. It is analogous to the use of the word "dance" as in "May I have this dance?" One *has* the dance only when one is dancing. Unlike the dance (which one ceases to have when dancing ceases), the knowledge or understanding that Krishnamurti spoke of leaves an effect on the one who had engaged in them. Even though such knowledge or understanding is not fixed, the impact of its presence is permanent. Hence, Krishnamurti would claim that action in contradiction to understanding necessarily means that the understanding had never been present.

These characteristics of "real knowing" help answer our third question about education: What facilitates the needed learning, acquisition, or development? Knowledge of riding a bicycle can only come about from experiencing the riding of a bicycle. Knowledge of the number of miles between the earth and the sun cannot come about through experience. It can only come about through abstraction. Every form of knowledge has a way of its coming into being that is determined by its nature. The question naturally follows, "What facilitates this form of knowledge?"

## WHAT FACILITATES THE NEEDED LEARNING, ACQUISITION, OR DEVELOPMENT

As usual, when wanting to discuss something subtle, Krishnamurti would often use the negative approach — what it isn't. Hence, he often presented as *not* facilitating the needed learning a long list of factors he felt plagued conventional learning: competition, fear, self-aggrandizement, pre-determined outcomes, etc. Amongst the most important that doesn't facilitate the needed learning is anything causal. In particular, Krishnamurti held that important learning could not be caused, it could only be invited and Krishnamurti often spoke of "leaving the door open" for it to come in. This is important as it means that such learning is not a result of human agency.

In trying to understand Krishnamurti's view of what can be done to facilitate the needed learning, we can distinguish two categories: material factors and human factors. Both of these are a consequence of human agency, and this may be the fullest extent of what any educator can think of doing.

## MATERIAL FACTORS THAT FACILITATE THE NEEDED LEARNING

In the material domain, there are four aspects that Krishnamurti frequently emphasized: (1) aesthetics, (2) atmosphere, (3) nature, and (4) a place of silence.

The schools Krishnamurti founded were deliberately located in very beautiful places. Krishnamurti felt that beauty is important, not just because it is pleasing, but because sensitivity to beauty is related to being religious and is indispensable to the healthy growth of a child. He told the students in one of his schools in India:

> To be religious is to be sensitive to reality. Your total being —
> body, mind, and heart — is sensitive to beauty and ugliness, to
> the donkey tied to a post, to the poverty and filth in this town, to
> laughter and tears, to everything about you. From this sensitiv-
> ity for the whole of existence springs goodness, love.... 
> (Krishnamurti, 1964)

Krishnamurti often spoke to the students and staff of his schools about the aesthetics with which they dressed — not the fashionableness or expense of their clothing, but the sensitivity they brought to what they wore — and the aesthetics of their movements — not affected or studied movement, but their kinesthetic awareness and sensitivity. Similarly he advocated good food — not lavish, expensive, or sophisticated cuisine — but fresh, tasty, and healthy food. The aesthetic tone of the environment has its own effect on the students, communicating qualities and awakening capacities that no didacticism can. There is a relationship between beauty and truth which has been acknowledged through history and which Krishnamurti felt has to be respected in education. Paying lip service to sensitivity and beauty in environments which give very little care to aesthetics is to teach a very strong lesson in hypocrisy.

Aesthetics are part of what generates the atmosphere of a school, but what is lived by the people in a place is even more responsible for an atmosphere than physical objects, and this puts another burden on the educator. A place may carry an atmosphere, but it is the people who create it or destroy it. Places with atmospheres that at one time were special but which were destroyed through neglect, incompetence or corrupt behavior are unfortunately common throughout history. Krishnamurti often cited great cathedrals or temples that became tourist industries or money making enterprises and so lost any sense of religiousness. They became lifeless and without meaning even though they maintained all the physical appearance of their former selves.

Krishnamurti felt that a relationship with nature had important implications for a relationship to the sacred and to living sanely. He felt that having a real contact with nature was part of "the healing of the mind" (Krishnamurti, 1987, p. 9) and that learning how to have that kind of contact was fundamental to having a real contact with everything else.

> If you establish a relationship with it [nature] then you have relationship with mankind.... But if you have no relationship with the living things on this earth you may lose whatever relationship you have with humanity, with human beings. (ibid.)

As well as contact with nature, Krishnamurti felt that contact with silence was important, and not just for adults but for students as well. He did not prescribe structured or practiced silences as in many meditative religions. Krishnamurti advocated talking to the students about what was available to the human mind in silence, providing a place where silence was possible, and having opportunities during the day when a student could be silent if he or she wished. In his own talks with students he would often encourage students to have "a quiet mind so that your mind becomes religious" (Krishnamurti, 1981a). Interestingly, Krishnamurti asked that places for silence in his schools be placed, not on the periphery of the main activities, but in the center as a *sanctum sanctorum* whose spirit would generate the rest of the school.

## HUMAN FACTORS THAT FACILITATE THE NEEDED LEARNING

Human factors are by far the most important facilitators of the learning Krishnamurti felt was important for Ultimacy. Understanding and knowing are individual actions and responsibilities in the sense that they take place within the individual. However, most of the materials that go into these individual processes are social constructions. A person may come to one's own understanding of something (even of something entirely internal like emotions) but one's thoughts and even language for thinking about that thing are social constructions. Certainly education must be construed as a social activity. To restrict this very large topic to the subject of this book it must be asked, "In Krishnamurti's view, do the social factors of education have a spiritual aspect?" The answer, I believe, is that they do, and that there are two main categories in which to see this: 1) the nature of the exchange between the teacher and the student, and 2) the nature of the educator.

Krishnamurti held that the relationship between the teacher and the student was of primary importance, even more important than what the teacher might ostensibly be teaching. This relationship is to be characterized by love, sensitivity, and care on both sides, but it is obviously the responsibility of the teacher to generate and sustain such a relationship. This may seem a fairly commonplace aspiration, but in examining what Krishnamurti meant by these terms his views show how radical he was. He insisted, for instance, that love, sensitivity and care necessarily lead the educator to give maximum freedom to the student for it was only in freedom that a child can fully develop. Such freedom is not to be a consequence of learning to conform to socially sanctioned conduct, but is a fundamental part of the pedagogic relationship from the start. "Freedom is at the beginning, it is not something to be gained at the end" (Krishnamurti, 1953b, p. 114).

Another aspect of the correct pedagogic relationship for Krishnamurti was the absence of hierarchy. There is, of course, a necessary functional hierarchy; someone must make decisions, a math teacher will know more about mathematics, etc. — but this does not imply *psychological* hierarchy. If each person has to discover self-knowledge for oneself and each person must have one's own unmediated insight into truth, there cannot be any psychological authority. Consequently, when it comes to learning the truly important things in life (as opposed to academics which have only a relative significance) the teacher and the student are both learning. Krishnamurti often spoke of such mutual learning or "being in the same boat" as fundamental to the right pedagogic relationship. As such, Krishnamurti often described the right pedagogic discourse as dialogue or discussing together as equals.

Krishnamurti also held that the *nature* of the teacher rather than the *actions* of the teacher are key to facilitating the needed learning. Teachers teach what they *are* far more than what they *say* or *do*. The teacher must be an active learner about oneself and the deeper issues of life (i.e., religious) if one wants the students to be such learners, and therefore religious. As mentioned above, the teacher does not do X to beget Y in the students. Rather, X begets X, and often in a mysterious way. This is not, as is often expressed, modeling, as modeling implies imitation, and this denies freedom and authenticity. It is more akin to the formation of crystals, in which a solution prone to crystallization needs a single crystal to initiate the process — the subsequent crystals don't model themselves on the first crystal, but the process of crystal formation is triggered by the first crystal. It is in this way that Krishnamurti felt a love of learning the important things of life spreads, as well as compassion, sensitivity, and the beauty of living a religious life.

Krishnamurti frequently said such things as "the right kind of educator is deeply and truly religious" (Krishnamurti, 1953b, p. 111). He held that communication springing from a deeply religious person looking deeply and honestly at substantive issues communicates much more than any words that are used. Perhaps this explains the enthrallment of many people in the audiences of his talks who frequently expressed that they felt they had learned a great deal of great importance without being able to express exactly what it was they learned. These people were either suffering from a mass self-delusion or Krishnamurti was practicing what he claimed was necessary in education, and people were showing the effects of a different but important kind of learning.

That Krishnamurti cared about education is incontrovertible. That he saw education as a religious activity is just as certain. What may be difficult for many people to understand is that for Krishnamurti education is principally about a form of learning that is not an accumulation of knowledge, and leading a religious life has nothing to do with any religion. For Krishnamurti, the sacred *is*; it is in the present and it can be perceived by sensitivity to and seeing correctly that which is present, including the self and all that distorts our perception of what is here and now. Krishnamurti held that such sensitivity and correct seeing is the way in which the significance of life could be discovered, and that education exists in order to help people (the educator as well as the educated) discover this significance.

## References

Krishnamurti, J. (1948, September 26). *5th Public Talk,* Poona. Unpublished manuscript.

Krishnamurti, J. (1953a, January 31). *3rd Public Talk,* Poona. Unpublished manuscript.

Krishnamurti, J. (1953b). *Education and the Significance of Life*. London: Victor Gollancz.

Krishnamurti, J. (1964). *This Matter of Culture*. London: Victor Gollancz.

Krishnamurti, J. (1974). *On Education*. Pondicherry, India: All India Press.

Krishnamurti, J. (1975, January, 26). *2nd Public Talk.* Bombay. Unpublished manuscript.

Krishnamurti, J. (1981a, November 19). *2nd Talk to Students,* Rajghat. Unpublished manuscript.

Krishnamurti, J. (1981b). *Letters to the Schools.* Vol. 1. Den Haag, Holland: Mirananda.

Krishnamurti, J. (1985). *Letters to the Schools.* Vol. 2. Den Haag, Holland: Mirananda.

Krishnamurti, J. (1987). *Krishnamurti to Himself.* London: Victor Gollancz.

# CHAPTER 8

# Ravindranath Tagore

## Education for Spiritual Fulfillment

### Takuya Kaneda

The human soul, confined in its limitation, has also dreamt of millennium, and striven for a spiritual emancipation which seems impossible of attainment, and yet it feels its reverence for some everpresent source of inspiration in which all its experience of the true, the good and beautiful finds its reality. (Tagore, 1931, pp. 236-237)

The first year of the 20th century, a famous Indian poet, Ravindranath Tagore, inaugurated an experimental school to realize his dream of the ideal education at "Santiniketan" (The abode of peace) in Bolpur, Bengal. In the beginning, the poet's school consisted of only five teachers holding classes under mango trees, but by 1922 it had expanded into a large educational institution which included all levels from a primary school to an international university, "Visva-Bharati." For the span of a full hundred years his spirit of education has been sustained to the present; myriads of students have studied at Santiniketan and entered the outer world supported by their marvelous experiences of school life.

I have encountered many of these former students. They speak passionately about their memories of school days and with unconditional admiration of Tagore's educational ideas and practices. In education, it is very important to plant a seed deeply in a student's spirit. That tiny seed, which may not be visible immediately, will flower after he/she grows up. Thus the final effect cannot necessarily be measured in a short period or by statistical analysis. If the depth of influence on a student's spirit is any measure of success in education, over these hundred years

Santiniketan has surely validated the educational philosophy of Ravindranath Tagore.

I had two opportunities to visit Santiniketan, one in 1976 and again in 1986. The following passage is a part of my diary about visiting Santiniketan:

> I took a train from Howrah Station in Calcutta for Bolpur. The old building of the station showed the light and shadow of the British colonial period. The train left the noisy city of Calcutta and soon the dusty scenery changed to the beautiful scenery of golden rice fields. After a slow but comfortable journey, I arrived at Bolpur station and took a cycle rickshaw for Santiniketan. Instead of a traffic jam, holy cows were walking in the center of the street. A big banyan tree was giving its gentle shade to a farmer wearing his off white cotton clothes, who was taking an earthen cup of tea. He seemed very simple but so satisfied.

> Birds were singing loudly in this vast open space. After a ride along tall palm trees in the hot wind of Bengal, the birds' songs suddenly changed to a delicate melody of sitar. I found myself at the gate of Santiniketan. My whole body began to feel "Santi," peacefulness, in the beautiful campus of the school. Several groups of students were studying under the shade of mango trees. The scene reminded me of an ancient ashram for learning in the forest.

To know the birth of this poet's school, it is necessary to trace back to Tagore's childhood.

## THE EARLY YEARS OF TAGORE

Ravindranath Tagore was born in 1861 to an aristocratic family in Calcutta. His father, Devendranath Tagore, was a spiritual seeker and an active leader of the Brahmo Samaj, a group supporting the reformist movement in Hinduism. He published a Bengali monthly magazine to awaken people's consciousness about religion during the British colonial time. Devendranath devoted his life to spiritual pursuits. His austere character deeply influenced his son, Ravindranath. He was sent to school but the rigid school education did not fit him. He was a boy of sensitivity who began writing poems when he was only eight years old.

In 1873, it was the first time for him to visit Santiniketan, which his father had bought for a retreat. The wonderful natural environment attracted him. Then his father took him on a tour of holy places in the Himalayas. Together they stayed in places that people in ancient times believed to be the actual abodes of the gods and goddesses. The sacred scenery deeply impressed him. He remembered this journey vividly and wrote about the invitation from the forest to hold communion with Nature: "I had the good fortune of answering this invitation when as a boy of ten I stood alone on the Himalayas under the shade of great deodars, awed by the dignity of life's first-born aristocracy, by its sturdy fortitude that was terrible as well as courteous" (1961, p. 291). This clearly showed his spiritual relationship to Nature. So it was that Ravindranath grew up in a very spiritual yet unconventional atmosphere.

When they returned to Calcutta, he tried to go to school again but could not continue it. After leaving school, he was taught at home by private tutors and by his brothers. Tagore criticized the modern school system as being too much like a factory. The modern educational system was developed to support industrial growth. Productivity and efficiency were the major concerns in both factories and schools. Therefore in such an education, the spiritual growth of students was neglected altogether. He recalled his school days: "In the usual course I was sent to school, but possibly my suffering was unusual, greater than that of most other children. The non-civilized in me was sensitive: it had a great thirst for colour, for music, for the movement of life" (Tagore & Elmhirst, 1961, p. 53).

These negative memories of his school days motivated him to be seriously concerned about education and to start his own school. Although he refused to accept any creed authorized by some scripture or organization, he gradually entered into the world of mystery within the depth of existence. He wrote about his spiritual experience in his youth:

> When I was eighteen, a sudden spring breeze of religious experience came to my life for the first time and passed away leaving in my memory a direct message of spiritual reality. One day while I stood watching at early dawn the sun sending out its rays from behind the trees, I suddenly felt as if some ancient mist had in a mo-

ment lifted from my sight, and the morning light on the face of the world revealed an inner radiance of joy. (1931, pp. 93-94)

After having such an unusual experience of transpersonal consciousness, he deepened his spiritual insight still further.

## EDUCATION AND RELIGION

Tagore wrote many essays to highlight the importance of spirituality in education. Throughout all of them, his expressed idea of education was filled with religious words and metaphors. In a sense, education and religion were synonymous for him. At this point, it is necessary to note that his concept of "religion" was different from that held by the West. In Hinduism, "dharma" is usually translated into English as "religion," but it is not the same concept as the Western definition of religion found in Christianity. Originally, "dharma" means right action in life. Education, something that illustrates the way of life, is naturally regarded as a part of "dharma" for Hindus. Traditionally, they thought that education was a part of religion. Tagore stated, "In ancient India the school was there where was the life itself" (1917, p. 128).

The present India is a secular nation and the government system of school education is not based on religious principles. However, religious customs are still intricately woven in to Indian daily life and it seems very difficult to separate religion from secular life. In other words, there is no Western concept of the secular against religion in Hinduism because "dharma," religion, is life itself for Hindus. On the contrary, in the modern West, education became secular and independent from religious authorities although many old educational institutions were established under Christianity. Modern education systems were developed in accordance with the process of secularizing schools from churches in the West, where it resulted in ignorance of spirituality in education.

## BUDDHA AND BAULS

Tagore asserted that the best wisdom, disciplines, literature and art, all the teachings of the noblest teachers of humanity for ages, had been created for spiritual life. He admired the Buddha, whose teaching was also born in the stream of profound wisdom of ancient India, as "the first of those who declared salvation to all men, without distinction, as by right man's own" (1922, p. 69). He emphasized that the teaching of Bud-

dha was "neither in texts of Scripture, nor in religious practices sancti-
fied by ages, but through the voice of a living man and the love that
flowed from a human heart" (p. 69). This passage indicates his cardinal
idea that religion should not depend on any authority.

He compared Buddhism, that had developed a system of metaphys-
ics, to the simple folk religion of Bauls, pointing out the fundamental
unity in them. Bauls are traditional religious singers in Bengal. They are
wanderers moving from village to village. They live a very simple nomadic life in obscurity, singing devotional songs with a one-stringed instrument, the *ektara*. Tagore loved the Bauls, who did not have their own
scriptures and temples. They sang:

> Temples and mosques obstruct thy path,
> and I fail to hear thy call or to move,
> when the teachers and priest angrily crowd round me.
>
> (Tagore, 1931, p. 111)

But yet, they expressed their feeling of the divinity of human personality from the depth of their souls. Tagore was enchanted by their unconventional ideas on spirituality. He introduced a song of the Bauls which
likened the spiritual fulfillment to the blossoming of a bud:

> The opening spirit has overtaken thee,
> Canst thou remain a bud any longer?
>
> (Tagore, 1922, p. 76)

This process of blossoming could imply the way of spiritual education.

## THE OBJECT OF EDUCATION

Tagore defined the object of education as to give the unity of truth and
continued:

> Formerly when life was simple all the different elements of man
> were in complete harmony. But when there came the separation of
> the intellect from the spiritual and physical, school education put
> its entire emphasis on the intellect and the physical side of man. We
> devote our sole attention to giving children information, not know-
> ing that by this emphasis we are accentuating a break between the
> intellectual, physical and the spiritual life. (1917, p. 126)

Tagore's idea of education developed from the tradition of Hinduism, but his idea was not limited to the narrow meaning of Hinduism. He had been to Europe and the United States several times and deeply understood Western culture as well as his own. He attempted to pursue universal truth beyond the differences between East and West. Hinduism is likely to imply exclusive religious customs in a particular region yet the original philosophy of Hinduism was actually quite universal. The name, Hindu, was derived from a term used by outsiders to imply the place where people maintained the special spiritual beliefs and practices based on the Vedas and the Upanishads, the sacred ancient literature of India. The indigenous inhabitants did not have any consciousness that they themselves were exclusively Hindus. They thought that the fundamental idea of their religion was universal although they practiced their own religious customs. In this idea of universal religion, all religions were the same in their spiritual pursuit for the truth beyond differences in religious customs, which were as various as languages and which also differed from place to place. The solidification of the concept of Hinduism was developed as part of a reaction to encroaching Islam and a result of the emergence of nationalism during British colonialism. Tagore, however, followed not the narrow orthodox doctrines of Hinduism but its original philosophy of a universal religion, the essence of the Upanishads; he applied it to his school by emphasizing the essential role of spiritual growth in education.

Tagore simply mentioned spirituality as follows:

> I believe in a spiritual world — not as anything separate from this world — but as its innermost truth. With the breath we draw we must always feel this truth, that we are living in God. Born in this great world, full of the mystery of the infinite, we cannot accept our existence as a momentary outburst of chance, drifting on the current matter towards an eternal nowhere. (1917, p. 126)

He claimed that spiritual reality was missed "by our incessant habit of ignoring it from childhood" (p. 127). To fulfill spiritual growth in education, Tagore proposed an entirely different picture of school from ordinary modern schools. This idea stemmed from an educational custom in ancient India.

## ANCIENT IDEA OF LEARNING

There was an idea of four different stages of life in ancient India. The first stage is called "Brahmacharya," the period of discipline and education. "Garhasthya" is the second period of life, in which one has a spouse and raises children to fulfill family and social life. "Vanaprasthya" is the third period of life when one concentrates on spiritual life in the forest after fulfillment of family and social duties. "Sannyasa" is the last period of life. In this period, it is necessary to abandon material necessities, to lead an austere life, and to seek a spiritual path. The first stage of Brahmacharya was very important to establish the physical, mental and spiritual base on which the following phases of life could be solidly built.

Tagore regarded this Brahmacharya as an ideal form of education for young students. When he reached 40 in 1901, he started his ideal education center at a remote and peaceful place, Santiniketan, in Bolpur of Bengal. This beautiful, natural setting had been previously chosen by the poet's father, Devendranath, as a retreat for spiritual pursuit. He had named it Santiniketan, "the abode of peace." The school was literally an "ashram" at the stage of Brahmacharya, that point of life in which it was essential for young students to live with a master in the forest. Living in the forest gave students the opportunity to encounter experiences which could hardly be found in ordinary daily life. Tagore explained the relationship between "forest" and the ancient people in India as follows:

> The forest entered into a close living relationship with their work and leisure, with their daily necessities and contemplations. They could not think of other surroundings as separate or inimical. So the view of truth, which these men found, did not make manifest the difference, but rather the unity of all things. They uttered their faith in these words: *"Yadidam kinch sarvam prana ejati nihsratam"* (All that is vibrates with life, having come out from life). (1922, pp. 47-48)

Tagore tried to make students isolated from the busy city life for their spiritual growth. He explained the reason: "The four elements of earth, water, air, and fire form a whole and are instinct with the universal soul — this knowledge cannot be gained at a school in town. A school in town is a factory which can only teach us to regard the world as a machine" (1961, p. 73). He repeatedly emphasized the importance of simple living:

This we can attain during our childhood by daily living in a place where the truth of the spiritual world is not obscured by a crowd of necessities assuming artificial importance; where life is simple, surrounded by fullness of leisure, by ample space and pure air and profound peace of nature; and where men live with a perfect faith in the eternal life before them. (Tagore, 1917, p. 135)

Such a simple life was an essential part of the stage of Brahmacharya, when the teachers and their students had to live together as family members. Tagore mentioned that book-learning had not been regarded as the most important part of education in ancient India and pointed out that this idea could be sometimes found in the present traditional schools of orthodox Hindu learning. He explained: "They are surrounded by an atmosphere of culture, and the teachers are dedicated to their vocation. They live a simple life, without any material interest or luxury to distract their minds, and with plenty of time and opportunity for absorbing into their nature the things they learn." (1961, p. 70).

Santiniketan was the place where he attempted to realize his ideal. At Santiniketan, students got up very early in the morning, sometimes before sunrise. Then they took exercises and Vedic chanting. After breakfast, all students and teachers assembled and sang a song. Morning classes, lunch, afternoon classes and games continued. After ablutions they started evening prayer. Then they relaxed and ate dinner together. Following a song in chorus, they went to bed. Ravindranath thought that this simple living in accordance with the rhythm of Nature was a very important discipline for students' spiritual growth as well as their mental and physical development. This discipline was not forced and students felt that it was very natural.

## THE IMPORTANCE OF NATURE IN EDUCATION

Tagore praised the ineffable beauty of Nature in his poems and emphasized that the natural environment was very important for education as in the ancient forest school. He thought that students needed to feel the breath of earth as flowers needed the sunlight and fresh air. His idea on Nature in education was described as follows: "We can grow into full manhood only if we have been nursed by earth and water, sky and air, and nourished by them as by our mother's breasts" (1961, p. 73). This idea could be traced to the worship of Nature in the Vedic period of India, where numerous gods and goddess were derived from Nature such as the sun, sky, rain, earth and so on. For Tagore, Nature was the source of education as well as religion. The natural environment of Santiniketan chosen for the school was very suitable for students to touch, feel, and be aware of the mysterious power of Nature through breathing in the fresh air and walking barefoot on the surface of the mother earth. Tagore (1922) repeatedly emphasized the importance of Nature:

> India holds sacred, and counts as places of pilgrimage, all spots which display a special beauty or splendor of nature. These had no original attraction on account of any special fitness for cultivation or settlement. Here, man is free, not to look upon them as a source of supply of his necessities, but to realize his soul beyond himself. (p. 62)

My diary on Santiniketan continued:

> Most of the students were living together in the campus. I saw many students studying under big trees and heard their voices mixed with birds' chirping. While they took a class, they could feel the mysterious power through the ground and the wind. Once Tagore criticized the modern school where the students were the same as parrots in the small cage. Here at Santiniketan, students seemed like birds flying freely in the blue sky.

Tagore (1931) insisted :

> The first stage of my realization was through a feeling of intimacy with Nature — not that Nature which had its channel of information for our mind and physical relationship with our living body, but that which satisfies our personality with manifestations that makes our life rich and stimulates our imagination in the harmony of forms, colors, sounds and movements. (p. 18)

His idea on Nature was closely linked to the concept of aesthetic sensibility, a type of responsiveness he considered to be essential to cultivate in students.

## AESTHETIC SENSIBILITY

Flowering of aesthetic sensibility was a very important part of Tagore's school. Traditionally, the five senses were never ignored in Hinduism. People tried to grasp spiritual truth through seeing pictures of

the gods and goddesses, touching the sacred statues, listening to devotional songs, tasting the sweetness of the offering, and smelling the scent
of incense. The physical world perceived by our senses is not the ultimate object of spiritual pursuit. However, when we concentrate on
sharpening our sensitivity and feel the beauty of lights, colors, forms and
sounds, we are able to access the door toward the spiritual universe. Aesthetic sensibility does not mean mere sensual reaction to outward appearance but spiritual correspondence to our inner soul.

Regarding aesthetic sensibility, Tagore (1915) stressed the importance
of the joy of beauty: "Truth is everywhere, therefore everything is the object of our knowledge. Beauty is omnipresent, therefore everything is capable of giving joy" (p. 138). This joy is not separable from our sense of
beauty. He emphasized the function of our sense of beauty to extend our
consciousness. In his idea, there is no distinction between beauty and ug-
liness as strong lights cannot be separated from shadows. He insisted
that it was possible to realize harmony in the universe through our sense
of beauty. The following sentences show the core of his thought on
beauty which is related to unity or harmony:

> As we become conscious of the harmony in our soul, our appre-
> hension of the blissfulness of the spirit of the world becomes
> universal, and the expression of beauty in our life moves in
> goodness and love towards the infinite. This is the ultimate ob-
> ject of our existence, that we must ever know that "beauty is
> truth, truth is beauty"; we must realize the whole world in love,
> for love gives it birth, sustains it, and takes it back to its bosom.
> (p. 141)

His emphasis of the joy of beauty encouraged multiform activities of
art and music at Santiniketan.

## ART AND MUSIC IN EDUCATION

Tagore's own experience of performing and of creating various arts
underscored how deeply he felt aesthetic sensibility connected to the joy
of beauty. He is generally known as a poet who received the Nobel Prize
for literature in 1913 for his work, *Gitanjali*, but his talent was not limited
to the field of poetry. He also created beautiful music and paintings. He
was a man of multiple talents, much like Leonardo da Vinci in Renais-
sance Italy. He demonstrated prodigious creativity in music, dramatics,
drawing, painting as well as poetry and literature. He deeply loved mu-

sic, regarding it as the purest form of art. He also became interested in the art of drawing and painting as early as his twenties. His works were not representative but filled with sentiment and delicacy. He created picturesque poems like a painter and produced melancholic paintings like a poet. His works were widely exhibited in Europe and America and he achieved a good reputation as a painter.

Tagore, who had experienced both art and music by himself, mentioned their distinction: "In the pictorial, plastic and literary arts, the object and our feelings with regard to it are closely associated, like the rose and its perfumes. In music, the feeling distilled in sound becomes itself an independent object" (1931, p. 141). His own creative experiences in the various fields of arts suggested to him the idea that artistic activities should have an important role in education. Familiar with the Western arts, he wrote many poems in English. However, his idea of art was not based on the modern concept of art established after the 19th century in the West. His description of art leads us to spiritual aspects of art.

Tagore wrote an essay titled "What is Art?" In this essay, intentionally, he did not answer the question as to what art is because the particular definition of art might limit the infinite reality of art. Art exists in the world of our feeling and emotion. In contrast to science, the mystery of art cannot be objectively analyzed or measured. He continued his idea with this comparison: "The scientist seeks an impersonal principle of unification, which can be applied to all things" (1917, pp. 23-24). On the other hand, "the artist finds out the unique, the individual, which yet is in the heart of the universe" (p. 24). In addition, he pointed out that the East believed in the soul of the universe while the West did not. In the East, artistic realization is the same thing as meditation. This Eastern faith in the universal soul is connected to an idea that "Truth, Power, Beauty lie in Simplicity, where it is transparent, where things do not obstruct the inner vision" (p. 25). Only such Simplicity in life can make it possible to realize "a positive Truth which, though invisible, is more real than the gross and the numerous" (p. 25).

Tagore mentioned the unity between the world and ourselves in art: "In art we express the delight of this unity by which this world is realized as humanly significant to us." Regarding our artistic nature, he also stated that: "The urging of our artistic nature is to realize the manifestation of personality in the world of appearance, the reality of existence which is in harmony with the real within us. Where this harmony is not deeply felt, there we are aliens and perpetually homesick. For man by nature is an artist" (1931, p. 132). He further commented,

> In the world of art, our consciousness being freed from the tan-
> gle of self interest, we gain an unobstructed vision of unity, the
> incarnation of the real, which is a joy forever. As in the world of
> art, so in the spiritual world, our soul waits for its freedom from
> the ego to reach that disinterested joy which is the source and
> goal of creation. (pp. 183 - 184)

For Tagore, who found the divinity within ourselves, artistic creation was related to the creation of the universe. His idea of creation was de-rived from the Upanishads. One of the ancient treatises declared:

> Where there is creation there is progress. Where there is no cre-
> ation there is no progress: know the nature of creation. Where
> there is joy there is creation. Where there is no joy there is no cre-
> ation: know the nature of joy. Where there is the Infinite there is
> joy. There is no joy in the finite. It was thought that "One of the
> tasks of education is to reveal the joy of the Infinite which is the
> joy of love." (Mascaro, 1965, p. 32)

Tagore applied this idea in his experimental school. He endeavored to make his school filled with such a joy. The school life at Santiniketan was accentuated by occasional festivals filled with colorful art and music. The campus was decorated with traditional auspicious designs and stu-dents enjoyed their art, songs, dances, and dramas during the festivals. Traditionally, not only Hinduism but also other religions had various festivals, when people could have a special opportunity to be aware of spirituality through art and music that was not experienced in ordinary daily life.

Tagore attempted to bring this function of festival into school life. Art and music in relation to joy have played a vital role of awakening the stu-dent's sensitivities toward spirituality in Tagore's school.

In the present Santiniketan, Kala Bhavana, or College of Art, is very famous all over India. In the primary school curriculum, activities of art, music and plays are highly encouraged as essential to students' holistic development. Students can take various classes of art and craft such as painting, paper craft, clay work, woodwork, metal work, dyeing, and weaving in each well equipped studio. The weaving class is related to a rich tradition of textiles in Bengal. At the first stage, junior students learn the basic skill with paper and then proceed to the next step to master the technique of weaving. The art teachers who live with and keep close relations with the students are also very active as artists in their own fields. This peaceful place, which is isolated from busy city life, seems to be an ideal environment to concentrate on their creative work. The artist teachers are often inspired by students' innocent imaginations and keen sensitivities at the same time that they stimulate students' creativity. All the results of the art classes are crystallized in seasonal festivals, when students create their original costumes and stage sets. Art and craft are integrated with dance and drama in the occasion. Then students can realize the joy of creation, which is essential for spiritual fulfillment.

## FOR THE FUTURE

What can we learn from the educational ideas and practices of Ravindranath Tagore, who initiated his school one hundred years ago? First of all, it is very important to remember that for him, the aim of education was to facilitate spiritual growth. There is no doubt that Tagore's educational idea was rooted in the wisdom of the Upanishads of ancient India. However, his philosophy was not limited to the narrow sense of Hinduism and he never depended on any authorized doctrine, scripture, and organization. He was always pursuing the universal truth beyond it, irrespective of time and place. Therefore, it is possible to apply his philosophy to our contemporary context of education. It is also important that Ravindranath was not only an idealist but also a man of practice. He himself did singing and painting as well as writing numerous poems and essays. He opened his own school and talked to the students himself constantly. Through his own experience, he repeatedly emphasized the necessity of living a simple life, of fostering a close relationship between students and Nature, and of encouraging students' artistic activities as an essential part of their holistic development. It is possible to try these things in our classrooms in many different ways. However, it should be remembered that any emphasis on Nature or encouragement of artistic activities will be very superficial if we are not aware of spiritual fulfillment in education.

This is the last page of my diary on Santiniketan:

> After observing classes under the mango trees, I decided to stay at the guesthouse of the school. The room was very simple like an ashram for meditation. After sunset, I went out for a walk. The cool

evening air was so fresh. In the white moonlight, a tall Baul appeared in a long robe of rags. Suddenly, he began to sing a devotional song. His beautiful voice rose from the depth of his soul, echoing throughout the vast campus and resonating in my heart. At that very instant, the current of time seemed to stop. Bauls might have sung in the same way hundreds of years ago.

Tagore must have walked this path and heard their songs. A hundred years is nothing for the Infinite. I really felt Tagore's spirit was alive here in Santiniketan.

### REFERENCES

Mascaro, J. (1965). *The Upanishads* (Translation from the Sanskrit with an introduction). Middlesex: Penguin Books.

Tagore, R. (1915). *Sadhana: The Realisation of Life*. New York: Macmillan.

Tagore, R. (1917). *Personality*. London: Macmillan.

Tagore, R. (1922). *Creative Unity*. London: Macmillan.

Tagore, R. (1931). *The Religion of Man*. London: Allen & Unwin.

Tagore, R. (1961). *Towards Universal Man*. New York: Asia Publishing House.

Tagore, R., & Elmhirst, L. K. (1961). *Ravindranath Tagore: Pioneer in Education*. London: John Murray.

### NOTES

I had an opportunity to stay at J. Krishnamurti's Rishi Valley School in India as a visiting teacher during the second term of 1999. J. Krishnamurti did not refer to Ravindranath Tagore's school. However, there were many similarities between the both schools such as their emphasis on Nature, beauty and simple living together with students and teachers. Some art teachers of Rishi Valley School studied their art at Santiniketan. This suggests a link between Ravindranath Tagore and J. Krishnamurti in education.

I wish to acknowledge Dr. Janet Montgomery for reading this manuscript in an early version.

# CHAPTER 9

# Martin Buber

## Education as Holistic Encounter and Dialogue

## Atsuhiko Yoshida

The primary word I-Thou can be spoken only with the whole being.... All real living is encounter. (Buber, 1923/1962, p. 85)

Only in this whole being, in all his spontaneity can the educator truly affect the whole being of his pupil.... It is not the educational intention but it is the encounter which is educationally fruitful. (Buber, 1939/1962, pp. 819 and 820)

Many of us experience an encounter in life that is spoken of in the following manner: "If I had not met her, my life would have been a totally different one." "The encounter with him transformed my self." Encounter is an essential event in the process of becoming more fully human. In education, the transformative effect of encounter cannot be underestimated. Since, however, encounter is not something that can be intentionally programmed, its significance has not been discussed enough in the theory and practice of education. I believe, in spite of the fact that we cannot be prepared for encounters, which by their very nature are unforeseen, the educator can be aware of the profundity of encounter. The educator needs to be open to encounter. Such awareness and openness create a difference in the relationship with learners.

Martin Buber is the first philosopher-educationalist to delve into encounter in such spiritual depth. As the title of his autobiography *Encounter* (Buber, 1960/1986) shows, Buber, who was a holistic educator as much as religious philosopher, lived out his philosophy of encounter. In this essay, I would like to elucidate his attitude toward spirituality and illuminate the significance of his educational philosophy that is strongly relevant for us today. The best way to do so, I think, is to review the growth of his thought in relation to crucial events that happened in his life.

## THE FORMATIVE YEARS OF BUBER'S PHILOSOPHY

Buber was born in Vienna in 1878 and brought up as a Jew in Poland and Hungary. During a historical time of intolerance and holocaust, he stayed in Germany until 1938 to continue educational activity and spiritual resistance. After this, he emigrated to Israel, where his life focused on inter-faith dialogue, including dialogue between Jews and Arabs, until his death in 1965. Buber's philosophy and educational activity were the result of his ceaseless response to the cataclysmic 20th century, and they are gaining increasing importance as we search for new spirituality for the 21$^{st}$ century, an era of postmodern pluralism and intensified interethnic conflict. My hope is to carve out some of the uniqueness of Buber's spiritual holistic thought and educational practice.

## MIS-ENCOUNTER WITH 'MOTHER':
## THE ERA OF LOST HOME

Buber's first experience of encounter was, in fact, a mis-encounter, when at the age of four he realized he had no mother. Without any explanation of his parents' divorce, Buber was left in the care of his grandparents. As a child, he did not doubt that his mother would return. One day, however, when he was playing with his neighbor's daughter on the balcony, she said, "No, she will never come back."

> I know that I remained silent, but also that I cherished no doubt of the truth of the spoken words. It remained fixed in me; from year to year it cleaved ever more to my heart, but after more than ten years I had begun to perceive it as something that concerned not only me, but all human beings. (1960/1986, p. 10)

Buber felt that this mis-encounter with mother was something we shared as a human species. This mis-encounter with mother meant not only the increasing divorce rate and numbers of dysfunctional families but also a lost sense of home, which is a characteristic of modern societies. It also points to the severed relations between human beings and the earth that is our mother. Namely, it is a loss of connection with the "mother" that gave birth to us and nurtured us. Buber termed this situation *Vergegnung*.

> Later I once made up the word 'Vergegnung' — 'mismeeting' or 'miscounter' to designate the failure of a real encounter between man and man. (p. 10)

In a sense, we all are estranged from "mother," from the roots of life. The beginning of Buber's spiritual quest was to recover this primary connection, which had been severed. His philosophy of encounter was not simply romantic naivete. The loss of his primary relationship to his mother led to his concern for modern estrangement in which every kind of connectedness is being severed.

## THE PRIMAL EXPERIENCE OF ENCOUNTER

In the grandparents' farm where Buber spent his childhood, there was a stable. In that stable, he had a favorite horse which he used to feed. Between the horse and himself, Buber experienced an innocent and tiny event, which however had great influence on the later formation of his philosophy. When the boy Martin entered the stable, the horse always raised its neck and moved its ears. The horse softly whinnied, as if to say that it loved him very much. The boy, too, loved the horse and would stroke its body gently. "When I stroked the mighty mane, and felt the life beneath my hand, it was as though the vital life-force bordered on my skin" (1960/1986, p. 25). Through the stroking hand, the life of the horse and the life of the boy resonated with each other. They were indeed one. That was how the boy always felt.

One day, while Martin was stroking the horse, he noticed how interesting it was. At that moment, he became self-conscious, i.e. conscious of his hand stroking the horse. Then, quite suddenly, something had shifted in a definite way. The movement of the stroking hand was there, as usual, but the friendly horse no longer was there. The next day, the boy wanted to caress the horse's neck, but it did not raise its head. That was a scary experience. The boy felt that he had betrayed the relationship. This experience pierced his heart and was not resolved for a long time.

The difference was between before and after he became conscious of his own curiosity and stroking hand; this difference marked the two different kinds of relationships in which a person relates to the other or to the world. From the objective perspective the act of stroking stayed the same; however, the relationship was changed according to how the heart was connecting. This experience served as a germ to the development of Buber's thought. Decades after, Buber(1923/1962) created the two terms "I and Thou" and "I and It," which represent the two different ways of relating. His major work, *I and Thou*, which had a profound influence on 20th century philosophy, begins with the following remark: "To man the world is twofold, in accordance with his twofold attitude" (p. 79).

Using the example of the event that Buber experienced with the horse, let me explain now the two kinds of relations. The relation in which the horse and the boy were fused in overflowing vitality and united as a whole is the "I and Thou" relationship. On the other hand, once the boy became conscious that it was interesting, the horse turned into the means by which he attained this enjoyment, and that ruined the experience, and made it selfish. The horse became "It," and the "I and Thou" relationship collapsed. There was no more vital exchange. The stroking hands of which he became conscious became the medium that set apart the horse and the boy. The relationship ceased to be a direct and mutual one as the horse was objectivized.

The "I and Thou" is the holistic, direct, mutual relationship with no subject/object separation. The "I and It" is the mediated, one-sided, instrumental relationship in which the subject and object are divided.

> The primary word I-Thou can be spoken only with the whole being. Concentration and fusion into the whole being can never take place through my agency, nor can it ever take place without me. I become through my relation to the Thou; as I become I, I say Thou. All real living is encounter. (1923/1962, p. 85)

Such "I-Thou" relationships are nothing but encounter. In modern societies, I-Thou relations tend to shift to I-It relationships, and once this shift has occurred, it is difficult to recover the I-Thou relationship. This situation points to what is beyond Buber's personal experience. It is a historical problem of our time. It is the problem of modernity where everything tends to be the object of conscious control, deriving from the prevailing instrumental rationalism.

In modern educational systems, also, the one to be educated is often treated as "It." There is less and less opportunity in which the student is encountered as "Thou." Later in the essay, I will focus more on education. Before turning to education, I will discuss Buber's youthful days, especially in respect to religious and spiritual matters.

## Antipathy to Missionary Activity and Affinity for Mystical Experience

Having learned reading and writing from his grandmother, Buber began school at the age of ten. It was a Polish school in the Austro-Hungarian Empire. At eight o'clock every morning, he had to participate in a Christian service. As one of the teachers stepped up on the pulpit, with a big cross on the wall, all the seated students stood up in unison. The teachers and Polish students solemnly made the cross on their chest and said Christian prayers aloud. During that time, Buber and the other Jews had to close their eyes and remain standing. From the age of ten, this ritual was repeated every single morning, for eight years.

There was no obvious persecution of Jews at the school. But, Buber says:

> ... the obligatory daily standing in the room resounding with strange service affected me worse than an act of intolerance could have affected me.... My antipathy to all missionary activity is rooted in that time. Not merely against the Christian to the Jews, but against all missionizing among men who have a faith with roots of its own. (1960/1989, p. 21)

Through the eight-year experience of the morning service in his youth, Buber began to reject all missionary activity. The antipathy was against missionary activity, not against all that is religious. Here we see the development of Buber's subtle relationship to "religion." Buber is known as a religious philosopher. He is highly respected as a scholar of the religious revolutionary movement known as Chasidism, and as a translator of the Old Testament into German. He was one of the most famous scholars of Judeo-Christianity in the world. In spite of that, the orthodox Jewish community considered him to be a heretic.

Chasidism, which inspired Buber in his early years, emphasized one's inner and direct communion along with service for others in daily life, rather than the sturdy ritualism that prevailed in orthodox Judaism. Buber was not satisfied with the narrow sense of religion and the frameworks of religious organizations. He made an effort to dialogue with Christians and people of other faiths. He even says that the self-righteous exclusivistic tendency of religion is "the source of human vice"(1952/1963, p. 744). Buber decided not to engage in any missionary activity. But spirituality, or that which resides at the core of various religions, was important to him. In fact, Buber had deep insight into spiritual experience that gives the primal vitality to all that is religious.

In his college life, Buber took part in social revolutionary movements in Vienna, Leipzig, and Berlin. He frequented the meetings of a socialist club and gave lectures. He became one of the leaders in the Zionist movement, which arose in those days. In the midst of this stormy activist life, however, Buber gradually came to question these political and social movements. Cultural and interior concerns were growing. By 1904, he had stopped all political activity and immersed himself in interior and scholastic work.

The themes of his work centered on mysticism such as Chasidism, Taoism, and the work of Nicolaus Cusanus and Jacob Boehme. In 1909, Buber (1909/1921) published *Confession of Ecstasy,* the analects of mystic experience from the East and West, ancient and contemporary. Buber himself engaged in spiritual practice including meditation. Through spiritual practice, he had an ecstatic experience in which the self was dissolved into communion with God. These were the kind of experiences that lie at the heart of religion, before religious organizations develop. His concerns, then, turned from social political movements to exploration of his own interiority and the mystical. Then, there came an awakening event, which he called 'conversion.'

## Conversion from Mysticism to Dialogue

It was one morning in 1914. Buber was 36 years old. That morning started with the ecstatic moment in which the self was felt dissolved. Before the overwhelming ecstasy subdued, a strange young man visited Buber to ask for his advice. It was not unusual in those days for a young man to visit Buber to seek spiritual insight. That morning, he warmly welcomed the young man, but the remnant of the early morning's mystical ambience was still there and kept him from engaging in the conversation fully. The urgency of the young man, whose heart was asking about matters of life and death, did not reach Buber.

Not after long, Buber heard the news of the young man. He had died in World War I, which began that year. Buber was in despair. He realized that the young man had been led to him by destiny at a time of vital importance in his life, and how he might have responded to him. Buber regretted from the depth of his heart that he was absent-minded and did not respond to the young man's request.

This event changed Buber's attitude toward the "religious." Thus, it was a "conversion." Buber (1930/1962) says;

> Since then I have given up the 'religious' which is nothing but the exception, extraction, exaltation, ecstasy; or it has given me up. I possess nothing but the everyday out of which I am never taken. The mystery is no longer disclosed, it has escaped or it has made its dwelling here where everything happens as it happens. I know no fullness but from being equal to it, yet I know that in the claim I am claimed and may respond in responsibility, and know who speaks and demands a response. (p. 187)

Buber's attitude toward the "religious" was transformed. He no longer considered withdrawing from daily worldly affairs to experience mystical ecstasy in the non-ordinary time and space known as the "religious." What is truly religious does not arise in non-ordinary secluded time and space where the sacred is cut off from the mundane. What is truly religious is not to distance the other that would come in daily life, but to respond to the other that is in front of me, and to stay responsible in the dialogue.

> If that is religious then it is just *all*, simply all that is lived in its possibility of dialogue. Here is space also for religion's highest form.... You are not swallowed up in a fullness without obligation, you are willed for the life of communion. (1930/1962, p. 187)

In other words;

> "Faith" is not a feeling in the soul of man but an entrance into reality, an entrance into *holistic* reality without reduction and curtailment. (1953/1962, p. 505)

Religion, then, means to live vital reality as a whole, and to live the vital whole as reality. "Holiness" lies nowhere other than in living the wholeness of holistic reality. Holiness does not exist in specially designated time and space that is isolated from ordinary life. Reality, to Buber, consists of dialogue. Only in those moments when I am open to the other is encounter bestowed as grace.

This conversion determined Buber's philosophy and educational practice in his later life. His major work, *I and Thou*, was written several years after his conversion experience. The work is founded on the boy's feeling of oneness with the horse, in which the border of the self was melted down. But, the center of the work is encounter with the other as Thou, not the mystical ecstasy. Buber (1936/1962), in *The Question to the Single One*, argued against Kierkegaard's thought that the individual can only as "the single one" enter communion with God. Instead, he proposed that dialogue "between man and man"[1] is the base unit of communion. "Between" is a keyword in Buber. He even created the term "between-humanity" (*Zwishenmenshlichen*). Buber(1947/1962) says:

> The space in which human beings exist genuinely as human beings has not been captured in concept. I would like to name it 'the sphere of the between.' (p. 405)

In this way, Buber's philosophy developed indeed to be distinct from other religious and existential philosophers. His is the philosophy of encounter and dialogue in between one being and another, and it has been asking us to understand the religious and spiritual in "the sphere of the between."

As Buber tried to live out his philosophy, it was natural that he increasingly involved himself in educational activity, and we turn now to his philosophy of education.

## EDUCATION AS HOLISTIC ENCOUNTER AND DIALOGUE

The birth of a baby is the precise moment of encounter with a new life. Between heaven and the earth, into this existing world, brand new life springs up. Life never repeats itself. The baby has a face, figure, and characteristics that are uniquely different from any other life that has ever existed. She has a soul that wishes to grow in a unique manner. In that moment of birth, the world becomes something different from what it has been. Today, in many places, an uncountable number of new lives have been initiated. The world renews itself ceaselessly, welcoming the reality of the newborn.

> ... [A] creative event if there was one, newness rising up, primal potential might. This potentiality, streaming unconquered, however, much of it is squandered, is the 'reality child': the phenomenon of uniqueness, which is more than just begetting and birth, this grace of beginning again and ever again. (Buber, 1926/1962, p. 787)

Although we tend to forget this "reality child" among the busy-ness of daily activity, says Buber, we should always remember it vividly. What an amazing mystery! What beautiful grace! What else is more ful-filling and a precious engagement than helping the bestowed reality of a child grow so as to unfold its potentiality? Education is nothing but this engagement of helping the "reality child." It is conscious participation in the actualizing force which creates the new ceaselessly and which gave birth to me and to you. Education is the engagement through which one is allowed to take part in the creation of heaven and earth. It is spiritual and holy engagement.

The key words in Buber's educational philosophy are "the actualiz-ing force" and "the primal reality." The source of his educational activity is this unique vision of reality and its spiritual roots.

> The other need only be opened out in this potentiality of his; more-over, this opening out takes place not essentially by teaching but by encounter, by existential communion between someone that is in actual being and someone that is in a process of becoming.... The educator sees every personal life as engaged in such a process of ac-tualization. He has come to see himself as a helper of the actualiz-ing forces. (Buber, 1954/1962, p. 281, 282)

The spiritual force that substantively actualizes reality is at work in "the reality child" and in the soul of the child. The work of education is to assist and facilitate the actualizing force as it is unfolding through the child's self.

What can the educator do to gain insight into the actualizing force in the child? First and foremost, the educator needs to encounter the child who is in front of him or her at the very moment and embrace the child as a whole. In other words, he or she needs to appreciate the child as "Thou" and not as "It."

In modern education, we have forgotten to perceive the child as a whole. We analyze the body, feeling, and intelligence, and tend to think that each segment can be developed separately. The standard images of the child and his or her developmental stages are set, and we see the child only by comparing to those standards.

In contrast with such an analytical or reductionist viewpoint, Buber (1954/1962) calls the way in which the educator should realize the actu-alizing spiritual force "awareness." This awareness is no less than to ex-perience the child as a whole, the wholeness of the child.

> To be aware of a thing or being means, in quite general terms, to
> experience it as a whole and yet at the same time without reduc-
> tion or abstraction, in all its concreteness. To be aware of a man,
> therefore, means in particular to perceive his wholeness as a per-
> son determined by the spirit; it means to perceive the dynamic
> center which stamps his every utterance, action, and attitude
> with the recognizable sign of uniqueness. (p. 278)

Here is Buber's holistic view of the human being. To be aware of the
wholeness of the personality is to be aware of the dynamic center of the
holy spirit. To perceive the wholeness of the child means to perceive the
dynamic center that is at work in him or her. And, that is expressed in the
child's each and every movement in a very unique manner. These are the
profound meanings of personality when it is carried into the spiritual dimension.

I would like to emphasize how primal the educational engagement
was for Buber in his spiritual life, after the "conversion." For Buber, spiritual practice is not the self-satisfying practice of the single person, but
encounter and dialogue with the other that is "Thou." Only in the relationship with "Thou" is awareness of the actualizing spiritual force possible. This attitude necessarily led Buber to assist such actualization,
which is the process of education. Buber's life was the process of unfolding dialogue after dialogue as he encountered each person, and through
the other's actualization of the self, he also realized his self. In that sense,
his life itself was education.

Having understood this background of Buber's own growth, I will
now discuss the educational activity that he actually involved himself in
as well as his educational thought.

## BEYOND EITHER COMPULSION OR FREEDOM

> At the opposite pole from compulsion there stands not freedom
> but communion. (Buber, 1926/1962, p. 795)

Buber taught at Liberal Jewish Academy in Frankfurt, which was
founded in 1920, and he gradually became the leader of the school. In
1930's, under the Nazi regime, he resigned the professorship at Frankfurt University and established the Jewish Adult Education Center. He
stayed in Germany until 1938 to continue educational activity in spite of
the increasing intolerance.

In the 1920's, educational reform movements appeared in various parts of the world including Germany. In Europe, the new educational trend flourished with key words such as "freedom," "creativity of the child," and "art education." International conferences were held. For example, the English organization which published the journal *The New Era* (to which A. S. Neill was a collaborator) held the first international educational conference in France. The second one was in Switzerland, and the third at Heidelberg in Germany in 1925.

Buber was the keynote speaker at this third international educational conference, where approximately 450 people participated from 30 nations. The conference organizers considered that Buber's educational practice and philosophy were not traditional and had affinity with their new focus. Of course, Buber agreed with their intention to reform traditional education. However, he had certain disagreements with the new movement. In the keynote speech at the conference, Buber (1926/1962) proposed a third alternative that is beyond the dichotomies of "the traditional and new," "the teacher-centered and child-centered," "compulsion and freedom."

Certainly, on one hand, Buber opposed compulsive education that pours knowledge from the teacher into students as if through a funnel. "The education of the whole person is to be built up on the natural activity of the self"(p. 789). He respected the spontaneous activity of students. On the other hand, however, Buber questioned the "liberalist," who argued that the educator should intervene as little as possible to let the students grow, emphasizing their autonomy and spontaneity. The "liberalist" respected the student's autonomy and argued for freedom from compulsive constraints. However, Buber thought that, even though the educator should wait for the students to learn independently, no spontaneous learning would emerge if their connection to the other was weakened and relations severed.

Without any relation to anyone, no spontaneity arises. Where there is rich connection with the world and the other, spontaneous independence grows. In creating the relationships that foster the student's spontaneity, the educator's way of being plays an important role. It is often said that freedom is not a matter of "leaving them alone." Thus, the necessity of some sort of relation is acknowledged. If it is neither compulsion nor leaving the students alone, the question is *how* should the educator relate to students? The keywords, such as "freedom" and "child-centered," do not clarify how the educator should relate to students.[2]

## Dialogue as Holistic Response

Buber (1926/1962) focuses on the relationship, that is, the way in which the educator relates to the students. As he puts it, "The hidden influence proceeding from wholeness of being has the integrating holistic power.... Relationships educate the child" (p. 795). Buber's philosophy emphasizes the educator's active role and responsibility to weave holistic relationships with the students. What is the quality of such holistic relationships? "The relation in education is one of genuine dialogue" (p. 803). Simply stated, the relationship that the educator should have with the learners is "dialogical relation." For Buber, dialogical relation meant responding to the call or query of the child. When the child is claiming my attention, I need to focus from the heart, listen, and respond to the best of my capacity. To the child who is quietly waiting, I need to speak. To respond to "the child lying with half-closed eyes, waiting with tense soul for its mother to speak to it,"(p. 792) is the responsibility of the adult, and it is the essence of Buber's "dialogue."

Genuine dialogue is a holistic response. The significance of dialogue as response is not limited to the content of what is spoken. What is more important is the fact that it is an encounter of beings as whole persons. Dialogue is "affirmation," "confirmation," and "acceptance" of being as a whole. It "make[s] the other present as a whole and a unique being, as the person that he is" (1954/1962, p. 285). A human being cannot confirm the meanings of one's presence alone. The holistic dialogue that is deepened with the other makes affirmation possible.

Needless to say, "such a confirmation does not mean approval; but no matter in what I am against the other, by accepting him as my partner in genuine dialogue I have affirmed him as a person" (*ibid.*). Therefore, the educator may give a firm "no" to the other's action or opinion. Those are the cases in which the educator affirms the child's presence by saying "no" to the action or opinion. In other words, the educator says no because he is affirming the child's presence. Buber says:

> [I]n the great faithfulness which is the climate of genuine dialogue, what I have to say at any one time already has in me the character of something that wishes to be uttered. (p. 285)

"Something that wishes to be uttered" must be expressed regardless of whether it is for or against the other person. Such utterance is not, in fact, utterance of my opinion. It is neither my opinion nor the other's; it is beyond both. "Something that wishes to be uttered" is born *between* myself and the other and is uttered through me. The genuine subject of the utterance is "the sphere of the between."

The educator is present as the deliverer of something that wishes to be uttered which is coming forth from the depth of the between.

## SPIRITUALITY, THE GENUINE SUBJECT IN EDUCATION

It is now obvious that this deepened dialogue is neither compulsion to impose oneself nor leaving students alone to let them do as they like. I wonder, however, if it is not too arrogant for an individual, who is also no more than another human being, to affirm and confirm the other's presence. To answer this question, Buber (1939/1962) lists humility as the most important quality of the educator. Moreover, he says, "a man can be arrogant without wishing to impose himself on others, and it is not enough to be modest in order to help another unfold" (1954/1962, p. 283).

What is essential is the awareness that it is not I as a human being that confirms and educates the other. It is the primal force, which is actualizing between the other and myself, that unfolds the other through encounter and dialogue. The primal force is not of my own. It is beyond I. The humility demanded from the educator is toward this force emerging from holy spirit. The educator should be humbly aware that she is only a channel through which the actualizing force is working, but nonetheless, *she* is responsible to respond to the child.

In Buber's educational philosophy, the subject in education is not the educator. Therefore, it is not teacher-centered. And, since the subject in education is not the child, it is not child-centered, either. In Buber, the genuine subject in education as encounter is that "actualizing force" itself, and "the primal reality" or "spirit" as its source. When the educator has deep faith in such spirituality and humbly tries to be a channel through which it can unfold, the primal spiritual force becomes the genuine subject in the educational engagement (see Buber,1935/1962, p. 810).

When education is vigorously realized in holistic encounter and dialogue, both the one who educates and the one educated learn to be aware of and trust the spiritual force that is actualizing through them. Both sides learn, through the deepening communion, what should be placed at the center of this dynamic educational process. We would like to call that something "spirituality in education." And, all that has been discussed is Buber's way of bringing spirituality into the heart of education.

## NOTES

1. *Between Man and Man* is adopted as the title for the English collection of Buber's works. Buber, 1947, trans. by R. G. Smith

2. Regarding the third vision beyond freedom and compulsion, I have discussed it thoroughly in my article that delved into the dialogue between Carl Rogers and Buber. Please refer to Yoshida, A. (1994). Beyond Freedom and Compulsion: Reflections on the Buber-Rogers Dialogue. *Holistic Education Review* 7(1): 4-10.

## REFERENCES

Buber, M. (Ed.). (1909/1921). *Ekstatische Konfessionen*. Leipzig: Insel Verlag.

Buber, M. (1962). *Werke Erster Band: Schriften zur Philosophie*. Munich and Heidelberg: Koesel Verlag and Verlag Lambert Schneider.

Buber, M. (1923/1962). *Ich und Du*. In *Werke* (pp. 77-170).

Buber, M. (1926/1962). *Über das Erzieherische*. In *Werke* (pp. 787-808).

Buber, M. (1930/1962). *Zwiesprache*. In *Werke* (pp. 171-214).

Buber, M. (1935/1962). *Bildung und Weltanschauung*. In *Werke* (pp. 809-816).

Buber, M. (1936/1962). *Die Frage an den Einzelnen*. In *Werke* (pp. 215-265).

Buber, M. (1939/1962). *Über Charaktererziehung*. In *Werke* (pp. 817-832).

Buber, M. (1947/1962). *Das Problem des Menschen*. In *Werke* (pp. 307-407).

Buber, M. (1953/1962). *Gottesfinsternis: Betrachtung zur Beziehung zwischen Religion und Philosophie*. In *Werke* (pp. 503-603).

Buber, M. (1954/1962). *Elemente des Zwischenmenschlichen*. In *Werke* (pp. 267-290).

Buber, M. (1952/1963). *Die chassidische Botschaft*. In *Werke Dritter Band: Schriften zum Chassidismus* (pp. 739-894). Munich and Heidelberg: Koesel Verlag and Verlag Lambert Schneider.

Buber, M. (1960/1986). *Begegnung: Autobiographische Fragmente*. Heidelberg: Verlag Lambert Schneider.

## Materials consulted about the English translation of Buber's works

Buber, M. (1923/1970). *I and Thou* (W. Kaufmann, Trans.). New York: Scribner.

Buber, M. (1947). *Between Man and Man* (R. G. Smith, Trans.). New York: Macmillan.

Buber, M. (1965). *The Knowledge of Man* (M. Friedman, Ed. and Trans.) New York: Harper & Row.

Schilpp, P. A., & Friedman, M. (Ed., and Trans.). (1967). *The Philosophy of Martin Buber*. Illinois and London: Open Court and Cambridge University Press.

## Acknowledgement

Special thanks to Yoshiko Matsuda for translating and Roger Prentice for revising this essay originally written in Japanese.

# CHAPTER 10

# Aldous Huxley

## A Quest for the Perennial Education

### Yoshiharu Nakagawa

> Education, insofar as it is not merely vocational, aims at recon-
> ciling the individual with himself, with his fellows, with society
> as a whole, with the nature of which he and his society are but a
> part, and with the immanent and transcendent spirit within
> which nature has its being. (Aldous Huxley, 1992, p. 101)

Aldous Huxley is widely regarded as a great writer and thinker of the
twentieth century. However, it is less known that he made significant
contributions to the development of contemporary holistic education.
He pioneered and deliberated ideas of holistic education in his conception of actualizing "human potentialities" through his extensive inquiries into diverse fields of knowledge and practice.

Huxley also valued spirituality in education. He was a spiritual
seeker who explored various spiritual paths from both Eastern and
Western traditions. These explorations led him to his views of the "perennial philosophy" upon which he built his work in holistic and spiritual education. In a sense, one could call Huxley's approach to education
"perennial education."

Briefly reviewing Huxley's biography and ideas on education, this
chapter will examine his contribution to the development of spirituality
in education.

#### THE LIFE OF ALDOUS HUXLEY

Aldous Huxley was born in 1894 in England and spent his youth
there. Then, as a middle-aged man, he moved to the United States in

1937, and settled in California and died there in 1963. Huxley came from a well-known scholarly family. His grandfather, Thomas Henry Huxley, was a prominent evolutionist and educator who contributed to the development of science education. His father, Leonard Huxley, was a Classics scholar, teacher, biographer, and editor of *Cornhill Magazine*. His mother, Julia Frances Arnold, the granddaughter of Dr. Thomas Arnold of Rugby and the niece of Matthew Arnold, was also an educator who founded a girls' school, but who died when Aldous Huxley was fourteen years old. His elder brother, Sir Julian Huxley, was a biologist and the first secretary of UNESCO.

Aldous Huxley attended Eton, a prestigious "public school" of England, and then Oxford. Although originally interested in medicine, at seventeen years old he had trouble with his eyesight, causing near-blindness for months, thereby forcing him to change his focus of study to literature. During the course of his life he continued to be very conscious of his physical health, which led to his involvement in psychophysical trainings such as the Bates Method (see Huxley, 1943/1985) and the Alexander Technique.

After a short period of teaching at Eton, Huxley also began writing and publishing novels, verse, stories, and essays, among other works. His early novels, in his twenties and thirties, included *Crome Yellow* (1921), *Point Counter Point* (1928), and *Brave New World* (1932), all of which commanded wide-spread acclaim.

Towards the end of his thirties, he began a new phase in his life. Huxley traveled in Central America, started to learn the Alexander Technique and the Bates Method, and committed himself to the peace movement. At 43, he moved to the United States with his friend, Gerald Heard, and settled down in southern California out of concern for his health. Huxley's important works from this transitory period included a novel *Eyeless in Gaza* (1936) and a collection of essays *Ends and Means* (1937).

In California, he initiated a life-long friendship with Jiddu Krishnamurti, when they met in 1938 (see Lutyens, 1983). Krishnamurti was also concerned with education, and he began the Oak Grove School in 1975 at Ojai, California, along with other schools. In many respects, Huxley and Krishnamurti's ideas on education were closely related, especially regarding the purpose of education and the emphasis upon the importance of awareness.

In 1945, at the age of 51, Huxley published *The Perennial Philosophy*, a classical study of mysticism. At 59, he pioneered the first mescalin experiment with Dr. Osmond, and published the experience in *The Doors of Perception* in 1954. In 1955 his first wife, Maria, died of cancer, and the next year Huxley married Laura Archera, an Italian-born musician and psychotherapist. During his last years, Laura contributed to his work through her expertise in psychotherapy. Huxley published important collections of essays *Adonis and the Alphabet* in 1956, and *Brave New World Revisited* in 1958.

At the age of 62 Huxley delivered a series of lectures at the University of California, Santa Barbara, which were later published as *The Human Situation* (1977), edited by Piero Ferrucci, the nephew of Laura Huxley. In his last years, despite a serious illness, Huxley traveled around the United States among other places, giving lectures that dealt with topics on "human potentialities." These activities had a considerable influence upon the emergence of the so-called "human potential movement." For instance, Walter Anderson (1983) reports that Michael Murphy and Richard Price asked Huxley about their plan to start the Esalen Institute, a birthplace of this movement (pp. 10-13). In 1961 a disastrous fire destroyed Huxley's library and all of his works, except the manuscript of his last novel, which was published the following year. This novel, *Island*, describes an ideal society in which people are able to realize their potentialities to the full extent. It is definitely Huxley's most comprehensive work containing the essential elements of his philosophy. Reading this book can still inspire us and give ideas for a holistic way of living. Fortunately, it also has large sections on education.

In 1963 Aldous Huxley, a twentieth century mystic, died at the age of 69. Throughout his life Huxley was a critical thinker, examining and identifying the discoveries of humankind. Since his death diverse movements of personal and cultural transformation have arisen, including humanistic and transpersonal psychologies, deep ecology, holistic healing, and holistic education. In this respect, many of Huxley's ideas have been actualized.

## ACTUALIZING HUMAN POTENTIALITIES

Despite his great concern for education, unfortunately Huxley did not leave us systematic descriptions on education, which has been a barrier to knowing his educational ideas. This may be one of the reasons that, as far as I am aware, few educational programs have been established based on his ideas. Therefore, it is our challenge to implement what he proposed. To accomplish this, we have to reconstruct a framework of his educational thought from various writings.

According to Huxley, the primary purpose of education is actualizing "human potentialities." Education is "[f]or actualization, for being turned into full-blown human beings" (1962, p. 202). Huxley's comprehensive view of education as a life-long process begins with proper nurturing and care of infants. In terms of this topic he refers to the influence of conditioning and the family system. In the elementary stage of education, Huxley recommends that children have "nonverbal" methods of education to cultivate one's wholeness. He presents a unique curriculum, called "nonverbal humanities," that embraces diverse methods developed in psychology, psychotherapy, body-mind trainings, and contemplative traditions.

Huxley's view of human potentialities includes a strong emphasis on spirituality. The ultimate goal of actualization is attaining spiritual enlightenment, primarily undertaken during adolescence and adulthood as a part of higher education. He celebrates practicing rites of passage in youth, so as to experience a glimpse of transcendence, and the art of awareness and contemplation for adults. In addition to this, being a "bridge-builder" between different fields, Huxley associates contemplative traditions with school curricula.

## BEYOND BRAVE NEW WORLD

In one of his earlier works, an anti-utopian novel *Brave New World*, Huxley (1932/1955) cautions us against the danger of conditioning and manipulating young children. This novel describes a totalitarian society whose members are controlled by psychological manipulation with scientific devices. He describes two methods of education (see chapter 2); namely, "neo-Pavlovian conditioning" and "hypnopaedia." They are devices designed to condition children to a given society on an unconscious level.

Neo-Pavlovian conditioning gives children negative stimuli to induce particular responses against the positive. The "Neo-Pavlovian Conditioning Room" contains flowers and books located in front of babies. During conditioning sessions, as crawling babies reach for either the flowers or the books, an explosive alarm goes off at the order of the room's "Director," along with a simultaneous "mild electric shock" sent through the floor. The Director says: "They'll grow up with what the psychologists used to call an 'instinctive' hatred of books and flowers. Reflexes unalterably conditioned. They'll be safe from books and botany all their lives" (p. 29). This results in the babies' learning to shrink away from nature and thought in horror.

The other method, hypnopaedia, or "sleep-teaching," is used as a tool of "moral education" by imprinting suggestive words during sleep. It is a refined system of conditioning; that is, "wordless conditioning is crude and wholesale; cannot bring home the finer distinctions, cannot inculcate the more complex courses of behaviour. For that there must be words, but words without reason. In brief, hypnopaedia" (p. 33). The Director regards hypnopaedia as "[t]he greatest moralizing and socializing force of all time" (p. 33) and insists:

> Till at last the child's mind *is* these suggestions, and the sum of the suggestions *is* the child's mind. And not the child's mind only. The adult's mind too — all his life long. The mind that judges and desires and decides — made up of these suggestions. But all these suggestions are *our* suggestions! (p. 34)

The grotesque picture described in *Brave New World* is not merely a fictional view, but rather an exaggeration of our highly industrialized society in which manipulation through conditioning by means of technology is quite commonplace. In 1958, twenty-six years after *Brave New World*, having witnessed real-world examples of conditioning, Huxley (1958/1965) published *Brave New World Revisited*, in which he recorded the growth of "mind-manipulation" technology including propaganda, selling, brainwashing, subconscious persuasion, and hypnopaedia. In a pessimistic tone he wrote, "The prophecies made in 1931 are coming true much sooner than I thought they would" (p. 4). An excerpt shows his fear of "Big Government" and "Big Business":

> In the world we live in … vast impersonal forces are making for the centralization of power and a regimented society. The genetic standardization of individuals is still impossible; but Big Government and Big Business already possess, or will very soon possess, all the techniques for mind-manipulation described in *Brave New World*.… Lacking the ability to impose genetic uniformity upon embryos, the rulers of tomorrow's over-populated and over-organized world will try to impose social and cultural uniformity upon adults and their children. To achieve this end,

they will (unless prevented) make use of all the mind-manipulating techniques at their disposal and will not hesitate to reinforce these methods of non-rational persuasion by economic coercion and threats of physical violence. (1958/1965, p. 103)

This statement conveys Huxley's realist perspective of the dangers and threats of our industrialized technological society. This realist attitude continued to exist into his last novel, *Island*. Although this is a novel about a utopian society, it does not offer only an optimistic view of society, but also considers the real dangers of industrialization.

In *Brave New World Revisited*, Huxley (1958/1965) promotes "an education for freedom" to prevent "social and cultural uniformity." He argues, "If this kind of tyranny is to be avoided, we must begin without delay to educate ourselves and our children for freedom and self-government" (pp. 103-104). Education for freedom involves several practical methods of de-conditioning.

For example, he refers to "the art of dissociation" as an antidote to "persuasion-by-association." "The propagandist arbitrarily associates his chosen product, candidate or cause with some idea, some image of a person or thing which most people, in a given culture, unquestioningly regard as good" (p. 81). This type of conditioning associates one event with another, more socially favorable event, to force people to accept the former. The art of dissociation is an attempt to dissociate associations of these events. In *Ends and Means* Huxley (1937) says:

> The art of dissociating ideas should have a place in every curriculum. Young people must be trained to consider the problems of government, international politics, religion and the like in isolation from the pleasant images, with which a particular solution of these problems has been associated, more or less deliberately, by those whose interest it is to make the public think, feel and judge in a certain way. (pp. 217-218)

In later years the art of de-conditioning plays an important role in his approach to education. It forms a prerequisite step to the education for human potentialities by reducing and releasing undesirable and harmful conditionings.

## Our Ultimate Investment

Huxley holds the idea that "two thirds" of all sorrow and misery in human life originates from the improper ways we live and we can avoid it by creating better systems, including education. The seeds of misery are sowed in the early years of life, and this brings to light the importance of preventive systems for childcare. For this purpose, Huxley proposes two methods in *Island*.

One method is "positive" conditioning that gives infant positive experiences necessary for him or her to live on earth with trust and love. An infant is an absorbent being that needs positive experiences to have a foundation for healthy development. Positive conditioning not only gives him or her a basic trust in life, but also prevents traumatic experiences. However, if a child does have these harmful experiences, positive conditioning allows the child to heal them in their initial stages.

Unlike in *Brave New World*, in *Island* Huxley (1962) promotes the use of "Pavlov purely for a good purpose," namely, "Pavlov for friendliness and trust and compassion" (p. 190). The formulation is this: "Food plus caress plus contact plus 'good' equals love. And love equals pleasure, love equals satisfaction" (p. 190). Recognizing this method's origin in indigenous childcare, Huxley describes it as follows:

> This technique was one of their happiest discoveries. Stroke the baby while you're feeding him; it doubles his pleasure. Then, while he's sucking and being caressed, introduce him to the animal or person you want him to love. Rub his body against theirs; let there be a warm physical contact between child and love-object. At the same time repeat some word like 'good.' (p. 189)

The other method is to create an enlarged family system called "MAC," or Mutual Adoption Club. According to his definition:

> Every MAC consists of anything from fifteen to twenty-five assorted couples. Newly elected brides and bridegrooms, old timers with growing children, grandparents and great-grandparents — everybody in the club adopts everyone else. Besides our own blood relations, we all have our quota of deputy mothers, deputy fathers, deputy aunts and uncles, deputy brothers and sisters, deputy babies and toddlers and teen-agers. (1962, p. 90)

Unlike ordinary, compulsory families, MAC is "[n]ot exclusive ... and not predestined, not compulsory. An inclusive, unpredestined and voluntary family" (p. 90). Under these circumstances, children have additional parents, and the parents, additional children. This allows both to avoid undesirable experiences and, at the same time, provides a nurturing and healing environment. In Huxley's view, a large part of our behavioral problems stem from the traditional family system.

> In your predestined and exclusive families children, as you say, serve a long prison term under a single set of parental jailers. These parental jailers may, of course, be good, wise, and intelligent. In that case the little prisoners will emerge more or less unscathed. But in point of fact most of your parental jailers are *not* conspicuously good, wise or intelligent. They're apt to be well-meaning but stupid, or not well-meaning and frivolous, or else neurotic, or occasionally downright malevolent, or frankly insane. (p. 92)

By restructuring the family system, Huxley believes one can avoid the development of behavioral problems. If a child feels unhappy in his or her first family, MAC permits other families to do the best for him or her, meanwhile his or her parents seek therapy from other members of their MAC (p. 93). A MAC is a caring community in which a child has interactions with enough people to develop in a healthy way.

> Here the children grow up in a world that's a working model of society at large, a small-scale but accurate version of the environment in which they're going to have to live when they're grown up. 'Holy,' 'Healthy,' 'whole' — they all come from the same root and carry different overtones of the same meaning. Etymologically and in fact, our kind of family, the inclusive and voluntary kind, is the genuine holy family. (p. 92)

Huxley's wife, Laura Huxley, has tried to implement his ideas on childcare. To do so, she founded an organization in 1977 called "Our Ultimate Investment," dedicated to "the nurturing of the possible human." Laura Huxley (1993) says, "The concept is that much of the predicament of the human situation begins not only in infancy, not only before birth.... but also in the physical, psychological, and spiritual preparation of the couple *before* conception" (p. 259). In other words, the message of Our Ultimate Investment is that if we are loved before the beginning — if a human being is a loving thought in its parents' mind before conception — if the focus of the couple is to improve their physical and mental health and their relationship before conception — the child will be a healthier, kinder, more capable human being on all levels. Certainly the improvement on physical and mental health would be enormous. (L. Huxley, 1994, p. 17)

Laura Huxley (1987/1992), with the help of Piero Ferrucci, gives us a comprehensive view of childbirth from pre-natal to post-natal periods within the following five stages: prelude to conception, conscious conception, reverence for life (pregnancy), O nobly born (the moment of birth), meeting the world (the first days and years). One of her attempts is to create an educational program for young people, introducing the "prelude to conception" phase. In this program, teens are invited to be with small children so as to gain a hands-on perspective of what it means to have a child.

Another program relating to "the first days and years" is "project caressing" for both babies and older people. The purpose of this program is to satisfy babies' need to be touched and for lonely, older people to be able to fulfill their own need to give themselves to others. Evidently Laura's projects owe much to Huxley's ideas of positive conditioning and the MAC family structure. In 1994 Aldous Huxley's centennial celebration took place in Los Angeles, together with an international conference entitled "Children: Our Ultimate Investment," showing his enduring legacy.

## THE NONVERBAL HUMANITIES

Now let us take a look at Huxley's ideas of holistic curriculum in elementary education. His ideas appear in *Adonis and the Alphabet* (with the very important chapter "The Education of an Amphibian"), *Island* (Chapter 13), *The Doors of Perception*, and *The Human Situation*, as well as articles including "Human Potentialities" and "Education on the Nonverbal Level," among others.

Huxley calls his ideas of holistic curriculum "the nonverbal humanities." Unlike conventional humanities that have favored the training of verbal faculties, the nonverbal humanities attempt to explore the nonverbal aspects of human being. Huxley maintains that a human being is an "amphibian," which exists simultaneously in the world of words and symbols and in the world of "immediate experience." And he stresses the importance of an attempt to "make the best of both worlds":

> Whether we like it or not, we are amphibians, living simultaneously in the world of experience and the world of notions, in the world of direct apprehension of Nature, God and ourselves, and the world of abstract, verbalized knowledge about these primary facts. Our business as human beings is to make the best of both these worlds. (1956, pp. 14-15)

Unfortunately, these two worlds are severely separated and imbalanced in society today. Language is undoubtedly an essential element of being human, thus Huxley (1956) defines humans as *homo loquax* (p. 10), or the loquacious one. However, the acquirement of language has disturbed the nonverbal world of immediate experience: "Language, it is evident, has its Gresham's Law. Bad words tend to drive out good words, and words in general, the good as well as the bad, tend to drive out immediate experience and our memories of immediate experience"(1956, p. 13). Humans perceive things through the filter of language and live in a world of meanings, which inevitably separates them from the world of immediate experience.

Huxley's notion of language agrees with recent findings in various disciplines regarding language — linguistics, semantics, structuralism, hermeneutics, and philosophy of language. These disciplines find that the world we live in is not a natural, biological, objective world but is a symbolic world constructed by language. Symbolic articulation of things through language makes our world as it is. However, for Huxley this refers to the verbal half of our amphibian nature. If we identified ourselves exclusively with this half, we would be enclosed in the world of language. This is why Huxley finds it necessary to limit the domination of language by cultivating a sound "skepticism" toward language. "Discouraging children from taking words too seriously, teaching them to analyze whatever they hear or read — this is an integral part of the school curriculum" (1962, p. 147).

On the basis of perennial philosophy, Huxley maintains that the world of language is not the only reality but an intermediate layer of the total reality. Thus we can explore realities deeper than the world of language through proper methods. In *The Doors of Perception* Huxley (1960) proposes:

> We can never dispense with language and the other symbol sys-
> tems; for it is by means of them, and only by their means, that we
> have raised ourselves above the brutes, to the level of human be-
> ings. But we can easily become the victims as well as the benefi-
> ciaries of these systems. We must learn how to handle words
> effectively; but at the same time we must preserve and, if neces-
> sary, intensify our ability to look at the world directly and not
> through that half-opaque medium of concepts, which distorts
> every given fact into the all too familiar likeness of some generic
> label or explanatory abstraction. (p. 59)

The central task of the nonverbal humanities is to raise our ability to look
at the world directly.

As a whole, education has made every effort to develop the verbal aspect of human abilities, failing to embrace education on the nonverbal
level. "Every child is educated in a particular language and (formulated
in terms of that language's syntax and vocabulary) in a set of basic notions about the world, himself and other people.… In civilized societies
of the Western type, this verbal and notional education is systematic and
intensive" (1965, p. 35). According to Huxley (1960), this holds true to every discipline: "Literary or scientific, liberal or specialist, all our education is predominantly verbal" (p. 59).

To counter this imbalance, Huxley emphasizes the importance of
training students on the nonverbal level. "What is needed, if more of the
potentialities of more people are to be actualized, is a training on the
nonverbal levels of our whole being as systematic as the training now
given to children and adults on the verbal level" (1965, p. 37).

According to Huxley (1956), the possible methods of the nonverbal
humanities include: "Training of the kinesthetic sense. Training of the
special senses. Training of memory. Training in control of the autonomic
nervous system. Training for spiritual insight" (p. 19). Concretely
Huxley uses the Alexander Technique for kinesthetic training, the Bates
Method for visual training, the Jacobson method of relaxation for training in the control of one's autonomic nervous system, and the traditions
of contemplation for spiritual training. He also refers to training of perception and awareness, such as Gestalt Therapy, the Vittoz Method, and
Tantric meditations (see Huxley, 1965, 1969). Furthermore, in *Island* he
uses techniques such as visualization and body movement for emotional
transformation. Using a wide variety of methods from many different

fields shows Huxley's intention "to make the best of both worlds — the Oriental and the European, the ancient and the modern" (1962, p. 129).

## THE ALEXANDER TECHNIQUE

The Alexander Technique has a special place in Huxley's life as well as the nonverbal humanities. His involvement in this method gave him a crucial key with which to restructure education in both theory and practice. A study by Frank Pierce Jones (1976/1979) reports that Huxley began practicing the Alexander Technique in 1935 with the founder, Frederick Matthias Alexander, out of concern for his physical health. But soon he realized that it affected not only his physical, but also his mental condition. In his letter to Hubert Benoit, he wrote as follows:

> This, as I know by experience, is an exceedingly valuable technique … practising this awareness makes it possible for the physical organism to function as it ought to function, thus improving the general state of physical and mental health. (cited in L. Huxley, 1981/1987, p. vii)

In *Ends and Means*, Huxley (1937) celebrated the Alexander Technique as a form of body-mind education that helps with the spiritual realization of "non-attachment" (pp. 219-224). Furthermore, in his novel *Eyeless in Gaza* (1936), he described F. M. Alexander as Dr. Miller (e.g., Jones, 1976/1979, 1987). It is said that his enthusiasm in the participation of this technique lasted until he died.

It is important to remember that F. M. Alexander designed this technique as a way of re-education working directly on body-mind when he discovered it in the early years of the twentieth century. Alexander regarded the method as a way for improving "the use of the self," or of the psychophysical organism as a whole. In Huxley's words, it is "a technique for the proper use of the self, a method for the creative conscious control of the whole psychophysical organism" (1978, p. 150). The Alexander Technique re-educates the self in an attempt to regain its proper use. According to Laura Huxley (1981/1987, p. vi), it is a method of "unlearning," for the misuse of the self is learned as a habitual pattern and can be unlearned through a re-educational process. This method requires us to raise the conscious control of our use, for the misuse is automated in subconscious patterns of behavior. To re-educate the misuse of the self, it is necessary to "inhibit" the misuse while simultaneously "directing" the proper use in accordance with the "primary control" of the organism by the teacher's help.

The Alexander Technique gave Huxley a new perspective on education, an education that takes place on the nonverbal level with a special emphasis on raising consciousness to the daily use of body-mind. It is important to note that Huxley discovered John Dewey's involvement in this method. Dewey had already practiced this method under Alexander since 1914 and regarded it as an essential contribution to education in general. In an "Introduction" to the work of Alexander, Dewey (1923/1985) recognized that "the method is not one of remedy; it is one of constructive education" (p. xxxiii). Dewey (1932/1984) later went as far as to say, "It [the technique of Mr. Alexander] provides ... the conditions for the central direction of all special educational processes. It bears the same relation to education that education itself bears to all other human activities" (p. xix). Huxley (1956) comments on Dewey's statements:

> These are strong words; for Dewey was convinced that man's only hope lies in education. But just as education is absolutely necessary to the world at large, so Alexander's methods of training the psycho-physical instrument are absolutely necessary to education. Schooling without proper training of the psycho-physical instrument cannot, in the very nature of things, do more than a limited amount of good and may, in the process of doing that limited amount of good, do the child a great deal of harm by systematically engraining his habits of improper use. (p. 21)

Unfortunately, Dewey's voice was ignored, even by progressive educators, as Huxley (1956) puts it:

> It is a most curious fact that of the literally millions of educators who, for two generations, have so constantly appealed to Dewey's authority, only an infinitesimal handful has ever bothered to look into the method which Dewey himself regarded as absolutely fundamental to any effective system of education. (p. 21)

It took almost half a century until this method became available in larger circles. However, still today it is necessary for those who are working in educational fields to pay more attention to the voices of Dewey and Huxley, for current education is missing a deeper understanding of body-mind approaches like the Alexander Technique.

## THE NOT-SELVES

The non-verbal humanities encompass a wide range of methods including therapeutic and psychological methods, body-mind approaches, and spiritual disciplines. They are not, however, an arbitrary collection of different methods but are arranged in association with the multidimensional structure of the human being. Huxley conceives a theory of the human being that involves not only the conscious self, or the verbal level, but also unconscious, deeper layers of what he calls the "not-selves." "Every human being is a conscious self; but, below the threshold of consciousness every human being is also a not-self — or, more precisely, he is five or six merging but clearly distinguishable not-selves" (1956, pp. 16-17).

The not-selves exist in multiple dimensions from the surface to the deeper levels. They are, (a) the "personal not-self," or "the subconscious," comprised of habits, conditioned reflexes, repressed impulses, past memories and other personal experiences; (b) the "vegetative soul" in charge of the physiological functions of the body; (c) the not-self that inhabits the world of insights and inspiration; (d) the not-self dwelling in the symbolic realm of Jungian archetypes; (e) the "mysterious" not-self that has visionary experience; (f) the "universal Not-Self," or the ultimate reality (1956, pp. 17-18).

These concepts of the not-selves are based on perennial philosophy as much as modern psychology. They detail what Huxley (1946) calls "autology" in *The Perennial Philosophy*. It means "the science, not of the personal ego, but of that eternal Self in the depth of particular, individualized selves, and identical with, or at least akin to, the divine Ground" (pp. 7-8). The practice of the perennial philosophy is concerned with exploration into the not-selves by the way of psychological and spiritual disciplines with the ultimate aim of identifying the universal Not-Self.

> To know the ultimate Not-Self, which transcends the other not-selves and the ego, but which is yet closer than breathing, nearer than hands and feet — this is the consummation of human life, the end and ultimate purpose of individual existence. (1956, p. 33)

Each method of the nonverbal humanities helps us explore the not-selves in one way or another. The first problem one faces is that the conscious ego and the subconscious layer of "the personal not-self" (inappropriate habits, neurosis caused by repressed emotions, and other conditioned behaviors) tend to obstruct the deeper not-selves.

> Man ... is a self associated with not-selves. By developing bad habits, the conscious ego and the personal sub-conscious interfere with the normal functioning of the deeper not-selves, from which we receive the animal grace of physical health and the spiritual grace of insight. (1956, p. 23)

It often happens that the surface dimensions of the ego and the subconscious repress the other deeper dimensions because of our exclusive identification with them. It is necessary to work on the surface layers to dissolve barriers the ego and the personal subconscious have created, which is one of the essential functions of the nonverbal humanities:

> That which must be relaxed is the ego and the personal subconscious, that which must be active is the vegetative soul and the not-selves which lie beyond it. The physiological and spiritual not-selves with which we are associated cannot do their work effectively until the ego and personal subconscious learn to let go. (1956, pp. 23-24)

The methods in the nonverbal humanities serve as an "art of combining relaxation with activity" in which the ego and the personal subconscious are relaxed and, at the same time, the vegetative soul and the deeper not-selves are activated.

## ISLAND

*Island* provides rich examples of the nonverbal humanities. Huxley (1962) summarizes his ideas in the following:

> What we give the children is simultaneously a training in perceiving and imagining, a training in applied physiology and psychology, a training in practical ethics and practical religion, a training in the proper use of language, and a training in self-knowledge. In a word, a training of the whole mind-body in all its aspects. (p. 208)

Three more methods are added to our discussion. To teach the differences between the verbal and nonverbal dimensions, there is a method in Huxley's curriculum, called "Elementary Applied Philosophy," which teaches differences between symbols and events (or what is going on in each person) in experiential ways (1962, pp. 214-217). As Huxley (1977) puts it in *The Human Situation,* "any development of awareness must go hand in hand with the development of our knowledge of language and concepts. If we are going to be aware of our direct experience, we must also be aware of the relationship between direct experience and the world of symbols and language and concepts in which we live" (p. 249). In this respect, he says, "twentieth-century developments in linguistics in general and in semantics should find their way into education on every level" (p. 249).

The novel describes that even in a class such as botany conceptual learning is related to receptive perception in "bridge-building lessons" (pp. 217-221). A flower is looked at not only in an analytical and scientific manner but also in alert passiveness and receptivity without labeling or categorizing.

> Everything from dissected frogs to the spiral nebulae, it all gets looked at receptively as well as conceptually, as a fact of aesthetic or spiritual experience as well as in terms of science or history or economics. Training in receptivity is the complement and antidote to training in analysis and symbol-manipulation. Both kinds of training are absolutely indispensable. (p. 219)

In his article, "Education on the Nonverbal Level," Huxley (1969) states, "Systematic training of perception should be an essential element in all education" (p. 156). He discerns two modes of perception, one as "a highly conceptualized, stereotyped, utilitarian, and even scientific mode" and the other as "a receptive, more or less unconceptualized, aesthetic and 'spiritual' mode of perceiving" (p. 156). He places his emphasis on the latter, which he calls "wise passiveness," borrowing Wordsworth's concept from his *Expostulation and Reply* and *The Tables Turned.* Wise passiveness is a condition for creativity, spiritual insight, and happiness. "Watching and receiving in a state of perfect ease or wise passiveness is an art which can be cultivated and should be taught on every educational level from the most elementary to the most advanced" (pp. 159-160).

The second method is expressive movement called "Rakshasi Hornpipe," which is "a device for letting off those dangerous heads of steam raised by anger and frustration" (1962, p. 222). In a class of this expressive dance movement, the teacher encourages the students to release their negative emotions through furious movement with shouting. This is a method of emotional transformation like Reichian therapy such as Bioenergetics. As to this method, Huxley accepts Laura Huxley's ideas on her approach to psychotherapy. He writes the following in an "Introduction" to Laura's *You Are Not the Target*:

> I discovered that some of the clearest and most practical answers to certain of my questions were being given by my wife in the "Recipes for Living and Loving".... Some of her recipes (for example, those for the Transformation of Energy) have found their way, almost unmodified, into my phantasy. Others have been changed and developed to suit the needs of my imaginary society and to fit into its peculiar culture. (1963/1994, pp. xii-xiii)

The third method is training in imagination and visualization called "Elementary Practical Psychology." Huxley recognizes the importance of visualization in healing and education. It is interesting to note how Huxley came to know of Robert Assagioli's Psychosynthesis. Laura Huxley (1982) writes that she met Assagioli in 1954 for the first time, and in 1963 Assagioli sent a letter to her in appreciation for her book. Then Aldous Huxley sent him his *Island* with this inscription: "To Robert Assagioli, in the hope that he may find something to interest him in this utopian essay on psychosynthesis" (cited in L. Huxley, 1982, p. 12). After Huxley's death, Laura's nephew, Piero Ferrucci, studied under and later collaborated with Assagioli to then become a representative theorist of Psychosynthesis.

## RITES OF PASSAGE

Huxley (1962) regards cultivating spirituality as a matter of higher education: "Individuals in their transcendent unity are the affair of higher education. That begins in adolescence and is given concurrently with advanced elementary education" (p. 202). The main training in the higher education is the art of awareness, which I will discuss later. Beside this Huxley pays special attention to rites of passage for youth as an initiation from childhood to adulthood. He is most likely influenced by traditions of native cultures. For him, rites of passage are extraordinary moments in which young people are invited to have a glimpse of transcendence.

*Island* describes a group of young people's expedition into the mountains. Their journey has three stages, "the yoga of danger," "the yoga of the summit," and "the yoga of jungle." The yoga of danger is an ordeal of climbing which gives them direct experience of life and death. "An ordeal that helps them to understand the world they'll have to live in, helps them to realize the omnipresence of death, the essential precariousness of all existence" (p. 159). Faced with the real threat of death, they are able to realize their full potentialities. In the second stage, or the yoga of summit, after their climbing, "the yoga of rest and letting go, the yoga of complete and total receptiveness" (p. 165) takes place. Here they are open to "formless, wordless Not-Thought" in the eternal moment. This story describes that these young people are going to have a beautiful taste of transcendental unity in the universe with the aid of the "*moksha*-medicine," a kind of psychedelic medicine. They then go down to the jungle, whose danger gives them vivid experiences of a life that includes both beauty and horror. At this third stage there is a "reconciliation," or a fusion, in which beauty is made one with horror.

The experience of rites of passage is important for us because the modern world has almost completely lost them. Our society today gives rise to difficult situations for young people to go through in their transformative process. Rites of passage have long been devices to offer opportunities in which everyone can transform his or her life during critical moments of transition. It is interesting to note that some holistic educators have recently begun to implement rites of passage into their practices (e.g., Kessler, 2000; Luvmour, 1993).

## THE ART OF AWARENESS

To practice the art of awareness in every aspect of living forms the key component of higher education for youths and adults. Huxley (1962) calls it "the yoga of everyday living":

> It's through awareness, complete and constant awareness, that we transform it [concrete materialism] into concrete spirituality. Be fully aware of what you're doing, and work becomes the yoga of work, play becomes the yoga of play, everyday living becomes the yoga of everyday living. (p. 149)

*Island* involves scenes in which a bird repeatedly calls "attention" to wake up people for the importance of this practice. Awareness is meant to notice that which is taking place in the present moment without any interventions of the mind, such as interpretation, judgment, comparison, etc. Awareness in this sense is alternately called "attention," "mindfulness," "witness," or "observation" in the contemplative disciplines. The practice of awareness is a foundation of contemplation, especially in the traditions of Eastern philosophy.

*Island* has philosophical fragments called "Notes on What's what" in which Huxley (1962) addresses essential parts of his philosophy. In terms of awareness he states:

> Good Being is in the knowledge of who in fact one is in relation to *all* experiences; so be aware — aware in every context, at all times and whatever, creditable or discreditable, pleasant or un- pleasant, you may be doing or suffering. This is the only genuine yoga, the only spiritual exercise worth practising. (p. 40)

These statements seem to reflect what Krishnamurti meant in his con- cept of "choiceless awareness." In his *The First and Last Freedom*, Krishnamurti (1954/1975) said, "To know ourselves means to know our relationship with the world.... What it [the understanding of relation- ship to the whole] demands is awareness to meet life as a whole" (p. 94). Huxley (1954/1975) comments on choiceless awareness in his foreword to this book as follows:

> Through this choiceless awareness, as it penetrates the succes- sive layers of the ego and its associated sub-conscious, will come love and understanding, but of another order than that with which we are ordinarily familiar. This choiceless awareness — at every moment and in all the circumstances of life — is the only effective meditation. (p. 17)

Generally speaking, the contemplative traditions expect that cease- less practice of awareness will bring about a radical transformation of consciousness, leading to a great awakening or enlightenment. Huxley (1962) holds this opinion: "Everybody's job — enlightenment. Which means, here and now, the preliminary job of practising all the yogas of in- creased awareness" (p. 236). In "Notes on What's what" he says:

> The more a man knows about himself in relation to every kind of experience, the greater his chance of suddenly, one fine morn- ing, realizing who in fact he is — or rather Who (capital W) in Fact (capital F) "he" (between quotation marks) Is (capital I). (p. 40)

He describes the state of consciousness in enlightenment as follows: "Ultimately and essentially there was only a luminous bliss, only a knowledge-less understanding, only union with unity in a limitless, undifferentiated awareness" (p. 263).

Furthermore, in accordance with the teachings of *The Tibetan Book of the Dead*, Huxley (1962) introduces what he calls "the yogas of living and dying" for dying people: "Going on being aware — it's the whole art of dying" (p. 239).

> We help them to go on practising the art of living even while they're dying. Knowing who in fact one is, being conscious of the universal and impersonal life that lives itself through each of us—that's the art of living, and that's what one can help the dying to go on practising. To the very end. Maybe beyond the end. (p. 239)

In *Island*, an old woman in her dying phase is guided by an experienced therapist into the world of clear light. This also happened for Aldous Huxley himself, with the aid of his wife Laura (e.g., L. Huxley, 1968/1991, pp. 295-308). She writes that "Aldous died as he lived, doing his best to develop fully in himself one of the essentials he recommended to others: *Awareness*" (p. 295). Interestingly, individuals like Ram Dass and Stephen Levine further developed Huxley's ideas on dying in their social movement of "conscious dying."

## THE BRIDGE BUILDER

We have seen what areas Aldous Huxley explored concerning holistic and spiritual education. Huxley regarded spirituality as an issue for higher education. However, it is more important to acknowledge the connections he made between spiritual disciplines and other methods of the nonverbal humanities. Every method of the nonverbal humanities has a certain relevance to spiritual cultivation. This is what distinguishes Huxley's contribution to our understanding of spirituality in education.

For example, when speaking of visualization Huxley (1962) remarks:

> What those children you saw here were being taught is a very simple technique—a technique that we'll develop later on into a method of liberation. Not complete liberation, of course.... This technique won't lead you to the discovery of your Buddha Nature: but it may help you to prepare for that discover —help you by liberating you

from the hauntings of your own painful memories, your remorses, your causeless anxieties about the future. (p. 225)

Getting rid of negative conditioning through visualization can be a preparatory phase leading to spiritual cultivation.

Huxley also sees the Alexander Technique as an elementary practice for contemplation, for it is the art of raising "elementary awareness." "Education in elementary awareness will have to include techniques for improving awareness of internal events and techniques for improving awareness of external events as these are revealed by our organs of sense" (1969, p. 155). The Alexander Technique is a way with which to enhance elementary awareness of one's kinesthetic sense. This is important because "[t]he kinesthetic sense is the main line of communication between the conscious self and the personal subconscious on the one hand and the vegetative soul on the other" (1956, p. 19).

It is through his association of this body-mind training with contemplation that Huxley provides us with a comprehensive view of *the education of awareness* from the elemental to the highest levels. Surprisingly, in his article on the Alexander Technique, "End-Gaining and Means-Whereby" (original work published in 1941), Huxley (1978) combines this technique with "the mystic's technique of transcending personality in a progressive awareness of ultimate reality" (p. 150) and conceives "a totally new type of education."

> Be that as it may, the fact remains that Alexander's technique for the conscious mastery of the primary control is now available, and that it can be combined in the most fruitful way with the technique of the mystics for transcending personality through increasing awareness of ultimate reality. It is now possible to conceive of a totally new type of education affecting the entire range of human activity, from physiological, through the intellectual, moral, and practical, to the spiritual — an education which, by teaching them the proper use of the self, would preserve children and adults from most of the diseases and evil habits that now afflict them; an education whose training in inhibition and conscious control would provide men and women with the psychophysical means for behaving rationally and morally; an education which in its upper reaches, would make possible the experience of ultimate reality. (1978, p. 152)

Huxley thus finds essential connections between psychophysical methods and spiritual cultivation. It is his genius as the *pontifex*, or the bridge builder, that provides such an integral vision of education.

## References

Alexander, F. M. (1923/1985). *Constructive Conscious Control of the Individual*. Long Beach, CA: Centerline Press.

Alexander, F. M. (1932/1984). *The Use of the Self*. Long Beach, CA: Centerline Press.

Anderson, W. T. (1983). *The Upstart Spring: Esalen and the American Awakening*. Reading, MA: Addison-Wesley.

Bedford, S. (1973/1987). *Aldous Huxley: A Biography. Vol. One. The Apparent Stability 1894-1939*. London: Paladin Grafton Books.

Bedford, S. (1974/1987). *Aldous Huxley: A Biography. Vol. Two. The Turning Points 1939-1963*. London: Paladin Grafton Books.

Dewey, J. (1923/1985). Introduction. In F. M. Alexander, *Constructive Conscious Control of the Individual* (pp. xxi-xxxiii). Long Beach, CA: Centerline Press.

Dewey, J. (1932/1984). Introduction. In F. M. Alexander, *The Use of the Self* (pp. viii-xix). Long Beach, CA: Centerline Press.

Huxley, A. (1932/1955). *Brave New World*. Harmondsworth, England: Penguin Books.

Huxley, A. (1937). *Ends and Means: An Inquiry into the Nature of Ideals and into the Methods Employed for their Realization*. London: Chatto and Windus.

Huxley, A. (1943/1985). *The Art of Seeing*. London: Triad Grafton.

Huxley, A. (1946). *The Perennial Philosophy*. London: Chatto & Windus.

Huxley, A. (1954/1975). Foreword. In J. Krishnamurti, *The First and Last Freedom*. San Francisco: HarperCollins

Huxley, A. (1956). *Adonis and the Alphabet*. London: Chatto & Windus.

Huxley, A. (1958/1965). *Brave New World Revisited*. New York: Harper & Row, Perennial Library.

Huxley, A. (1960). *The Doors of Perception* and *Heaven and Hell*. London: Chatto & Windus.

Huxley, A. (1962). *Island*. London: Chatto & Windus.

Huxley, A. (1963/1994). Introduction. In L. A. Huxley, *You Are Not the Target* (pp. xi-xiv). New York: Farrar, Straus and Company.

Huxley, A. (1965). Human potentialities. In R. E. Farson (Ed.), *Science and Human Affairs* (pp. 32-44). Palo Alto, CA: Science and Behavior Books.

Huxley, A. (1969). Education on the nonverbal level. In H. Chiang & A. H. Maslow (Eds.), *The Healthy Personality: Readings* (pp. 150-165). New York: Van Nostrand Reinhold.

Huxley, A. (1977). *The Human Situation: Lectures at Santa Barbara* (P. Ferrucci, Ed). London: Chatto & Windus.

Huxley, A. (1978). End-gaining and means-whereby. In W. Barlow (Ed.), *More Talk of Alexander* (pp. 149-153). London: Victor Gollacz.

Huxley, A. (1992). *Huxley and God: Essays* (J. H. Bridgeman, Ed.). San Francisco: HarperCollins.

Huxley, L. A. (1963/1994). *You Are Not the Target*. New York: Farrar, Straus and Company.

Huxley, L. (1968/1991). *This Timeless Moment: A Personal View of Aldous Huxley*. San Francisco: Mercury House.

Huxley, L. (1981/1987). Foreword to new edition. In M. Gelb, *Body learning: An Introduction to the Alexander Technique*. London: Aurum Press.

Huxley, L. (1982). Foreword. In P. Ferrucci, *What We May Be: Techniques for Psychological and Spiritual Growth Through Psychosynthesis* (pp. 11-13). Los Angeles: Jeremy P. Tarcher.

Huxley, L. (1993). Bridging heaven and earth. In D. J. Brown & R. M. Novick (Eds.), *Mavericks of the Mind: Conversations for the New Millennium* (pp. 240-260). Freedom, CA: The Crossing Press.

Huxley, L. (1994). An interview with Laura Huxley. *Island Views, 1* (3), 1, 14-17.

Huxley, L., & Ferrucci, P. (1987/1992). *The Child of your Dreams*. Rochester, VT: Destiny Books.

Jones, F. P. (1976/1979). *Body Awareness in Action: A Study of the Alexander Technique*. New York: Schocken Books.

Jones, F. P. (1987). Aldous Huxley and F. Matthias Alexander. *The Alexander Review, 2*(2), 11-22.

Kessler, R. (2000). *The Soul of Education: Helping Students Find Connection, Compassion, and Character at School*. Alexandria, VA: Association for Supervision and Curriculum Development.

Krishnamurti, J. (1954/1975). *The First and Last Freedom*. San Francisco: HarperCollins.

Lutyens, M. (1983). *Krishnamurti: The Years of Fulfillment*. New York: Avon Books.

Luvmour, J. & S. (1993). *Natural Learning Rhythms: Discovering How and When Your Child Learns.* Berkeley, CA. Celestial Arts.

Nakagawa, Y. (2000). *Education for Awakening: An Eastern Approach to Holistic Education.* Brandon, VT: The Foundation for Educational Renewal.

# CHAPTER 11

# Being What We Are

## Thomas Merton's Spirituality of Education

### Thomas Del Prete

Thomas Merton was a monk from 1941 to 1968 at the Abbey of Gethsemani in Kentucky, a Catholic Christian monastery heir to a contemplative tradition begun in the twelfth century. During that time he was also a teacher, spiritual writer, peace advocate, poet, and literary essayist, a key figure in opening East-West religious dialogue, and extraordinary correspondent and journal writer. In 1965 he began living full-time as a hermit on his monastery's grounds. He published over fifty-five books before his death in 1968; many more, including seven volumes of journals, have been published posthumously.

In a talk that he gave during a rare trip away from his monastery, in 1968, Merton remarks, "My dear brothers, we are already one.... What we have to be is what we are" (Merton, 1975, p. 308). The three parts of this message — understanding what we are, learning to be what we are, and realizing our fundamental unity — aptly frame Merton's spirituality of education.

Merton understood that our real identity is inherent in us, something deeper than what he called the "social" or "illusory" self, something "ultimate and indestructible" yet at the same time dynamic, creatively developed and uniquely expressed in our ordinary selves (Merton, 1963; Merton, 1979, p. 5). To know "what we are," we must come to understand that the source of freedom and meaning in our lives, indeed, life itself is in the very "ground of [our] own being" — "the hidden ground of love" (Merton, 1961, pp. 32-39; 1968a, p.114; 1979, p. 5).

To say that it is inherent does not mean that our true identity is easily realized. Ironically, we have to *be* what we already *are*. That we must learn to do so suggests something of our own blindness and the need for a certain inner capacity and understanding. In Merton's spirituality of education the activation and development of our inner capacity to understand and live fully as our real selves is the central concern.

Finally, though deeply personal, the process of inner transformation that leads to self-discovery is simultaneously a process of discovering our deep relatedness to others. "I must look for my identity, somehow, not only in God but in other[s]," Merton writes (Merton, 1961, p. 51). To be what we are requires that we realize our oneness, our existence in an "original unity" intimated in Eastern as well as Western religion (Merton, 1975, pp. 307-8).

Each of these themes — that our personal identity is embedded dynamically in love in our own being, that discovering ourselves is a process of inner realization that leads us to be what we already are, and that we are most fully ourselves when we live in awareness and response to a hidden relatedness — forms a distinct dimension of Merton's spirituality of education. His spirituality of the person illuminates "what we are." His spirituality of learning and growth suggests what it means to become what we are. His spirituality of relatedness is the basis for understanding what he means when he says, "We are already one."

## WHAT WE ARE: MERTON'S SPIRITUALITY OF THE PERSON

As Merton states it, "The purpose of education is to show a person how to define himself authentically and spontaneously in relation to his world — not to impose a prefabricated definition of the world, still less an arbitrary definition of the individual himself…" (Merton, 1979, pp. 3-4). We cannot live genuinely and truly free, making the choices that freedom affords, learning what we have to offer to the contemporary world and how to make our personal contribution valid, unless we know "who it is that chooses" (Merton, 1979, p.4).

Even as Merton identifies self-discovery as the fundamental purpose of education, however, he wraps the notion of self in irony and paradox. As he puts it, "Learning to be oneself means … learning to die in order to live. It means discovering in the ground of one's being a 'self' which is ultimate and indestructible, which not only survives the destruction of all other more superficial selves but finds its identity affirmed and clarified by their destruction" (Merton, 1979, p. 5).

To discover oneself means seeking "the very self that finds," not, as we are culturally disposed to think, to find something outside ourselves — some marker of identity — that we can name (Merton, 1979, p. 4). For Merton, the "very self that finds" is the indivisible or whole, albeit "inner" self. The whole self cannot define itself; to do so presumes that it can be both whole and regard itself as if there is some other perspective outside the whole — a self-contradiction. Our real identity is beyond "essence" and "beyond all ego … and a consciousness that transcends all division, all separation" (Merton, 1979, p. 9). To discover oneself means breaking through to a new consciousness and realization of our own wholeness.

Merton expresses this idea much differently in his essay, "Day of a Stranger" (Merton, 1981a). More characteristic of his later writing as he sought new ways to communicate to his contemporaries within the Western cultural tradition, and influenced by his study of Eastern religion, he abandons the philosophical language of self and being for a more indirect and ironic style that suggests what we are as persons by challenging our perspective in a way that concepts cannot. He assumes the posture of "stranger" to confound the notion that he can give himself an identity. Thus he writes, "In an age where there is much talk about 'being yourself' I reserve to myself the right to forget about being myself, since in any case there is very little chance of my being anybody else. Rather it seems to me that when one is too intent on 'being himself' he runs the risk of impersonating a shadow" (Merton, 1981a, p. 31). His description of his life as a hermit living in a monastic community also defies the expected response to "what do you do?" — "What I wear is pants. What I do is live. How I pray is breathe" (Merton, 1981a, p. 41). Merton in this instance is not simply confronting social expectation as a declaration of his individuality. He has dissolved the duality of mind and self, or self and image of self in a testimony to his own being. His is a *lived* wholeness. He apprehends his own living wholeness and the importance of safeguarding it in an age habituated to inner division — to a divided consciousness of self. In his journal he writes simply, "It comes close to being real" (Merton, 1997, p. 169).

Merton confounds cultural expectations similarly in response to a request from an author to say how he had become a "success," recording that he replied, "If I had a message to my contemporaries … it was surely this: Be anything you like, be madmen, drunks, and bastards of every shape and form, but at all costs avoid one thing: success" (Merton, 1979, p. 11). He concludes, "... whatever you do, every act, however small, can teach you everything — provided you see *who* it is that is acting" [emphasis mine] (Merton, 1979, p. 14).

In renouncing the underlying cultural presumption of the West that we can create our own ultimate reality, Merton shifts discussion from a social or "prefabricated" and "arbitrary" ground to an inner and existential one. On a certain existential ground, we are defined — or discover ourselves — more "authentically and spontaneously" in relation to the world, not in social terms. Conceptual language cannot communicate adequately what that means.

In terms of the psychological as well as philosophical language that he often uses, Merton is underscoring the difference between what he designates variously as the "external," "divided," "social," "ego," or "false" self and the "true," "real," "authentic," "inmost," or "whole" self (Del Prete, 1990, pp. 34-51; Merton, 1961, 1963, 1968a, 1968d, 1979, 1983). He is confronting likewise the stubborn legacy of the modern, Cartesian worldview in Western culture that builds consciousness and meaning on the basis of inner and outer dualities — the dualities of mind and self, and self and world — and that projects an atomized view of the world, with each thing and person not only distinct, but separate and disconnected (Merton, 1968d, p. 22).

A worldview based on a divided and separate self labors under the illusion that we know ourselves as real from our own individual self-assertions and an affirmation of our own will (Del Prete, 1990, pp. 35-39; Merton, 1968a, pp. 23, 219). We end up seeking who we are outside ourselves in the visible imprints of our thoughts and actions, in the image that we think others want to see, or, drawn by the gravitational pull of commercial culture, in the false sense of reality gained in the pursuit of things as an end in itself. We seek ourselves as an object, a search that is "futile and self-contradictory"(Merton, 1979, p. 4). We lose contact with the integrity of our own inner depths (Merton, 1975, p. 317). In Merton's words, "Modern man believes he is fruitful and productive when his ego is aggressively affirmed, when he is visibly active, and when his action produces obvious results.... Only when our activity proceeds out of the ground in which we have consented to be dissolved does it have the divine fruitfulness of love and grace ... does it really reach others in true communion" (Merton, 1979, p. 23).

A post-modern reaction against the modernist or Cartesian worldview might suggest that our identities are constructed in relation to social and cultural environments, or co-constructed rather than individually determined. "Identity" in this sense is highly contextualized, as well as fluid and situational. It can have a profound impact on our lives, giving us a sense of place and meaning, for better or worse, in relation to others. Merton would not disagree with this conceptualization of how a sense of identity is formed and re-formed. What he would say, however, is that any identity constructed by us or by our social environment, or both, is not our most fundamental and true identity, but a provisional one that makes it more or less possible for us to find ourselves on a deeper level and identify ourselves authentically and spontaneously in relation to the world.

To add a twist of complexity to its paradoxical nature, Merton makes clear that while self-discovery should be the fundamental purpose of education, we cannot discover ourselves wholly on our own. As ultimately the "spark" of "the Absolute recognizing itself in me," our true selves are animated uniquely in each of us through God present in love directly and personally in our own being (Merton, 1961, pp. 39-40; Merton, 1979, p. 10). In the non-metaphysical and non-theological language that he used, particularly in comparative religious discussion, we "find" ourselves when the reality of the love that grounds our existence is realized within us. And what we find is as mysterious as it is utterly transforming; in our ordinary, everyday selves, as he says in one celebrated passage, we "are all walking around shining like the sun" (Merton, 1965c, p. 157).

The dissolution of ego and all false identity in the ground of being and of love is the inner transformation that animates our ordinary lives in love. We wear pants, we live, we breathe; we live our wholeness. In its Christian dimension, as Merton emphasizes, this transformation is fulfilled when we can say with St. Paul, "I live, now not I, but Christ lives in me" (Merton, 1955, p. 15; Merton, 1979, p. 22). Lived wholeness ultimately becomes lived theology — a living experience of Christian truth — in Merton's spirituality of the person (Merton, 1971, p. 198).

During one of the weekly conferences that he gave at Gethsemani Abbey, Merton links Christ with our real identity in an extraordinarily concrete and personal way. His ostensible topic is William Faulkner's "The Bear," but in his introduction he momentarily diverts to a concentrated reflection on becoming oneself (Del Prete, 1999; Merton, 1967). Note that in referring to "Louie" in the passage transcribed below, Merton is using the religious name by which he was known in the monastic community to refer to himself.

> There's only one thing for anybody to become in life — there's no point in becoming spiritual, a waste of time … you've come here [to the monastery] … to become yourself, to discover your complete identity, to be you … not something else other than you. The 'catch' to that of course is that our full identity as monks and as Christians is Christ, but it is Christ in each one of us, see, and the idea is … I have to become me in such a way that I am the Christ who can only be Christ in me. There is a 'Louie-Christ' which has to be brought into existence and hasn't matured yet…. Not just an abstract Christ but the Christ who can only be what he wants to be in us and he can't be in me what he is in anybody else. See, there is a unique realization of Christ which He wants to find in me and in each one of us. (Merton, 1967)

Merton's personalization of the meaning of self-discovery as the realization of Christ uniquely in each of us stands in radical contrast to the prevailing cultural tendency to make of ourselves a "project" or the fulfillment of an image, whether spiritual or otherwise (Merton, 1965d). To become what we are as persons is not only to become our ordinary, whole, real, naked, inmost self, but also and at once our unique "Christ-self" grounded in a hidden wholeness and hidden love, absolute, infinitely enlivening and creative, and all-encompassing.

## BECOMING WHAT WE ARE:
## MERTON'S SPIRITUALITY OF LEARNING

Merton writes that our learning must "dispose" us to the discovery of ourselves on the deepest possible level, and that the various disciplines of study should "provide ways or paths" for developing our capacity to ignite the spark that is "the flash of the Absolute recognizing itself in me" (Merton, 1979, p. 10). How does Merton suggest that we educate so as to activate our capacity to be what we are? Putting aside the question of particular monastic or spiritual practices such as daily prayer and manual work so as to make discussion pertinent to formal education in as broad a sense as possible, the answer is most evident in his spirituality of learning and in his teaching.

*Seeking the Truth*: As the end of education, true personal identity cannot be achieved without the development of some sense of freedom and
the ability to make choices from real possibilities, therefore the capacity
to judge and think (Merton, 1979, p. 3; 1994, p. 169). What this implies in
turn is not the absence of critical thinking and genuine thought, but the
determined application of it in a process of discerning what is real and
true, and a curriculum that will foster that process meaningfully, particularly as a safeguard against the insidious influence of various forms of
propaganda. Merton was grateful for his tutelage under teachers such as
Mark Van Doren from Columbia University precisely because they,
along with different books that he read and personal contacts that he
had, cultivated his sense of what was significant and how to determine it
(Del Prete, 1990, pp. 148-155; Merton, 1948, pp. 139-141).

The lasting impact of Merton's teaching mentors is evident in his own
advice to others as well as his sense of purpose as a teacher. Responding
to a college bookstore manager who asked him about the importance of
reading in college, he wrote, "I might mention … that the quality of the
books one reads and of the thoughts one 'buys' certainly does make a difference. The mere fact that an idea is new and exciting does not necessarily make it true. Truth is important and the whole purpose of thinking is
to be able to tell the difference between what is true and what only looks
good" (Merton, 1994, p. 169). Reflecting on his vocation in his journal, he
mused, "I am a writer, a student and a teacher as well as a contemplative
of sorts.… And the great thing in my life is, or should be, love of truth. I
know there is nothing more precious than the bond of charity created by
communicating and sharing the truth. This is really my whole life" (Merton, 1996b, p. 264).

"Truth" for Merton has several levels of meaning, each an aspect of
"the ultimate, hidden and definitive truth which is believed rather than
known," and each having a distinct epistemological dimension (Merton,
1971, p. 190). The "incarnate" truth is the truth of what we are as persons
(Merton, 1980a, p. 211). Thus Merton writes, "Life is, or should be, nothing but a struggle to seek truth: yet what we seek is really the truth that
we already possess" (Merton, 1965c, p. 184). The living truth that we embody, involving our whole, undivided selves, is known only through
love (Merton, 1985, p. 141). The counterpart to this embodied truth in the
natural world is the knowledge of things as they are. To know things
fully, as they are, we must know them whole, in their dynamic and total
being. In contrast, the "experimental" approach to learning in science

yields only a "provisional" truth (Merton, 1971, pp. 190, 203). The larger "definitive" truth, the reality of God at the center of our being, is the ground of all of the other dimensions of truth (Merton, 1971, p. 190).

The search for our inner truth — our true selves — "involves not only dialectic, but a long labor of acceptance, obedience, liberty and love" (Merton, 1965c, p. 184). The dialectic between opening to and experiencing our deepest reality, which is our true source of freedom, on the one hand, and recognizing the formative influence and limitations of self or socially constructed sources of identity, on the other, is a key process of growth in Merton's spirituality of education.

*An intuitive and interior way of knowing.* To activate and grow in our capacity to know the living dimensions of truth requires practice in an intuitive way of knowing that Merton views as natural, though neglected in Western society, as he explains in one of the weekly conferences that he taught as "Master of Novices" for ten years (Merton, 1988a). He begins by making an important distinction between the roles of reason and experience in arriving at "the natural knowledge of God," emphasizing that reason alone is not sufficient. One must develop first of all an awareness and experience of being. As he explains it, we have to become aware of our own existence, "to the fact that 'I am.'" Furthermore, we have to recognize in the experience of our own being — our own "isness" — the reality of all being. In Merton's words:

> There is this intuition of being, and not only a sense of one's own existence but a sense that everything exists.… The whole thing is … this very strong experience of 'isness' … If you deepen that … all that is, so to speak, becomes completely transparent … and you see … beyond all this being is Infinite Being. And very simply one sees that this Infinite Being is our Father, a person. This kind of realization … should be part of everybody's normal equipment (Merton, 1988a).

In his commentary to the novice monks, it is clear that Merton views an awareness of being, or ontological awareness, as much different from self-awareness. He makes this distinction more explicit elsewhere (Merton, 1968d). The intuition of being is not a self-reflexive act, should not be confused with "the subjective experience of the individual self" (Merton, 1968d, p. 23). To become aware of the reality of our own being, we must transcend, in an intuition of "Being," the consciousness of self as independent subject or object (Merton, 1968d, p. 24). To use nonmetaphysical language, we must intuit our inmost being in the hidden and infinite ground of love. (Merton, 1968d, p. 25)

Merton emphasizes the full scope of what it means to intuit our own being incisively in a passage from his journal that he prepared for publication:

> All being is from God.
>
> This is not simply an arbitrary and tendentious 'religious' affirmation … [it] implies the deepest respect for reality and for the being of everything that is…. [The] *direct intuition of the act of being*…is an act of contemplation and philosophical wisdom rather than the fruit of scientific analysis…. Such an intuition is simply an immediate grasp of one's own inexplicable personal reality in one's own incommunicable act of existing!
>
> One who has experienced the baffling, humbling, and liberating clarity of this immediate sense of what it means to *be* has in that very act experienced something of the presence of God. For God is present to me in the act of my own being…. (Merton, 1965c, pp. 220-221)

Shifting to a more prophetic voice, he adds, "The real root-sin of modern man is that, in ignoring and contemning being, and especially his own *being*, he has made his *existence* a disease and affliction" (Merton, 1965c, p. 221).

In emphasizing the importance of an intuitive way of knowing as the inner path to an awareness and experience of being, Merton is hardly setting up reason as a dangerous foil. As he notes in his conference with the novices, reason, oriented accordingly, can and should support intellectual formation dedicated to discerning what is real and true. An intuitive way of knowing, however, leads to another realm — a realm of inner experience that is beyond the conceptual and analytical, beyond even concepts such as true self and false self that reason, as much as it should try, can at best only allude to. Whereas a Western analytical mode — the modes of Aristotelian or scholastic philosophy, for instance — presumes a distance or capacity to stand apart from what is being considered, to intuit being means to apprehend with one's whole self in a direct, experiential, concrete way (Merton, 1968d, pp. 26-27). An intuitive awareness of being bridges the divide between self and mind, or self and reality, fostered by Western dualistic thinking; one enters into the realm of holistic experience, living truth and wisdom.

Ontological awareness and inner experience are central themes in Merton's spirituality of education. If, as Merton insists, education must dispose us to self-discovery, to the possibility of inner transformation in love, then it must help foster an inner openness, openness first of all to an experience of our own being and the integrity of our inner depths. For Merton that possibility is inherently real — "part of everybody's normal equipment." At the same time he sees much in our culture to confound the effort.

*Interior knowing, being and our cultural selves*: To develop an awareness of being requires a certain degree of openness beyond identity in a social and cultural sense, which in turn implies more than a superficial understanding of how these dimensions of our lives are formed (Merton, 1968b). As Merton writes in "The Need for a New Education," an essay that is addressing monastic practice, but which is rich with insight having broader significance, "Monks are intent on exploring the inner meaning of the Mystery of Christ in the world of our time and this requires some understanding of the world and of themselves as modern people, as well as a realization of and witness to the presence of Christ in the world" (Merton, 1971, p. 198).

Merton tried in various ways through the monastic curriculum to stimulate deep cultural understanding and a dynamic interplay between inner experience (as an experience of being) and culturally constructed modes of thinking and making meaning. In a pattern that became typical toward the end of his decade as Master of Novices in 1965, and afterwards when he gave weekly talks in his community, he drew from his own ever-widening studies to present new perspectives on themes pertinent to the formation of monks as whole persons, yet at first blush far removed from the traditional Trappist monastic curriculum, which focused on Biblical, monastic and Christian spiritual study (Del Prete, 1996). To take one example as representative, consider one of Merton's last conferences as Master of Novices on Bantu philosophy. The Bantu are located in central Africa, in what is now the Congo. The "primitive" Bantu view of the world was relevant precisely because it raised important questions about the presumptions underlying the modern Western worldview. As he explains in introducing the topic, "I am very interested in this whole question of primitive kinds of philosophy, and primitive outlooks on life and being … it's closer to the Bible, for example, than some of the stuff that we have with our post-Cartesian viewpoint" (Merton, 1965a).

Merton contrasts the Western cultural habit of standing back, of analyzing, judging, and categorizing from a distance with the more direct, immediate, and concrete Bantu apprehension of reality. Whereas the Western view of the relationship of self and world presumes the person is set over and against everything else, in a subject-object relationship, the Bantu are "right in the middle of everything." The deeply ingrained Western way of thinking is manifested in language constructions that presume an ability to separate out and make a judgement about what is (Merton uses "This is a quail" as an example). In contrast, the Bantu see themselves as one living force among many. They live with a sense of the world that might be described as inter-subjective, in which they see themselves as a living force seeking a kind of right relationship with other living forces. Their experience of these forces is very concrete (e.g., one's mother and father, whether alive or dead, are a permanent living force). Perceiving themselves as acted upon by other beings as well as acting, they do not exercise judgement with regard to what something is, but instead experience and live in acceptance and response to its active presence. Merton suggests that this way of knowing and experiencing the world has a Biblical analogy, as in Genesis when the well Abraham is digging is "the well of the seeing," Abraham in some very concrete sense being "under the eyes of God." It would be quite different if one were to say, "God is present," and even more abstract to refer to "the Presence of God."

For Merton, the Bantu way of knowing is intuitive, originating in a sense of interiority dulled in Western culture, and resulting in an "intuitive contact with reality" outside the realm of general Western experience. As he emphasizes, "… a very deep sense of interiority … is natural to man, and it's natural to primitive man, and it's natural to people in less civilized cultures than ours, because people in these simple primitive cultures are naturally interior. Our society is such that it has been systematically destroyed by the different modes we have for keeping people outside themselves all the time …the greatest problem, psychologically speaking, of our society is that people are prevented from getting inside…." (Merton, 1965a).

He puts it somewhat differently in another context during a taped conversation, "… one of the reasons why [our society] is sick is that it's completely from the top of the head. It's completely cerebral. It has utterly neglected everything to do with the rest of the human being; the whole person is reduced to a very small part of who and what the person is" (Merton, 1991, p. 48). This is not to say that Merton undervalues the Western mode of thinking — "The fact that we are able to abstract and analyze ... and work things out intellectually has made us free to do all sorts of things with our knowledge" (Merton, 1965a). But he makes clear that understanding the limitations of our own deeply ingrained cultural ways of seeing and experiencing the world is necessary if we are to open inner paths to understanding what we are.

Merton uses alternative cultural perspectives such as Bantu philosophy as pedagogical tools not only to engender deep cultural understanding, but also to foster a way of knowing grounded in experience and intuition. He reminds the novices in his talk on the Bantu that it is our manner of knowing that determines whether we come to experience, "what it means to be called by God and what it means to dwell in a place where God speaks to everybody" (1965a).

*Integrating intellect, study and spiritual life*: If in Merton's spirituality of learning there is an intimate relationship between who we are and how we know, between self-discovery and inner experience, what then is the role of intellect and study? How, in addition, are we to regard the natural as well as human world as subjects for study?

It is helpful to understand how traditional monastic learning was framed in order to understand how intellect and the life of the mind are integrated with intuition and experience in Merton's spirituality of learning. As Merton interprets St. Bernard of Clairvaux, founder of his Cistercian monastic order in the 12th century, "we study in order to love" (Merton, 1980b, p. 127). In the context of traditional monastic life, "study" was virtually synonymous with reading the Bible and the Fathers, or key early leaders, of the Church. The manner and purpose of monastic study differed from scholastic approaches, which emphasized the development of knowledge through the application of a rigorous and impersonal method of investigating a text or issue, with a protocol of posing and solving problems. Monastic education was not first and foremost focused on attaining insight in this speculative and deductive manner; it was more personalistic, concerned not with intellectual understanding (*"scientia"*) so much as experience, not with abstract truth so much as a concrete experience of living truth and wisdom (*"sapientia"*) (Leclercq, 1961, pp. 12-16).

Thus in monastic culture the practice known as "*lectio divina*" developed, during which one reads not simply to be able to say what has been written, but to comprehend the truth on a deep level; that is, to break through to spiritual awareness — to "enter into the wisdom and knowledge of God." Merton phrased it simply in a letter addressing the importance of book reading, "Traditionally, for a monk, reading is inseparable from *meditation*" (Merton, 1994, p. 165). *Lectio divina* leads beyond the "surface of things" to an assimilation of God's word, and a meditation on life and the meaning of our own lives; it leads finally to contemplative prayer. Monastic learning is meant always to be deeply personal, always potentially integrating and transformative, always pointing to the discovery of the "true self" as a matter of inner experience and love.

It is natural to ask whether the traditional orientation of monastic learning to inner experience and its emphasis on more meditative and intuitive modes of knowing is anti-intellectual. Certainly the question of what role the mind plays in monastic study concerned Merton as a young monk and novice monastic teacher. He wrote to Cistercian scholar Jean Leclercq of his interest in understanding St. Bernard's attitude towards learning, clearly seeking affirmation for his view that the pursuit of knowledge and the desire for wisdom were conjoined in Bernard, as a form of assurance that his own intellectual efforts aligned with Cistercian spiritual tradition (Merton, 1990, p. 24). As he clearly came to see, what is critical is a matter of means and ends, of how we use our minds and to what purpose (Merton, 1979, p. 11). The message he gave to his students in a monastic orientation guide is simple: "Our studies should mean something in our own lives." He oriented a young student similarly in a letter, "Do not study merely to pass exams or to please your teachers, but to find truth and to awaken deeper levels of life in yourself…"(Merton, 1989b, p. 335).

St. Bernard in his time, like Merton in his, had a keen awareness of how easy it is to subvert the personalistic end of education. Bernard commented directly on the potential for speculative and abstract knowing, fueled by pride, to become an end in itself — "Science puffeth up" (Merton, 1980b, p.126). We need only to reflect on the haunting record of desensitized doctors working for Nazi purposes in World War II, or on those swept up unthinkingly in the allure of power in the continued development of the technology of nuclear destruction to see the contemporary relevance of St. Bernard's insight (Lifton and Markusen, 1990). So that intellect would be harnessed to wisdom rather than pride, Bernard counseled simplicity in intellectual work, and learning to shed "all that is superfluous, unnecessary, indirect" in coming to know and love God (Merton, 1980b, p. 126).

In his effort to promote a manner of knowing that deepens inner experience and disposes one to become what we are, Merton was a monastic learner and teacher formed in the mold of St. Bernard. This connection is strikingly palpable in one instance of his teaching in which St. Bernard's work itself is the subject. Merton begins by assuring the novices that he does not intend to give a review of Bernard's work — that would be "like school" (Merton, 1988b). Nor is the point simply to decode the meaning of the words of the twelfth century Cistercian founder. He asks his students instead to attend not so much to the words as to their "implications," and to listen in their implications for the "resonances" and "echoes" of genuine inner experience. His pedagogy in this instance reveals his belief that language need not be viewed simply as a medium that encodes cultural meaning; it can also be a medium for expressing, or at least pointing to lived inner experience. Bernard communicated the kind of qualitative experience of reality that is both personal and universal, and that is vitally real and *present* across time. The key to unlocking the door to understanding that experience is to "transpose it into our time and our way of looking at things" (Merton, 1988b). The process of transposition is a central feature of Merton's spirituality of learning and his pedagogy.

To know in the manner that Merton endeavors to foster in his conference on Bernard is both an intellectual and intuitive act. The process of transposition requires an understanding of words as well as an intuitive grasp of their source and meaning in experience. Merton is concerned with developing a personal openness to a qualitative perception of reality, not simply knowing about and explaining in conceptual terms what someone else has experienced.

Merton's treatment of Bernard reflects the importance he places more generally on differentiating between knowledge that opens the possibility for inner experience and ideas divorced from experience. He was intent in his teaching on opening his students to the "echoes" and "resonances" of truth in deep personal experience using resources from the contemplative spiritual tradition such as Bernard's work (Merton, 1971, p. 180). He advises more generally that we learn from books through a certain manner of knowing only when they bring us into "contact with great persons, with [persons] who had more than their own share of humanity ... who were persons for the whole world and not for themselves alone" (Merton, 1956, p. 63).

For Merton, "Ideas and words are not the food of the intelligence, but truth. And not an abstract truth that feeds the mind alone ... [but] something that can be embraced and loved..." (Merton, 1956, p. 63). In keeping with monastic tradition, one must aspire in study to move from intellectual understanding to "sapiential" understanding — "a kind of understanding rooted in love" (Merton, 1971, p. 201). Such "loving knowledge" is a "contemplative knowledge, a fruit of a living and realizing faith ..." (Merton, 1971, p. 161). Karl Rahner, for whom love is the "full flower of knowledge," is illuminating in this regard: "Only the experience of knowledge's blooming into love has any power to work a transformation in me, in my very self" (Rahner, 1984, p. 29).

Merton evokes and enlarges a tradition of learning that seeks to unite knowledge with wisdom, love, and inner transformation. It was imperative for him as a learner and teacher not only to become attentive to the "echoes" and "resonances" of deep human experience and integrity, of living truth, but also to make them transparent and available to the present as seeds for the development of loving knowledge. It was in this way that he strove to make study serve the purpose of awakening deeper levels of life, an integrative, personalistic and "life-giving" approach essential for the formation of the whole person (Merton, 1962).

*Study in the Arts and Humanities*: As consistent with monastic tradition as he was in his sense of purpose as a teacher, and as gifted in fulfilling it, Merton expanded the boundaries of the traditional curriculum to encompass the arts and humanities as well as cultural studies such as the one on the Bantu. As a poet and literary essayist, and the son of a visual artist, he had a keen sense of the possibilities for the arts and humanities to represent deep human experience. Whether through the Bible, literature from Christian or non-Christian spiritual tradition, Aeschylus, Bernard, Blake, Chuang Tzu, Confucianism, Eckhart, Faulkner or others in the humanities, he read and taught from a wide variety of works whose authors "had more than their own share of humanity."

Examples such as his way of introducing St. Bernard abound in his teaching. One series of conferences in the Novitiate, for instance, is united by the theme of "wholeness." Bridging a discussion of Greek tragedy with a study of Chinese thought, he begins what he anticipates to be "a wild conference" (presumably because of the challenge to connect his subject matter with monastic education) by explaining:

> We're working on the wholeness of the development of man. Be-
> hind this whole idea of Greek tragedy is this idea of the wholeness
> of man, and what is in a whole … the idea that you have to make
> something out of your life. You can make a wholeness out of your
> life or not. Then, if this is true, you have to understand the principle
> of life. There is something to discover about life that one needs to
> know … if you find it and put it into practice, then you become a
> whole person. (Merton, 1965b)

Merton introduces the Confucian concept of wholeness as a symbolic
fourfold structure that is expressed variously in poetry, philosophy, lit-
urgy and religion (he mentions as an example the mandala design used
as a symbol of wholeness for the purpose of contemplation in Tibetan
Buddhism). Then he sets up the transposition that makes an understanding of an ancient Chinese philosophical tradition relevant for his monastic students, saying:

> The basic thesis I am working on to make this useful to us is that in
> these pagan philosophies and Chinese philosophies … what you
> have … is not simply a new answer. These are natural adumbra-
> tions … patterns calling for a fulfillment…. We as Christians
> should see not only the fact that this is very interesting and very
> wise … but a deeper link…. The fourfold structure, for example,
> has a fulfillment very obvious and very simple in First Corinthi-
> ans….This Confucian wholeness for us is going to have meaning
> insofar as this is something that is going to be fulfilled perfectly in
> Christ. (Merton, 1965b)

Using a Confucian concept, Merton characterizes the ancient Chinese
wisdom as "human-heartedness" seeking fulfillment. For Merton the
Christian dimension of this wisdom is Christ. Through the redemptive
love of Christ — through the grace of God — human-heartedness becomes divinely fulfilled.

Merton's conference on William Faulkner's "The Bear" stands apart
as an example of his teaching that links a non-sacred text to a theme of
spiritual import (Merton, 1967). Merton considered Faulkner's written
works among those he would call "sapiential" (denoting wisdom), literature characterized by a deep symbolic level of communication "directed … at … man's own understanding of himself" (Merton, 1981b, p.
100). In his journal, Merton describes "The Bear" as "Shattering, cleans-

ing, mind-changing and transforming myth ..."(Merton, 1997, p. 165). It represents the kind of literature that can bring the reader "into living participation with basic and universal human values which words can point to but cannot fully attain" (Merton, 1981b, p. 98).

For Merton, Faulkner's story inscribes a pattern of development towards self-discovery in a deep sense (Del Prete, 1999; Merton, 1981b, p. 106). Ike McCaslin, the protagonist in the story, grows up in the shadow of a bear that is the subject of a ritual hunt. Each successive year that the bear eludes its pursuers increases its mythic stature. One day Ike is led deeply into the forest that is the bear's home, encountering momentary signs of the bear, but not the animal itself. Along the way, Ike loses "his doubt and dread." Merton comments, "This is when you're really grooving in the spiritual life" (Merton, 1967). Ike also lets go of the guise and trappings of a hunter — his compass and watch — traveling on blind faith as it were, and outside the bounds of linear time into a seemingly timeless or eschatological realm. The bear is no longer quarry, in fact leads Ike back to where he has left his compass and watch. It is only at the point where he can regain his bearings — where he returns to himself, as it were — that he catches a glimpse of the bear, in an experience that Merton characterizes as a theophany.

Merton traces the steps that mark Ike's development, commenting:

> The degrees of awareness, the degrees of intimacy with which this man gets to know the bear ... is exactly like ... an ascent to mystical union in the study of [St. Bernard's] Canticle of Canticles ... it is exactly the same kind of pattern, and what that shows is that this ascent to perfect realization is not something purely outside of life that sort of bursts into it, but there is something built into life itself.... (Merton, 1967)

In drawing the analogy between Ike's pattern of development in relation to the bear and our innate capacity to discover who we are, Merton moves from a symbolic literary realm to one that is at once universal and personal. It is in this sense that he exemplifies a sapiential approach to teaching and learning.

Merton's development of the monastic curriculum and the evolution of his teaching practice reflect more than his own expanding intellectual horizons. They signify also the development of his capacity as a teacher to integrate the life of the mind and growth in spiritual awareness. His ability to use diverse sources such as Faulkner and Confucius, as well as the Bantu, to uncover and transpose into "our time and way of looking at things" the human experience of ultimate reality reifies *lectio divina*, more broadly, his spirituality of learning, as a pedagogical practice.

*Science, knowing and reality:* To say, as in Merton's cosmology, that God is intimated in all being "implies the deepest respect for reality and for the being of everything that is" (Merton, 1965c, p. 220). It also means "realizing ourselves as part of nature" (Merton, 1965c, p. 295). What does it mean to "know" the reality of which one is a part? How does one reconcile the seemingly antithetical scientific and intuitive or contemplative ways of knowing the reality of the physical and natural world?

In Merton's spirituality of learning one strives to attain a "qualitative perception of reality ... as a thing shining with the light of God" (Merton, 1965a). The "loving knowledge" that derives from this qualitative perception of reality consists more in a realization of the interconnectedness of the world in "the hidden ground of being" than in understanding, as in a more scientific mode of knowing, its discrete constituent parts and their functions or interrelationships.

Merton distinguished the qualitative and scientific ways of knowing reality in this way in his journal:

> [One] can know all about God's creation by examining its phenomena, by dissecting and experimenting and this is all good. But it is misleading because with this kind of knowledge you *do not really* know the beings you know. You only know about them. That is to say you create for yourself a knowledge based on your observations. What you observe is really as much the product of your knowledge as its cause. You take the thing not as it is but as you want to investigate it....
>
> There is something you cannot know about a wren by cutting it up in a laboratory and which you can only know if it remains fully and completely a wren, itself, and hops on your shoulder if it feels like it....
>
> I want not only to observe but to know living things, and this implies a dimension of primordial familiarity which is simple and primitive and religious and poor. (Merton, 1996a, p. 190)

Merton concludes his epistemological reflection by saying that the reality he needs is "the vestige of God in His creatures ... and in man's history and culture ..." (Merton, 1996a, p. 190).

The contemplative way of knowing results in what Merton calls "direct knowledge" (Merton, 1983, p. 122). In contrast to the scientific way, there is no distinction between means and ends in the contemplative way of knowing. Knowing intuitively, with the totality of one's own being, one instead becomes open and attentive to the "isness" that abounds in the world, to the momentary but concrete and immediate revelations of being that awaken us to our own aliveness.

In differentiating a contemplative way of knowing — knowing something whole, in its whole being as an intimation of the hidden ground of life — from a scientific one, Merton clearly did not set one over the other or discount science. What concerned him was the exclusion of a natural qualitative perception of reality in normal intellectual discourse and the perpetuation of a false separation of self from the world. So in a journal entry that begins with a simple noting of the "isness" of a meadowlark, he writes,

> The meadowlark, feeding and singing. Then the quiet, totally silent, dry, sun-drenched mid-morning of spring, under the climbing sun.... How absolutely central is the truth that we are first of all *part of nature*, though we are a very special part, that which is conscious of God ... it is man's own technocratic and self-centered 'worldliness' which is in reality a falsification and a perversion of natural perspectives, which separates him from the reality of creation.... (Merton, 1965c, p. 294)

It was through an encounter with quantum physics that Merton began to sense the possibility for an epistemological bridge and basis for dialogue between contemplative knowing and scientific knowing. His interest in quantum physics may have been piqued in the early sixties when he read Werner Heisenberg's *Physics and Philosophy*, which he termed "an exciting book" (Merton, 1996b, p. 322). Heisenberg led him to see the profound difference between the understanding of reality posited by quantum physics and the reality suggested by the modern scientific worldview of classical or Newtonian physics. The latter, grounded in a false duality of self and world, with the self as a detached observer, viewed reality as material and infinitely calculable. Quantum physics confounded that view. Matter in its most minute configurations — the sub-atomic world of mesons, neutrons, protons and electrons — defied precise measurement. This elusiveness was not simply the result of complex behavior or for lack of the right measuring tools; it was the very act of trying to measure sub-atomic particles that made them inaccessible. The startling revelation of quantum physics was that we affect what we are trying to observe at the sub-atomic level because we are part of it.

Known as the "Uncertainty Principle," what was discovered about the intimate relationship between knower and known in quantum physics aligned with Merton's intuitive and contemplative insight that we are part of nature. As Merton wrote in response to his reading of Heisenberg, "it leads to a fabulous new concept in nature *with ourselves in the midst of it*, and destroys the simple illusion of ourselves as detached and infallible observers" (Merton, 1996b, pp. 322-23). The implications of quantum physics for human consciousness of reality and how it is known were enormously significant to Merton. They suggested the possibility of dialogue that would bring qualitative and quantitative perceptions of reality into a much more complementary and mutually informing relationship. In Niels Bohr, Merton saw a person with whom that dialogue could be realized.

Bohr was one of those persons whom Merton called a "*sapiente*," one of the "truly wise" who had more than his own share of humanity and acted for the whole world more than for himself (Merton, 1971, p. 203). A key figure in the development of quantum physics and a strong voice in opposition to the unilateral application of that knowledge in the development of an atomic weapon, Bohr became one of Merton's "culture heroes" (Merton, 1997, p. 237). More than most of their contemporaries, men like Bohr "grasped all the consequences of their discoveries in a widely human way. As opposed to this kind of narrow scientism which sees only a short range and purely technical consequence" (Merton, 1997, p. 244). Bohr in particular "had the ability to translate his discoveries into a language relevant to everybody, to all humanity, and to the deepest and most critical problems of man then and there — here and now" (Merton, 1997, p. 244). Like Merton, though from a different intellectual and experiential base, Bohr could say, "We ... are part of Nature" (Moore, 1985, p. 181).

Bohr's effort to make quantum theory and the question of its application for destructive purposes a matter for public discourse during World War II ultimately failed. But in his effort Merton saw the possibility of addressing science and its manifestation in technology from a qualitative perception of reality, from a view of reality in which we are interconnected and integrally a part, thus which we should seek to control advisedly. Though Merton himself was not able to fulfill his sense of the possibility for this kind of dialogue, he saw clearly the potential for intellectual engagement that brings together the limited and provisional truth-seeking of science with the intuitive and experiential wisdom of the contemplative in a consciousness of reality as fundamentally whole rather than divided and atomized. In his words, "The qualitative, experiential, and personal values developed in monastic life should complement the objective, quantitative and experimental discoveries of science and their exploitation by technology and business ..." (Merton, 1971, p. 203).

We can know *about* things, but we also must *know* them — know them whole as something greater than what can be defined in terms of what can be measured, described, and manipulated, and in their mutuality with us as part of nature. Merton would have appreciated no doubt an example of these complementary forms of knowing joined in the work of another Nobel-prize winning scientist, Barbara McClintock. Recognized for her long-term study of the genetics of corn, McClintock said this about her approach: "You have to have a feeling for the organism" (Keller, 1983).

*Responding to love*: Merton reminded his monastic brothers that "Our real journey in life is interior: it is a matter of growth, deepening and of an even greater surrender to the action of love and grace in our hearts" (Merton, 1975, p. 296). In Merton's spirituality, as one attains a sense of being and an interior openness to love, one disengages from a futile drive for self-affirmation and moves towards an awareness of and response to love. True freedom and spontaneity — unlike the illusory forms contrived under false and "prefabricated" definitions of self — consist not in the fulfillment of self-will but in the realization of self in love. One becomes free insofar as one "surrenders to" love.

Our effort to respond to the dynamic of love in our own being is a central process of growth on the interior journey towards becoming what we are, and for Merton a key aspect of prayer (Merton, 1968c). This process of growth is complicated in the context of the social, cultural and political world. For Merton crossing the threshold between a life of self-assertion and one of response to love orients one to a certain way of being in the world. He counseled social activists such as James Forest who sought his guidance in the 1960s not to put their faith in their causes, action and results so much as direct themselves to people and their real needs (Merton, 1985, pp. 294-297). As he points out in a teaching conference, "God does not ask for great results from us, he asks for love from us

..." (1968c). Likewise, he saw as the purpose of nonviolence to "awaken [mutual] response" to truth, not to control (Merton, 1968a, p. 28). When action and the desire for results supplant a process of awakening and responding to the "incarnate" or living truths involved in social life, they degenerate into a "false drive for self-affirmation." The ever-present challenge is to learn to live by ever-present love (Merton, 1975, p. 333).

## WE ARE ALREADY ONE: MERTON'S SPIRITUALITY OF RELATEDNESS

The dynamic of becoming what we are has, then, several dimensions in Merton's spirituality of education. The dynamic of inner growth is a movement from a false or illusory individuality or "I" to a more authentic personal identity that is ultimately Christ realized uniquely within or one's "Christ-self." That overall development is stimulated in a dialectic involving an intuition of being and inner experience on the one hand, and an effort to understand our cultural consciousness and identity on the other. It likewise involves an increasing openness and response to the love that is the living truth of our being. Indeed, for Merton inner openness and response is vital for true prayer (Merton, 1968c).

In terms of intellectual life, one should study not "merely to pass exams and please your teachers, but to find truth and to awaken deeper levels of life in yourself" (Merton, 1989b, p. 335). Driven by this purpose, study for Merton involves in part delving beyond words to an understanding of the concrete and qualitative experience of life reflected in spiritual literature and the arts and humanities, a "sapiential" approach to teaching and learning. There is in this respect a dialectical movement between abstract knowledge and "loving knowledge," between knowing about things and people and having a direct, concrete knowledge rooted in love. In keeping with the monastic tradition of learning, for Merton love is the ultimate knowledge. It is through this "loving knowledge," which we come to know only in our totality as persons, that wisdom grows.

In intellectual endeavor, it is also critical to negotiate the difference between "quantitative" and "qualitative" perceptions of reality. The difference between learning as if the world and people are independent of one another, and with the consciousness of relatedness and being part of nature that Merton shared with the scientist Niels Bohr, among others, is profound, comparable to the difference between Merton's view of the partial or masked self and the whole self.

Beyond all of these dimensions of becoming what we are, the dynamic between self and other, between the illusion of individual separateness and the reality of spiritual relatedness, is a central theme. In his introduction to *No Man is an Island*, Merton writes that we cannot find ourselves in ourselves alone but only in and through others (1955, p. 14). Part of the paradox and mystery of self-discovery is that it entails other-discovery, or in the Christian formulation of St. Paul, as Merton emphasizes, realizing that " 'we are all members one of another'" (Merton, 1955, p. 14).

The mystery of self-discovery can be framed just as readily in nonmetaphysical and non-Christian terms in Merton's spirituality as the inner dynamic of love. The unique personal love that enables Merton to refer to himself as the "Louie-Christ" that has yet to mature is at once a universal love. As he writes, "The person is one in the unity of love" (Merton, 1979, p. 17). Having understood that, one realizes with Merton that "There are no strangers!" (Merton, 1965c, p. 158).

The false duality of self and other, reinforced in various ways by the discourse of individuality in our society, has a parallel inner division. As Merton contends, "[It is] the precise nature of our society ... to bring about ... division ... [and] alienation" from the love that is "the ground of all" (Merton, 1979, p. 17). To develop from a divided to a more integrated self, from a consciousness of separateness to one of relatedness, requires resolving the duality in the paradox and mystery of love. One must surrender to the inner dynamic of love that leads to an awareness of relatedness and to a realization that as persons we are "at one with everything in that *hidden ground of love* for which there can be no explanations" (Merton, 1985, p. 115).

Building our capacity for this depth and quality of personal experience, Merton's spirituality of learning enlarges as well the capacity for relatedness, but relatedness in a different sense than the kind of virtue promoted today by some forms of "character education." As he explains in one of his teaching conferences, it is more important as a person to become "related" than virtuous, and that means learning to "identify completely" with and value another as a person (Merton, 1966). In Merton's spirituality of education, relatedness is not only a key part of the dynamic of inner integration, it leads to a greater capacity to love and serve — "The identity of the person is fully realized only in a conscious and mature collaboration with others" (Merton, 1971, p. 76).

For Merton, our experience of and capacity for relatedness grow directly out of our recognition of what we are as persons. Merton expresses this idea in his introduction to the Japanese edition of *The Seven Storey Mountain*, both directly in his message and, important to note, indirectly in its language and form.

> ... if the Truth is to make me free, I must also let go my hold upon myself, and not retain the semblance of a self which is an object or a 'thing.' I too must be no-thing. And when I am no-thing, I am in the All, and Christ lives in me. But He who lives in me is in all those around me.

> ... My monastery is ... a place in which I disappear from the world as an object of interest in order to be everywhere in it by hiddenness and compassion. To exist everywhere I have to be No-one." (Merton, 1989a, pp. 64-65)

As "an object of interest," whether to himself or others, he is living in a false world of separateness; as a person he is connected to others through the hidden love that "is in all those around me" and must respond; response is inherent in love.

The passage illustrates as well his effort to communicate in a language and form that reaches across cultural boundaries. By blending expressions such as "no-thing" and "No-one" into his explanation of the paradox of losing oneself as an object in order to find oneself as a person, he acknowledges the influence of Zen Buddhism in Japanese culture, in particular the use of negation to point to a reality that cannot be captured directly and conceptually (Merton, 1968d, p. 10). In characterizing personal growth in terms of being present in the world through compassion he is no doubt trying consciously to connect to the Buddhist foundation of the culture as well. This represents a kind of cross-cultural and cross-religious communication that Merton strove to practice (Merton, 1971, pp. 199-200; 1975, pp. 314-317).

The capacity for relatedness and corresponding capacity for dialogue based on "spiritual communication" were intimately connected for Merton (Merton, 1971, pp. 307-308; pp. 314-315). Merton thus spoke of the necessity for "mutual understanding and spiritual communication between the North and the South [hemispheres]" (Merton, 1993, p. 233). After meeting Thich Nhat Hanh, a Vietnamese Buddhist monk he declared, "Nhat Hanh Is My Brother" (Merton, 1980a, pp. 263-264). Nhat

Hanh participated in a nonpolitical, person-oriented effort to understand conflict in his country during the war-torn 1960s, personifying for Merton how communication embedded in a deep experience of relatedness could make a difference in the well-being and wisdom of the world. For Merton, our development as whole persons and a deep understanding of the personal and universal in our human identity go hand in hand, leading ultimately to a "transcultural integration" or "universal consciousness" that is eschatological, in Christian terms "a rebirth into the transformed and redeemed time" (Merton, 1971, p. 216; 1975, p. 317; 1991, p. 69).

The dimensions and patterns of learning and growth implied in Merton's spirituality of education are unmistakable in his own life. He writes not only in a seemingly counter-cultural mode as a "stranger" who "wears pants" and avoids "success," but as a person who is fully alive in proportion as he is in solidarity with all others. For Merton, response to the reality of our spiritual unity took many forms: the exercise of his intellectual gifts as a teacher to open paths of inner growth for others or to protest the various degradations of humanity in his time; the conscious effort to develop a capacity for dialogue and transposition across religious traditions or cultural and historical experience, with the language of poetry or inner experience as the medium of communication; letters empathizing with others' struggles for authentic identity, communicated in a way that was accessible to them.

Merton embodies as learner and teacher a spirituality of education that engages us in finding ourselves on the deepest possible level so that we might become uniquely what we already are, and thus actualize in an authentic freedom our personal capacity to contribute to the world and to make our personal offering valid in and through the love that unites us all.

### REFERENCES

Del Prete, T. (1990). *Thomas Merton and the Education of the Whole Person*. Birmingham, AL: Religious Education Press.

Del Prete, T. (1996). Culture and the formation of personal identity: Dilemma and dialectic in Thomas Merton's teaching. In M. Downey (Ed.) *The Merton Annual*, Vol. 8. (pp. 105-121). Collegeville, MN: Liturgical Press.

Del Prete, T. (1999). Geography of nowhere: Living beyond boundaries. *The Merton Seasonal*, 24 (3), 3-8.

Keller, E. F. (1983). *A Feeling for the Organism: The Life and Work of Barbara McClintock*. San Francisco: W. H. Freeman.

Leclercq, J. (1961). *The Love of Learning and the Desire for God: A Study of Monastic Culture* (C. Misraki, Trans.). New York: Mentor Omega Books.

Lifton, R.J., & Markusen, E. (1990). *The Genocidal Mentality: Nazi Holocaust and Nuclear Threat*. New York: Basic Books.

Merton, T. (1948). *The Seven Storey Mountain*. New York: Harcourt Brace Jovanovich.

Merton, T. (1955). *No Man is an Island*. New York: Harcourt Brace Jovanovich.

Merton, T. (1955) *Lectio Divina*. Monastic orientation notes. Louisville, KY: Thomas Merton Center, Bellarmine College.

Merton, T. (1956). *Thoughts in Solitude*. New York: Farrar, Straus & Giroux.

Merton, T. (1960). *Our Monastic Observances*. Louisville, KY: Thomas Merton Center, Bellarmine College.

Merton, T. (1961). *New Seeds of Contemplation*. New York: New Directions.

Merton, T. (1962). *Liberal Arts — Good or Bad?* (Tape No. 43). Louisville, KY: Thomas Merton Center, Bellarmine College.

Merton, T. (1963). *Love and False Self in St. Paul* (Tape No. 85). Louisville, KY: Thomas Merton Center, Bellarmine College.

Merton, T. (1965a). *Bantu Philosophy* (Tape No. 220). Louisville, KY: Thomas Merton Center, Bellarmine College.

Merton, T. (1965b). *Chinese Thought* (Tape No. 216A). Louisville, KY: Thomas Merton Center, Bellarmine College.

Merton, T. (1965c). *Conjectures of a Guilty Bystander*. Garden City, NY: Image Books.

Merton, T. (1965d). *Freedom and Spontaneity* (Tape No. 230B). Louisville, KY: Thomas Merton Center, Bellarmine College.

Merton, T. (1966). *Christian Hope and Relatedness* (Tape No. 243B). Louisville, KY: Thomas Merton Center, Bellarmine College.

Merton, T. (1967). *The Bear* (Tape No. AA2079). Kansas City, MO: Credence Cassettes.

Merton, T. (1968a). *Faith and Violence*. Notre Dame, IN: University of Notre Dame Press.

Merton, T. (1968b). *Monastic Education* (Tape No. 306). Louisville, KY: Thomas Merton Center, Bellarmine College.

Merton, T. (1968c). *Sanctity* (Tape No. A3050). Kansas City, MO: Credence Cassettes.

Merton, T. (1968d). *Zen and the Birds of Appetite*. New York: New Directions.

Merton, T. (1971). *Contemplation in a World of Action* (N. Burton, Ed.). Garden City, NY: Doubleday & Company.

Merton, T. (1975). *The Asian Journal* (N. Burton, P. Hart, & J. Laughlin, Eds.). New York: New Directions.

Merton, T. (1979). *Love and Living*. (N. Burton & P. Hart, Eds.). New York: Harcourt Brace & Company.

Merton, T. (1980a). *The Nonviolent Alternative* (G. Zahn, Ed.). New York: Farrar, Straus & Giroux.

Merton, T. (1980b). *Thomas Merton on St. Bernard* (P. Hart, Ed.). Kalamazoo, MI: Cistercian Publications.

Merton, T. (1981a). *The Day of a Stranger* (R. Daggy, Ed.). Salt Lake City, UT: Gibbs M. Smith, Inc.

Merton, T. (1981b). *The Literary Essays of Thomas Merton* (P. Hart, Ed.). New York: New Directions.

Merton, T. (1983). The inner experience: Society and the inner self. *Cistercian Studies*, 13 (2), 121-134.

Merton, T. (1985). *The Hidden Ground of Love: The Letters of Thomas Merton on Religious Experience and Social Concerns* (W. Shannon, Ed.). New York: Farrar, Straus & Giroux.

Merton, T. (1988a). *Community and the Christian Life* (Tape No. AA2456). Kansas City, MO: Credence Cassettes.

Merton, T. (1988b). *Love Casts Out Fear* (Tape No. AA2134). Kansas City, MO: Credence Cassettes.

Merton, T. (1988c). *Prayer and the Active Life* (Tape No. A2120). Kansas City, MO: Credence Cassettes.

Merton, T. (1989a). *'Honorable Reader': Reflections on my Work* (R. Daggy, Ed.). New York: Crossroad Publishing Company.

Merton, T. (1989b). *The Road to Joy: The Letters of Thomas Merton to New and Old Friends* (R. Daggy, Ed.). New York: Farrar, Straus & Giroux.

Merton, T. (1990). *The School of Charity: Letters on Religious Renewal and Spiritual Direction* (P. Hart, Ed.). New York: Harcourt Brace Jovanovich.

Merton, T. (1991). *Preview of the Asian Journey* (W. Capps, Ed.). New York: The Crossroad Publishing Company.

Merton, T. (1993). *The Courage for Truth: Letters to Writers* (C. Bochen, Ed.). New York: Harcourt Brace & Company.

Merton, T. (1994). *Witness to Freedom: Letters in Times of Crisis* (W. Shannon, Ed.). New York: Farrar, Straus & Giroux.

Merton, T. (1996a). *A Search for Solitude: Journals*, Vol. 3: 1952-1960 (L. Cunningham, Ed.). San Francisco: HarperSanFrancisco.

Merton, T. (1996b). *Turning Toward the World: Journals*, Vol. 4: 1960-1963 (V. Kramer, Ed.) San Francisco: HarperSanFrancisco.

Merton, T. (1997). *Learning to Love: Journals*, Vol. 6: 1966-1967 (C. Bochen, Ed.). San Francisco: HarperSanFrancisco.

Moore, R. (1985). *Niels Bohr: The Man, His Science, and the World They Changed*. Cambridge, MA: MIT Press.

Rahner, K. (1984). *Encounters with Silence* (J. Demske, Trans.). Westminster, MD: Christian Classics.

## NOTE

This chapter has been published in *Catholic Education: A Journal of Inquiry and Practice*, Vol. 5, No. 2, December 2001, 157-180.

# CHAPTER 12

# Emerson, Thoreau, And Alcott

## Prophets for Holistic Learning

### John (Jack) P. Miller

Ralph Waldo Emerson, Henry David Thoreau, and Bronson Allcott were associated with the transcendentalist movement in 19th century America. Transcendentalism was not really a movement in the true sense of the term. Perhaps the only idea that linked people to this term was the belief that our best moments come when we listen to our consciences or the "still small voice" within rather than following the expectations of society. Other individuals associated with transcendentalism include Margaret Fuller and Walt Whitman.

Emerson and Henry Thoreau are among the most important writers in American letters. Bronson Alcott was a close friend to both of these men when they all lived in Concord and Alcott was the most interested in education. However, both Thoreau and Emerson were teachers and wrote about education. In this chapter I will explore the ideas of these three men and how their ideas are antecedents to holistic education.

#### EMERSON

Emerson was born in 1803 in Boston. His father, a minister, died when Emerson was eight. His mother managed to support the family so that Emerson and his brothers could go to school. Emerson studied at Harvard, and he too became a minister. He married shortly after beginning his Unitarian ministry, but his first wife died of tuberculosis less than 18 months later. He suffered many personal tragedies in his life including the death of his son but he did not alter his optimistic approach to life.

After the death of his first wife, Emerson resigned from his ministerial post in Boston. He felt that he could no longer conduct some of the rituals which he felt come in the way of religious and spiritual experience. He wrote once that "I like the silent church before the service begins, better than any preaching."

He then began a career as a writer and lecturer and earned his living through the lectures he gave all over the U.S. Although not a dynamic speaker, he spoke with such sincerity that James Russell Lowell wrote "I have heard some great speakers and some accomplished orators, but never any that so moved and persuaded me as he" (cited in McAleer, 1984, p. 493).

One lecture that stands out was one given at Harvard Divinity School in 1838. After this address it was to be 30 years before he was invited back to Harvard. McAleer (1984) summarizes the address:

> In strictly theological terms, the basic message of the Divinity ad-
> dress was that man by responding intuitively through nature to the
> moral sentiment expresses his divinity. Christ taught that "God in-
> carnates himself in man." Christian leaders have failed their
> fellowman because they have neglected to explore "the Moral Na-
> ture ... as the fountain of the established teaching in society." They
> have fossilized Christianity by putting too much emphasis on for-
> mal ritual. True faith is attained only when a man experiences a
> personal awareness of the Supreme Spirit dwelling within him. (p.
> 249)

Emerson was a reluctant activist. He did speak out against slavery, supported women's rights and opposed the expulsion of the Cherokee Indians from Georgia.

With regard to education Emerson taught school as young man. Howard Mumford Jones (1966) recounts his history as a teacher: "In 1821 he assisted his brother William in a girls' school in Roxbury, Massachu-setts, where he was shy and awkward but managed to impress. In 1825 he taught at Chelmsford, in 1826 again at Roxbury and a little later Cam-bridge." (p. 3)

A resident of Concord most of his life, he was virtually a permanent member of the local school committee. Emerson was deeply loved by people in his community. When his house burned down members of the community helped rebuild his home while he was away in Europe. He died in 1882.

His view of education was closely connected to his overall philosophy which was holistic in nature. Emerson (1990) wrote: "Nothing is quite beautiful alone, nothing but is beautiful in the whole. A single object is only so far beautiful as it suggests this universal grace" (p. 26). Emerson saw elements in relation to one another almost in a holographic sense. He wrote: "Each particle is a microcosm, and faithfully renders the likeness of the world ... so intimate is this unity that it is easily seen, it lies under the undermost garment of Nature and betrays its source in Universal Spirit" (1990, p. 37).

Emerson rejected atomistic and fragmented approaches. He felt that people were struggling with the problem of fragmentation when he wrote: "The reason the world lacks unity, and lies broken and in heaps, is because man is disunited with himself" (1990, p. 54). To address this problem Emerson wrote that the individual "should be instructed that the inward is more valuable than their outward estate"(p. 60). He also wrote: "In yourself is the law of all nature" (p. 99). Emerson here is in the tradition of the great mystics and of the other transcendentalists. Education for Emerson then should nurture and awaken students to this law within.

With the emphasis now on testing in our schools we can imagine Emerson would not be pleased with current educational priorities. Instead, Emerson called for schools and colleges to fire the imagination of the young. He wrote: "Colleges can only highly serve us when they aim not to drill but to create; when they gather from every ray of various genius to their hospitable halls, and by the concentrated fires set the hearts of their youth on flame" (1990, p. 88).

By setting the "hearts of their youth on flame" students will discover their destinies. Emerson believed that "Each man has his own calling.... There is one direction to every man in which unlimited space is open to him ... on that side all obstruction is taken away (p. 73). Education then should help each person find their own destiny or calling. How different this is from the career education that we hear about today where people must find a job to compete in the global economy.

Emerson's view of education is that it should nurture soul. The individual for Emerson is a reflection of that universal spirit, or Oversoul. Education then should allow for contemplation where the soul can witness from a more inclusive perspective.

We live on different planes or platforms. There is an external life, which is educated at school, taught to read, write, cipher and trade; taught to grasp all the boy can get, urging him to put himself forward, to make himself useful and agreeable in the world, to ride, run, argue and contend, unfold his talents, shine, conquer and possess.

But the inner life sits at home, and does not learn to do things nor values these feats at all. 'Tis quiet, wise perception. It loves truth, because it is itself real; it loves right, it knows nothing else; but it makes no progress; was as wise in our first memory of it as now; is just the same now in maturity and hereafter in age, as it was in youth. We have grown to manhood and womanhood; we have powers, connection, children, reputations, professions: this makes no account of them all. It lives in the great present; it makes the present great. This tranquil, well founded, wide-seeing soul is no express-rider, no attorney, no magistrate: it lies in the sun and broods on the world. (Cited in Geldard, p. 172)

Education then should provide opportunities for contemplation. In other contexts I have argued for a curriculum for the inner life which nurtures contemplation (Miller, 2000). Activities might include journal writing, autobiography, visualization, dreamwork and meditation.

Emerson saw learning in a holistic manner. He wrote once: "A painter told me that nobody could draw a tree without in some sort becoming a tree"(1990, p. 134). This sentence reminds me of Walt Whitman's view of learning that he expressed in one of his poems:

There was a child went forth every day,
And the first object he look'd upon, that object he became,
And that object became part of him for the da
  or certain part of the day,
Or for many years or stretching cycles of years
                (cited in Goleman et al., 1992)

Whitman then goes on to describe all the things in nature and life that the child encounters that become part of his or her being. In holistic learning all that we study or encounter becomes part of our being and not some piece of information which is quickly forgotten after the test. Learning is deeply integrated.

More important than any technique is the teacher's awareness of non-verbal communication. Emerson wrote: "The action of the soul is oftener in that which is felt and left unsaid than that which is said in conversation"(1990, p. 178). The teacher needs to be aware of his or her tone of voice and all the non-verbal messages that he or she sends to others. The presence of the teacher is central to Emerson's vision of education. He wrote: "The infallible index of true progress is the tone the man takes.... That which we are, we shall teach" (1990, p. 182). More specifically he encouraged the teacher in this way:

> By simple living, by an illimitable soul, you inspire, you correct, you instruct, you raise, you embellish all. By your own act you teach the beholder how to do the practicable. According to the depth from which you draw your life not only of your strenuous effort but of your manners and presence. (1966, p. 227)

How can the teacher seek such depth and presence? Again contemplative living is the principal means. This means living more in the present and also living and teaching more spontaneously. Emerson stated: "For practical success, there must not be too much design.... All good conversation, manners and action, come from a spontaneity which forgets usages and makes the moment great. Nature hates calculators, her methods are saltatory and impulsive" (pp. 237-8).

Emerson's ideas are close to the notion of the "teachable moment" where the teacher leaves the lesson plan and follows his or her intuition. I believe the Emersonian teacher has a plan but it is flexible and open. Teachers should be open with their own feelings. Emerson (1990) once wrote in reference to a preacher but I think it also applies to the teacher: "The preacher had lived in vain. He had not one word intimating that he had laughed or wept, was married or in love, had been commended, or cheated or chagrined. If he had ever lived and acted we were none the wiser for it" (p. 116).

At times teachers should not be afraid to reveal part of themselves and say something about their passions and interests. This allows the student to see the teacher as a human being and not just in the role of teacher.

## THOREAU

Emerson was both mentor and friend to Thoreau although their relationship cooled somewhat over the years. In conventional terms Thoreau's life can be viewed as a failure since he held no job and unlike Emerson his writing was not well known during his lifetime. After his death, however, he has become a central figure in American letters and social history because of *Walden* and his non-violent philosophy which influenced Tolstoy, Gandhi, and Martin Luther King.

Thoreau lived from 1817 to 1862 in Concord, Mass. He studied and graduated from Harvard in 1837. He said of his Harvard education that he was taught all the branches of learning but none of the roots. He taught school briefly during his student days and he took a teaching job in Concord after his graduation at a college preparatory school. Very early in his tenure there one of his supervisors requested that Thoreau use corporal punishment on the students since he felt that the students were too noisy. Thoreau then applied the cane to six students the next day. He was so upset by what he did that he resigned that evening.

Not deterred by this experience Thoreau started his own school in 1838. The school, the Concord Academy, had only four students but he was able to continue for a year so that there were enough students to continue and to hire his brother, John, to help teach the additional students who had enrolled. The school was traditional in many ways as the students studied academic subjects both in the morning and afternoon. However, a significant feature of the school was the field activities. Sanborn describes one of these activities in his early biography of Thoreau.

> Henry Thoreau called attention to a spot on the rivershore, where he fancied the Indians had made their fires, and perhaps had a fishing village.... "Do you see," said Henry, "anything here that would be likely to attract Indians to this spot?" One body said, "Why, here is the river for their fishing"; another pointed to the woodland near by, which could give them game. "Well, is there anything else?" pointing out a small rivulet that must come, he said, from a spring not far off, which could furnish water cooler than the river in the summer; and a hillside above it that would keep off the north and northwest wind in winter. Then, moving inland a little farther, and looking carefully about, he struck his spade several times, without result. Presently, when the boys began to think their young teacher and guide was mistaken, his spade struck a stone. Moving forward a foot or two, he set his space in again, stuck another stone, and began to dig in a circle. He soon uncovered the red, fire-marked stones of the long-disused Indian fireplace; thus proving that he had been right in his conjecture. Having settled the point, he care-

fully covered up his find and replaced the turf, -not wishing to have the domestic altar of the aborigines profaned by mere curiosity. (1917, p. 205-6)

Thoreau was able to use these field experiences to foster inquiry and observation. "Wisdom," he wrote, "does not inspect, but behold" (cited in Bickman, 1999, p. 60). He felt that by observing things close at hand we can gain the greatest understanding. Thoreau wrote: "I wish so to live ever as to derive my satisfactions and inspirations from the commonest events, every-day phenomena, so that what my senses perceive, my daily walk, the conversation of my neighbors, may inspire me, and I may dream of no heaven but that which lies about me" (in Bickman, 1999, p. 42). His descriptions of his experiences at Walden are evidence of his ability to draw so much from his daily observations. Thoreau felt that the "roots of letters are things" and "natural objects and phenomena." Language then is rooted in our experience with the natural world.

Thoreau believed in the value of direct experience. He once wrote in his journal: "We reason from our hands to our head." He also felt that learning should be embodied and not confined to the head: "A man thinks as well through his legs and arms as his brain. We exaggerate the importance and exclusiveness of the headquarters" (*Journal* XIII:69-70).

Thoreau felt that writing and speaking should flow naturally and not be overly encumbered by concern for grammar:

... the first requisite and rule is that expression shall be vital and natural.... Essentially your truest poetic sentence is as free and lawless as a lamb's bleat. The grammarian is often one who can neither cry or laugh, yet thinks that he can express human emotions. (*Journal* XI: 386)

The field studies example cited above also demonstrates how Thoreau saw the role of teacher as guide and mutual inquirer. He said that he felt that "We should seek to be fellow students with the pupil, and should learn of, as well as with him, if we would be most helpful to him." Thoreau was an advocate of continuous learning and adult education. This continuous learning was not a search for information but a deep connection to the cosmos. He wrote:

My desire for knowledge is intermittent but my desire to commune with the spirit of the universe — to be intoxicated even with the fumes, call it, of that divine nectar — to bear my head

through atmospheres and over heights unknown to my feet-is perennial & constant. (*Journal*, 3:185)

Thoreau was a man who grounded his thinking in experience with the
natural world but like Emerson and Alcott he was drawn to a higher vision.

## BRONSON ALCOTT

Alcott (1799-1888), a friend of both Emerson and Thoreau, devoted
much of his life to education. The father of the writer Louisa May Alcott,
he struggled throughout his life to support his family. Emerson frequently came to his aid. In the 1840's Alcott helped found two cooperative communities — Brook Farm and Fruitlands. Fruitlands was a
vegetarian community where the members even avoided wearing
leather shoes. This community barely lasted a year and could not make it
through the winter of 1844.

Alcott believed in the preexistence of the soul. He thus saw children as
coming into the world not as *tabula rasas* but as charged with a divine
mission. He wrote a manuscript entitled *Observations on the Spiritual
Nurture of My Children* based on the idea that each child has a soul which
needs to nurtured and developed. He observed his children and their behavior and then speculated on the reasons for their behavior. For example he wrote: "Anna is apt to *theorize* both for herself and Louisa; whereas
Louisa, intent solely on *practice*, is constantly demolishing Anna's ideal
castles and irritating her Spirit with Gothic rudeness. The one builds; the
other demolishes; and between the struggle of contrary forces, their tran-
quillity is disturbed …" (cited in Bedell, p. 83).

While Alcott lived in Philadelphia, he taught at the School of Human
Culture where he tried to nurture the spiritual development of the children. Although short lived, letters and documents from the school inspired Alcott's friend Elizabeth Peabody to help him start a new school
in Boston in 1834. Named the Temple School, it has its place in the history
of holistic education. Martin Bickman (1999) has written about the
school: "The education was what we would now call "holistic," since
skills like spelling, grammar, and vocabulary were integrated into larger
lessons on ethical and spiritual matters" (p. xxiii).

It was called the Temple School because it was housed in the two
rooms at the top of the Masonic Temple directly across from the Boston
Commons. Elizabeth Peabody was instrumental to the work of the
school. She helped recruit students, taught there, and also recorded

many of the "conversations" that Alcott held with the students. The school opened in September, 1834 and eighteen students were there the first day. The students were between the ages of 5 and 10 and came from some of the most famous families in Boston.

Alcott taught them both reading and writing simultaneously. He had them print the letters first before writing script "understanding — as no one had before him — that coordination between hand and eye in writing script was too difficult for young children to master" (Bedell, p. 94). In writing he wanted the students to express their thoughts and feelings and not just copy something from a book. In discussions Alcott also encouraged the students to stand up and speak out. One student stated "I never knew I had a mind till I came to this school" (Bedell, p. 96). Alcott did not use corporal punishment, a common practice at that time.

By the winter the enrollment had doubled. Elizabeth Peabody, who had first contracted to work just two hours a day now stayed for the entire school day and began keeping her record of the school. According to Bedell, "*The Record of a School* remains today probably the best exploration of Bronson Alcott's theories on education"(p. 102). Published in 1835 the book was part of larger movement of social change that included women's rights and antislavery activities. Bedell suggests that *Record of a School* became a "symbol of a whole new era in American thought" (p. 103). Alcott himself had never been happier or felt more fulfilled. He wrote that he had found "a unity and a fullness" in his existence.

The most unusual feature of the school was the series of conversations that Bronson held with students regarding spiritual matters. For example:

> MR. ALCOTT. *Now, does our spirit differ in any sense from God's spirit? Each may answer.*
>
> CHARLES. *(10-12 years old). God made our spirits.*
>
> MR. ALCOTT. *They differ from His then in being derived?*
>
> GEORGE K. *(7-10). They are not so good.*
>
> WILLIAM B. *(10-12). They have not so much power.*
>
> AUGUSTINE. *(7-10). I don't think our spirit does differ much.*
>
> CHARLES. *God is spirit, we are spirit and body.*
>
> JOSIAH. *(5 years old). He differs from us, as a king's body differs from ours. A king's body is arrayed with more goodness than ours.*
>
> EDWARD B. *(10-12). God's spirit is a million times larger than ours, and we come out of him as the drops of the ocean.*
>
> (Cited in Howell, p. xiii)

Another book entitled *Conversations with Children on the Gospels* was published in 1836. This book received very negative reviews. One writer called Alcott "either insane or half-witted" while preachers felt that the conversations showed no respect for Christ's divinity. These attacks and debts during an economic recession led to the closing of the school.

Later in his career Emerson helped get Alcott hired as superintendent for the Concord Schools. One of the projects he tried to undertake was to have Thoreau write a text on Concord's local history and geography. However, Thoreau died before the project could be completed.

## CONCLUSIONS

Alcott, Emerson, and Thoreau can be viewed as helping provide some of the foundations for holistic education today. Some of the key contributions include:

1. These thinkers developed the idea that within each person is a soul which needs to be respected and nurtured by the teacher and the educational environment. I believe that all three would echo Peabody's idea that "Education depends on its attitude toward soul." Emerson also wrote that "The one thing of value in the universe is the active soul" (1990, p. 10). Alcott in his teaching practiced this in his conservations which tried to draw forth the child's intuitive understandings.

2. All three individuals emphasized that the teacher should respect the child. Unlike many educators of the time who focused on controlling children, these three thinkers advised teachers to respect the intuitive wisdom of children. Emerson wrote of children: "They know truth from counterfeit as quick as the chemist does. They detect weakness in your eye and behavior a week before you open your mouth, have given you benefit of their opinion as quick as a wink" (1966, p. 214). Alcott's conversations with children were based on the assumption that within children was an innate wisdom that can be drawn out.

3. Another important principle was that experience was central to learning. Thoreau's field trips and again Alcott's conversations were based on this principle. Experience allows the learning to be integrated rather than just being transmission of information.

4 The teacher should work from his or her spiritual center. This is essential for contacting the intuitive wisdom of children. Alice Howell (1991) in commenting on Alcott's teaching states:

Alcott's secret, and I believe, his success consisted in his approach to children; he worked from his innermost center toward the same one he knew existed in each of them. A bond of trust, mutual respect, and affection was established at that level, so that the usual ego-to-ego tussle between teacher and student was avoided. (p. xxxii)

The vision offered by Alcott, Emerson, and Thoreau is an inspiring one and can also be seen as deeply holistic. Sometimes holistic educators are identified as "new age" with no roots in the past. The work of these three transcendentalists strongly counters that notion.

## REFERENCES

Bickman, M. (Ed.) (1999). *Uncommon Learning: Henry David Thoreau on Education.* Boston: Houghton Mifflin.

Bedell, M. (1980). *The Alcotts: Biography of a Family.* New York: Crown.

Emerson, R. W. (1990). *Selected Essays, Lectures and Poems* (R. Richardson, Ed.). New York: Bantam.

Geldard, R. (1993). *The Esoteric Emerson: The Spiritual Teachings of Ralph Waldo Emerson.* Hudson, NY. Lindisfarne Press.

Goleman, D., Kaufman, P., & Bay, M. (1992). *The Creative Spirit.* New York: Dutton.

Howell, A. (Ed.) (1991). *How Like an Angel Came I Down.* Hudson, NY: Lindisfarne Press.

Jones, H. M. (Ed.) (1966). *Emerson on Education: Selections.* New York: Teachers College Press

McALeer, J. J. (1984). *Ralph Waldo Emerson: Days of Encounter.* Boston: Little, Brown.

Miller, J. P. (2000). *Education and the Soul: Toward a Spiritual Curriculum.* Albany, NY: SUNY Press.

Sanborn, F. B. (1917). *The Life of Henry David Thoreau.* Boston: Houghton Mifflin.

Thoreau, H. D. (1906). *The Journals of Henry David Thoreau.* Vol. 1-14. Boston: Houghton Mifflin.

Thoreau, H. D. (1963). *Journal.* Princeton, NJ: Princeton University Press.

# CHAPTER 13

# A Spiritual Perspective In Education

## The Implications of the Work of J. G. Bennett

## Bob London

In choosing to write this chapter, I feel I have taken on a difficult task; that is, to try to summarize the implications for education of a spiritual perspective that is comprehensive and requires an experiential basis to be well understood. Additionally, J. G. Bennett has written little directly on education. At the same time, as a student and teacher in this tradition for over twenty-five years, as well as an educator for over thirty years, I believe that there are meaningful and significant implications for education that can be derived from this spiritual perspective. In considering how I could present this material in a way that would be useful for the educator without a background in this tradition, I realized that I could not present an in-depth summary of the theoretical framework for the educational implications, given the limitations of space. Therefore, I will first briefly give the reader a sense of the context of this chapter, including a short outline of the historical context of the work of J. G. Bennett, as well as my relationship to his work. Second, I will outline some of the basic terms and principles that underlie Bennett's theoretical framework. The purpose of this section is not to give a complete account of Bennett's conceptual framework, but rather to discuss the theory that is necessary to understand the implications of Bennett's work for education. In the major section of this chapter, I will identify five principles from Bennett's work and discuss the implications of those principles for educational practice. When appropriate, and particularly in discussing the first principle, I will try to connect the written material to the reader's experience.

## CONTEXT

J. G. Bennett was a student of G. I. Gurdjieff, a Russian mystic who lived from 1872 to 1949. Gurdjieff, in his book *Meetings with Remarkable Men* (1969), documents his early life searching for answers to the fundamental questions of life throughout remote regions of the world. Each chapter tells the story of one of the remarkable men and women that shared Gurdjieff's consuming interest in the deepest mysteries of life. His initial work with groups was during the time of the Bolshevik revolution and later, when conditions deteriorated in Russia, he moved his work to Europe, also including a trip to America. His work attracted the interest of a number of leading intellectuals of the period, including P. D. Ouspensky, Frank Lloyd Wright, Aldous Huxley, A. R. Orage and Maurice Nicoll. A number of books document this period, the most well known being *In Search of the Miraculous* (Ouspensky, 1949) which documents P. D. Ouspensky's work with Gurdjieff from 1915 to 1924.

J. G. Bennett was born in 1897 and identified a near death experience in 1918 as the beginning of his spiritual search (Bennett, 1974, p. 1). Bennett first met Gurdjieff in 1920 and was connected with him until Gurdjieff's death approximately 30 years later. Bennett also worked with or met many of the great spiritual teachers of the time. After over fifty years of his own search and over thirty years of working with groups on the ideas of Gurdjieff, Bennett decided to engage in an experiment to provide a more intense focus on spiritual transformation. In October 1971, Bennett started the first of what would be four ten-month residential courses with approximately ninety students at the Sherborne house in Sherborne, England. He directed the courses until his death in December 1974, during the fourth course. Shortly before his death, he initiated the establishment of a similar course in the United States in Claymont, West Virginia. A group primarily of students or teachers from the Sherborne courses initiated the first nine-month course at Claymont in 1975. In developing his program for the courses, Bennett saw the work of Gurdjieff as the foundation for his process but considered it implied by Gurdjieff that the particulars of a specific path need to change with differing conditions. Bennett (1974) stated, "I was not in the 'orthodox' group of Gurdjieff's followers [e.g., Ouspensky] who had set themselves to preserve his teaching 'without change or addition'" (p. 378), and "Fifty years of search had convinced me that Gurdjieff's method brought up to date and completed from other sources was the best available technique for giving just the training that the world needs" (p. v). Today, groups led primarily by students of the Sherborne or Claymont courses are generally called Gurdjieff/Bennett groups.

My own spiritual quest consciously began in 1972, initiated by two transpersonal experiences connected with courses in my doctoral program. In 1975, after completing my doctoral work, I joined a Bennett/Gurdjieff group in Boston facilitated by two graduates of Sherborne courses. I felt attracted to the comprehensiveness and consistency with my experience (and other teachings that I respected) of the theory, as well as the emphasis on applying the theory in our day-to-day life. In 1979, after four years in the Boston group, I took a nine month residential course at the Claymont Institute in West Virginia, which included training in the sacred movements of G. I. Gurdjieff, a series of morning exercises from Bennett for transforming energies, and a theoretical and practical study of the principles of spiritual psychology. Reflecting Bennett's openness to other spiritual traditions, the course included internationally known guest instructors such as Sonyal Rinpoche, Sheik Sulieman Dede, Venerable Dharmawara Mahathera, Dr. Edith Wallace, Sheikh Muzzafer Ozak and Bawa Muhaiyaddeen. The course was completed by 76 students from all over the world.

From 1982 to 1995, at the request of Pierre Elliot, I led Gurdjieff/Bennett spiritual growth groups for adults in New Haven, Connecticut. In 1995, I accepted a position as a professor at California State University, San Bernardino. Connected to starting that new position, in 1997, there was a major change in the focus of my professional life. After over 20 years of professional work with a focus on integrative approaches to teaching problem solving, primarily in the context of mathematics curriculum, a combination of events indicated to me that the time was appropriate to focus my professional work on identifying the implications of a spiritual perspective in education, and, indeed, that has been the focus of my professional work since then.

## TERMINOLOGY

When we discuss spirituality, many times we are discussing experiences that are either incomprehensible to us or not easily discussed given the subjective nature of the experiences. Even when we see commonalties in the "what and how" of our experiences, there may be fundamental differences in our explanations of the "why" of the experiences. To have a good understanding of such concepts, one needs to test the ideas with one's direct experience; this process allows an understanding that is rarely possible through just language. Therefore I will try to limit the terminology involving spirituality to the concepts necessary to understand the educational implications of Bennett's work, omit a discussion of certain philosophical issues, and, when possible, connect the terminology with the reader's experience (see London, 1998, or Bennett, 1961, for a fuller discussion of terminology). Also, I will capitalize some of the defined terminology to denote the usage implied by the definition.

For this chapter, three distinct yet interdependent components of our experience as humans will be defined (Spirit, Soul or Being, and Body or Function). It needs to be noted that I am not denying the possibility that at some level of being the three can be seen or experienced as one. In fact, Bennett (1961) is clear that we are capable of experiencing a basic unity of the three components. However, for understanding our ordinary experience, including our experience as educators, the division into three components seems useful.

The first component of our experience, the world of Function, is associated with the functioning of the material, or conditioned world; that is, the processes that are predictable, observable and objective. Function includes the ordinary workings of thinking, feeling and bodily movements — not what a person is, but rather what we do. It should be noted that this definition of the world of Function is meant to be consistent with the use of the word Body in the sense of Body, Spirit and Soul.

Second, we need to recognize that there is a component of our experience that cannot be reduced to the functioning of the conditioned material world that is a nonmaterial source of meaning and value for our lives. We will label this source as Spirit. Spirit, as we are defining it, is that which impels, or is the impetus for the action. The action itself is a functional process. It needs to be clear that we understand that Spirit is not something that can be observed in the same way as the functional world. We see thoughts like, 'I will do this thing' but that is just a function, something happening, and more often than not the thought fails to be actualized.

For the third component of our experience, we recognize the need for an instrument or a process to reconcile two otherwise incompatible worlds, the world of Function and the world of Spirit. We will label this component of our experience as Being. (It should be noted that Bennett

used both the word Being and Soul for this component of our experience.) Being is connected to both worlds; Being can be understood as the
instrument that allows our material body to receive and cooperate with
impulses whose source is the world of Spirit. One interpretation of Being
is that it is the instrument that allows Spirit to manifest itself in the
world.

Being is the component of our experiences that enables or undergoes
transformation, awakening or unfolding; therefore, Level of Being will
be defined as a measure of our general ability to reconcile the world of
Function and the world of Spirit. Level of Being can be seen as a measure
of our level of consciousness as reflected by the state of concentration, or
the state of availability, of energy. But energies are of different qualities
(Bennett, 1964) and there are different Levels of Being corresponding to
the quality of the energies that are concentrated (Bennett, 1961). In many
traditions, the highest Level of Being would indicate a way of being in
which there is no duality between the world of Function and the world of
Spirit, a world in which we are able to consistently cooperate with Spirit.
Similarly, many traditions would define a lower Level of Being as a way
of being in which we are driven mostly by impulses from the world of
Function (e.g., our ego, personality).

To clarify the difference between Function and Spirit, Bennett (1961)
defined essential impulses and existential impulses. An essential impulse has its source in Spirit and an existential impulse has its source in
existence (i.e., all that can be conceived as material, and is therefore fact).
It is realized that the use of the term impulse can be limiting in that it can
suggest the injection of force into a system versus an awakening to what
is already there. However, it seems to be the most appropriate term for
our work with the understanding that the actual "impulse" to act may be
a reaction (or interpretation) of our functional self to an awakening of
our essence, rather than a characteristic of what we actually experience
in the moment of awakening. In other words, sometimes we experience
an awakening in a moment (essential impulse) and then "interpret" that
impulse (a functional activity) to imply a certain action — the actual moment of awakening is from the world of Spirit, but the interpretation and
action taken (or not taken) is in the world of Function.

The term "cooperating with essential impulses" in this chapter is
meant to be consistent with terminology from a variety of spiritual approaches, for example, "cooperating with the Tao," "consenting to the
Dharma," "being sensitive to the reconciling force," "listening to higher

intuition," and "being an instrument of God's Will" (see London, 1998). It should be noted that our actions many times are motivated by a combination of essential and existential impulses. Finally, when the term Help is used in this chapter, it will indicate an essential impulse that is experienced as providing what is needed in a particular situation, typically experienced as an unexpected source of help.

## IMPLICATIONS OF THE TEACHINGS OF J. G. BENNETT FOR EDUCATION

I divided this section into five parts, each organized around a general principle of Bennett's work, and the implications of that principle for education. I tried to divide and order the principles in such a way that it can be reasonably well "digested" by the reader; however, it should be noted that many of the principles are interrelated and some of the organization is somewhat arbitrary.

## PRINCIPLE 1

**Spirit is a nonmaterial source participating in the emergence or evolution of the Universe that can connect us with meaning, value and purpose. When we cooperate with essential impulses, we allow Spirit to connect us with meaning, value and purpose. In other words, in the process of spiritual transformation, there is an emphasis on awakening or developing Being or Soul.**

Based primarily on my experiences, I am certain ("certain" seems an inappropriate word from a logical point of view, yet seems a better word than "convinced", "confident", etc.) of the involvement of Spirit in human evolution and certainly in my life. However, I am unclear of the exact nature and dynamics of the workings of Spirit; that is, I have had numerous experiences (and have second hand knowledge of many other experiences) which when taken together can only make one certain of the involvement of Spirit in our lives. Yet the timing, nature and dynamics of these experiences certainly elude my clear understanding. "The tao that can be told is not the eternal Tao. The name that can be named is not the eternal Name" (Mitchell, 1988, p.1). Bennett (1961) states the same principle thusly: "Human thought can only make contact with the latter [Spirit], and then only by way of signs and symbols, the full meaning of which must always transcend the limit of our power of understanding" (p. 69).

Despite this mysterious nature of Spirit, it seems important to *attempt* to clarify the nature and dynamics of the workings of Spirit and essential impulses in at least some of our experience, in order to establish a foundation for implementing the implications and principles that will be discussed later. Bennett (1975) made it clear that there were a variety of ways in which we can connect with Spirit in our life. Here, I will focus on one example of a type of connection we can make with Spirit; specifically, the type of experience that happens in a moment (in Bennett's terms outside the dimension of time). The result of this is an "impulse" to take a certain line of action, an insight or intuition into a problem or situation, or a "seeing" of what is needed in a certain situation. I will suggest that generally this type of experience has the following characteristics: (a) We do not cause the experience in the sense of causation in the world of Function — there may be a connection between the experience and our efforts or actions preceding the experience, but usually the experience seems unexpected and from another dimension than our ego or personality. (b) The experience does not cause an action; we decide whether to cooperate or not cooperate with the impulse. (c) Many times we do not see or understand the full significance of the experience, but do have the feeling that we are cooperating with something "bigger than us," what Bennett (1961) defines as the world of Value. (d) Sometimes the experience leads us in a direction that we would not have taken without the experience.

To clarify the explanation of this assumption, I will discuss what I believe are two examples of cooperating with essential impulses from my experience in teaching. Then I will suggest a few exercises that hopefully will allow the reader to connect the concept of essential impulses to her/his own experience.

The first example from my teaching involved a Calculus class. As part of a fellowship in the summer of 1984, I was introduced to a number of interesting mathematics problems. I decided to use some of the problems in my Calculus class. At the beginning of the school year I did not see the problems as a "curriculum" or as a significant addition to the course. I took a small portion of a class to introduce a problem, let them work on the problem outside of class for approximately two weeks, collected their solutions, and, after reading their work, spent a portion of a class discussing various solutions and the significance of the problem. Toward the end of the school year, the students had finished their work on the eighth problem. When I finished reading their papers I had the

sudden realization that they had made a quantum leap in their understanding of the process of problem solving. I have described this leap as
follows: "It is as if the student has been transformed mathematically! Instead of acting in all the ways that we normally attribute to most high
school students, the student acts similarly to a 'mathematically mature'
person" (London, 1989, p. 1). At the same time I "saw" what each student
needed to complete or solidify the leap and "saw" individual problems
to assign each student to help them complete the process. I can still picture most of the students in the class and the assignments I gave them.

What I want to emphasize is that it was this unexpected realization that
convinced me that I had stumbled onto something significant, not my
own previous work or the work of others. That experience encouraged me
to reflect (a functional process) on what it was I did that had been so successful. The result of this reflection was the development of a curriculum
of non-routine problems, which has been a major focus of my professional
career for over 15 years, and the topic of many professional presentations
and much writing — all connected to one moment in one class.

The second example illustrates the mysterious nature (from the point
of view of our Level of Being) of the workings of Spirit. Each year I taught
a problem solving class. Typically, the students in the class were not
"successful" students and typically took the course because it was the
only viable option to complete their mathematics requirement for graduation. I still recall with fondness the typical first day of class — as each
student entered the classroom, the other students would comment:
"You're in this class too!" I do not remember the context of the particular
class I want to discuss, perhaps because what happened had no rational
connection in my mind with the context. What is relevant to note is that
very rarely were all the students present.

The day before this class, spontaneously two "thoughts" occurred to
me, both in a persistent manner. First, I felt that the focus of the class
should be discussing with each individual student what type of person
they should eventually marry. Second, I had the clear feeling that every
student would be present for the class. From my point of view, there was
no logical reason why I should have such discussions with each student
— I had never had such discussions with even one student in the past
and there was no connection that I could see with the content of the
course. In addition, I was the type of teacher that would never initiate
such a topic. In fact, my interpretation, in hindsight, of the second
"thought" (i.e., that all the students would be present) is that it was

needed to "convince me" to actually carry out the first idea. Otherwise, I am sure I would have convinced myself that the idea was crazy and would not have done it.

In planning the class, I wrote down on a piece of paper in large print something to the effect: "I predict that today all the students will be present in class." My plan was to show the prediction to the students and use it as an introduction to the class, sharing what had happened. By the way, I had decided that if all the students were not present, I would not teach the lesson — that being evidence that the first thought was not legitimate. In addition, I thought some about each student and what I would say about the type of person they should marry.

By this point in my life, I had had enough experiences of this type that I was not surprised when all the students showed up. In planning the lesson, I could not imagine how the students would react to what I saw as a personal intrusion into their life — they were not the type of student that generally appreciated unsolicited advice! They reacted as if this idea made perfect sense and the lesson proceeded smoothly. What I believe is important to mention about this example is that there was no follow-up to this lesson, none of the students ever mentioned the conversations again, and I have no idea if the advice ever effected any of their decisions concerning marriage. In other words, even though I am convinced of the reality of the intuition and the need for actualizing the intuition, I have no sense of the significance of the "event" for me or the students, and I suspect that it had little, or nothing, to do with whom they actually married. At the same time, I am convinced that something was communicated between us that was significant — even though I could not understand the significance. Also, what I find important about this example, which is consistent with other experiences I have had, is that what was communicated to me during the experience was exactly what I needed to actualize the event; that is, the second thought that all the students would be present.

What I would readily admit is that there are other ways of interpreting these events other than what I am labeling as a spiritual perspective. However, from my point of view, the actual feelings associated with and the nature of the insights (as well as the occurrence in my life of many similar events) strongly convinces me that the reality of what happened is more consistent with what I am labeling as a spiritual perspective. I must add that at best I consider my explanation an approximation of what really happened — the workings of Spirit are a great mystery to me!

Consistent with the approach of Gurdjieff/Bennett, I do not suggest
that you accept my explanation as valid. You need to test this explanation with your experience. To facilitate that process, I will suggest six
questions that I have used in working with teachers (and others) to generate examples in the teacher's life of cooperating with essential impulses. I suggest that before asking yourself each question, you shut
your eyes and try to relax your body, then ask the question (or have
someone else ask the question) and try to visualize whatever experience
comes to mind. The first two are general questions that seem to frequently elicit examples: (a) Can you remember an experience in which
you felt nourished by Nature? and (b) Can you remember an experience
in which you felt nourished by Spirit?

The two above questions many times generate dramatic examples.
The next four questions generate somewhat more commonplace examples, involving points in the process of solving a significant problem
(one that requires a change in Level of Being) in which, according to
Bennett, Help is required from Spirit (see London, 1998 or Bennett, 1983):
Can you remember an experience (or perhaps four different experiences,
one for each question) in solving a problem in which (a) you felt a persistent urge to investigate a problem for no apparent rational reason, (b) an
unexpected event allowed you to actually start a project or pursue a solution to a problem, (c) a solution or way to a solution unexpectedly presented itself (e.g., the "aha" experience) or (d) at a certain point you
"knew" a problem was solved or you "knew" it was time to finish a project or work on a problem?

Before preceding with a discussion of the implications of this principle, it is important to mention a hazard associated with the idea of essential impulses; that is, there is not an objective method for verifying the
authenticity of an essential impulse. In other words, we can believe that
the source for the impulse to take a particular action is essential when, in
fact, it comes from our personality or ego, perhaps even from an un-
healthy part of our personality. However, in my opinion, this hazard
does not alter the reality of essential impulses and the significance of cooperating with essential impulses in our life. Therefore; in my practice, I
maintain a cautious attitude, discriminating among impulses that seem
clearly essential in nature, impulses that are clearly existential in nature,
and impulses that are unclear. In all cases, I try not to interpret the significance of the impulse (i.e., allow my personality to "jump in"), but rather
try to allow the impulse to work on me without interference. Also, even

in cases that seem clearly essential in nature, I "test" the impulse against my commonsense view of what is needed in my life or in the situation, and what is healthy. If an impulse seems inconsistent with what my logical mind or feelings see as healthy, I do not "cooperate" with the impulse in that moment, but rather, try to remain open to the possibility that at some later point the impulse may make more sense. Of course, I have found that this cautious attitude needs to be balanced with a willingness to take a reasonable risk that may feel uncomfortable from an intellectual or emotional point of view.

Perhaps the first implication of this principle is that our teaching can be more meaningful if we are more sensitive to essential impulses. For example, the work of Miller (1994) and Brown (1998) indicates that including a contemplative practice as part of teacher training can have a positive effect on a person's teaching. For example, Miller allowed teachers to select from a variety of contemplative practices (or create their own form) to practice as part of certain courses in education. Miller (1994) states that this requirement is based on the assumption that "teaching should come from the Self rather than the ego ... [and] that when we teach from the Self, we gradually experience more moments of communion with our students ... we experience moments of deep inner joy in teaching as we connect with our students in profound and subtle ways" (p. 122). I consider Miller's use of the term "Self" to be consistent with Bennett's use of the term "True Self," which from Bennett's point of view (1961) allows a connection with Spirit and, therefore, essential impulses.

A second implication of this principle is that it provides the foundation for a spiritual perspective in education by recognizing the existence of something greater in the Universe than our limited functional and material characteristics, and implies a mystery to life that we need to recognize and respect. For example, this principle implies that there is a mystery concerning what it means to create a school consistent with a spiritual perspective. Each school needs to be sensitive to what is actually needed to serve the needs of the students, staff, community, and so on. At times, this will not be consistent with what our "logical mind" would suggest but rather will require us to connect with a purpose beyond our rational understanding. In addition, the individual teacher needs to be sensitive in a grounded way to the spiritual — the mystery of life; the nonmaterial, nonverbal — and specifically to what is needed to nourish each child's natural spirituality and unfolding.

Third, this principle has implications for how we can more directly help students cooperate with essential impulses. Bennett (1961) implied that for the most part young children naturally cooperate with essential impulses and that this cooperation can build the foundation for later spiritual development. His work (1984b) supports the need to be sensitive to essential impulses, and although he clearly sees the period before adulthood as a time to prepare the child to live a healthy life on earth, he also clearly stresses the importance of not allowing the child to lose her/his connection with Spirit. In addition, Bennett (1984a) made it clear that Gurdjieff saw the "normal" educational process "as something almost entirely harmful to the essential nature of the child, and as resulting in an artificial being who has lost touch with his real self" (p. 66).

Consequently, Bennett (1984a, 1984d) suggested that a significant component of helping the student maintain her/his connection with Spirit is a form of non-doing; that is, we need to not allow our conditioned personality (versus essence) to become an instrument for disconnecting students from their essential nature. For example, we need to not interfere with students' natural tendency to connect with nature, express themselves creatively (e.g., through the arts), recognize and solve problems, and be aware of essential impulses.

In addition, there are some general approaches to curriculum that help many students to connect with their essential nature. These include strengthening students' connection to nature, integrating the arts as a way of connecting with our creativity, establishing ritual and celebrations as an integral component of the curriculum, allowing for meditative or quiet time, providing opportunities for students to discuss issues related to Spirit, and exposing students to nonlinear sources of meaning such as myths and fables. For example, to expose students to nonlinear sources of meaning, one elementary school created a five-day sequence that included telling the students a fairy tale, reading the fairy tale and showing pictures, having students make flannel board characters and scenery for the story, having the students create a puppet show or illustrate a scene from the story, and having the class act out the story. The principle is to allow students to naturally absorb the meaning (versus a more didactic approach) by experiencing the story in different ways. Similarly, for older students in my Calculus class, I would read the students three of my favorite Grimm's tales (Manheim, 1977) and then allow one student a week to select a favorite tale and read it to the class.

Although we never discussed the significance of the tales, it was clear that the tales affected at least some of the students.

Rachael Kessler (2000) shares an example of providing students an opportunity to discuss issues connected to spirituality in the context of a council meeting (a structured opportunity for students to speak on a topic without immediate reaction; see Zimmerman, 1996). She led the meeting with a group of high school seniors who had worked together for most of a semester. At one point the students were asked "'Would you be willing to each tell us a story about a time in your lives when your own spirit — whatever that means to you — was nourished?' ... Everybody has a story — a story that commands the full, riveted attention of each student in the room. Many stories are about nature or about a sense of belonging. Others are about the joy of creativity, the strength that comes through challenge or even suffering, the awe that comes from discovering faith in God" (p. 15).

## PRINCIPLE 2

**One component of the process of transformation is the successful resolution of a sequence of "problems" or "encounters" that naturally present themselves and require a change in the person's understanding (Level of Being). This type of unfolding includes "vertical" change, referring to a basic reorganization of one's way of seeing the world and "horizontal" change referring to applications of the new understanding to a variety of contexts.**

There is certainly much debate concerning the validity and implications of cognitive developmental theory as defined by Piaget and his followers, particularly concerning the universality and the perceived (by some) hierarchical nature of the stages. The wording of this principle does not support the "Piagetian view" or any other specific view. Rather, this principle recognizes that a significant component of our growth involves the healthy recognition and resolution of a sequence of "problems" or "encounters." In my opinion, Bennett's development of Gurdjieff's concepts of the triad, seven worlds and the enneagram offers an understanding of transformative growth that is both consistent with experience and the writings of others on this subject (e.g., Wilber, 1986, 1996, Flier, 1995, Steiner, 1995, Montessori, 1966 and Marshak, 1997), and addresses some of the concerns with "developmental approaches." (For the interested reader I suggest the following material: for triads, Bennett,

1993, pp. 36-62, for the seven worlds, Bennett, 1961, pp. 69-211, and for the enneagram, Bennett, 1983 or London, 1998). This work implies that: (a) The process that we generally label as spiritual transformation begins at birth (or before!) and involves gradual movement in the direction of increasing conscious cooperation with essential impulses. (b) The problems that students encounter as part of their "developmental" growth (e.g., Piagetian tasks) are connected to the problems that they might encounter in their spiritual quest later in life in the sense that a healthy resolution of the earlier developmental problems builds the foundation for addressing later problems connected with spiritual transformation. (c) Formal operational thinking (e.g., the scientific method, logical reasoning) has limitations that are not limitations for a higher stage of development. (d) Appropriate problems (and solutions) will naturally present themselves to the student if not interfered with by the student, the teacher or others. (e) The laws of the higher worlds are embedded (coexist) in the lower worlds; that is, no matter what a person's Level of Being, she/he can experience contact with essential impulses.

Bennett (1984a, 1984c) saw the developmental approaches of Montessori and Steiner as consistent with the teachings of Gurdjieff. While Bennett added little to the discussion of the specifics of the general stages through which a child progresses (probably appreciating the depth of Steiner's and Montessori's work), he did comment on the general approach to stimulating developmental growth; that is, presenting the student with a problem solving situation meaningful to the student and at the appropriate level of difficulty. Bennett (1984a) emphasized the difference between a "wordless" demonstration in which we present the student with a situation, and an attempt to "get something over" to the child. He made it clear that the latter approach was inappropriate, quoting Gurdjieff, "if you try to 'get something over' to them, you are only increasing the great weakness of man ... his suggestibility and his dependence on others. You must simply put them in front of situations where they are able to learn" (1984a, p. 75).

Bennett (1984a) cites an example of Gurdjieff presenting this type of situation to children in the context of teaching the student responsibility in taking decisions:

> He put a big tray on the floor and said to the children [approximately forty, ages 3 to 16], 'You can choose what you like, you can have either four silver dollars or one five dollar bill.' And the

children went and stood in front of it, and you could see that this was really a choice. The silver dollars were very beautiful, but the five-dollar bill would buy a little more. (p. 74)

Bennett (1984a) emphasizes that this type of action or "teaching" was used very infrequently with children by Gurdjieff, stating that Gurdjieff "said that if a child were constantly expected to make decisions.... This would only produce a state of nervousness, and even the failure to develop his own 'I'" (p. 73). In my opinion, the approach suggested by this example is consistent with a Piagetian approach to teaching; in fact, the example reminds me of the use of dilemmas suggested by Kohlberg's work applying Piagetian theory to moral development.

In summary, this approach to the process of transformation has the following general implications for teaching:

1. A central focus of education is to help each student recognize and resolve a series of problems that naturally present themselves to the student. Many of these problems are connected to developmental tasks or sensitive periods common to most, if not all, students in a given community and of a given age. We can plan activities that can help the students resolve these problems in a healthy way.

2. In addition, there are some problems that are unique for each human; each of us has a unique path. Teachers need to be sensitive to spontaneous opportunities for stimulating transformative growth unique to individual students.

3. Problems and conflict (in the appropriate context) are necessary and appropriate sources for opportunities for transformative growth. Education needs to help students see problems and conflict as a natural part of life and an opportunity for growth, and give the student the tools to effectively address problems and conflict.

4. Formal operational thinking should not be seen as the endpoint of the growth process. For example, when I shared Grimms' tales with my Calculus class, I introduced the concept that there were ways of understanding that were different from the linear methods they learned in mathematics.

## PRINCIPLE 3

**As adults, we need to realize our present situation; that includes the fact that we are *not* typically fully present and that we do not, in general, consciously cooperate with Spirit.**

According to Bennett (1983), a significant first step in the process of spiritual transformation as an adult is when we get a glimpse of our true condition and the implications of that condition; that is, in Gurdjieff's terminology, one realizes

> one's own nothingness; from that point everything can begin. So long as one is burdened by the illusion of having something — having something to protect, having some spiritual wealth, one cannot begin … one does not have anything of one's own, one has no "I," one is not awake. This realization represents the threshold of this work of ours. (p. 124-5)

In spiritual work, this is a difficult realization that must be understood experientially. For myself, I remember an exercise that I attempted while in a Gurdjieff/Bennett group: for a week, every hour on the hour (for ten hours of the day, e.g., 8 to 6), for one minute to put my attention on my hand. This had to be done exactly on the hour without the use of alarms. If we are capable of deciding to do (in the real sense of the word), then this task should be fairly easy. However, my experience and the experience of many others is that, in fact, the task is impossible in our present condition (e.g., even with the directions to try the exercise with our best efforts as an experiment, versus as a "significant" exercise, many times a day will pass without once remembering the exercise). Further, in attempting the task, one sees very clearly the utter mechanistic or automatic nature of our lives. This is a very shocking and sobering realization. I suggest this exercise as an experiment for the reader to attempt. Personally, I have attempted the exercise many times, each time, as a result, feeling clearer about my typical state of Being.

The implications of this principle will be discussed in connection with the next principle.

## PRINCIPLE 4

**The emphasis on cooperating with essential impulses does *not* imply that there is no need to make "human" efforts at understanding; rather, it is implied that right human efforts can create the conditions which open us to Help and allow us to cooperate with essential impulses.**

In my opinion, the importance of this assumption is key to understanding a spiritual perspective in education. So far the assumptions seem to imply a certain dependence on receptivity, coupled with an understanding of the inadequacy of our ordinary states. While it is clear that even well intentioned efforts are in many cases not effective, it does not follow that there is not a proper and important role for our efforts. Bennett (1975) describes well the relationship between efforts and receiving help:

> Working through efforts and working through receiving cannot substitute for each other.... Help is needed to begin something new and help is needed to bring this to completion, but without effort there is no action. The combination of the two sides in us ... is necessary to the wholeness of the Work. The Work is not something we do nor that is done to us; but we can *participate*.... This participation is sometimes a matter of efforts and at other times a matter of being receptive. (p. 13-14)

Bennett (1984b) explains the dynamics of our efforts and the possible effect on students:

> If I struggle with a defect ... in an honest way, I shall see a great deal more about myself than if I had not struggled; and it is the seeing that is more important, more effectual, than the actual change.... By *seeing*, man himself changes, and not merely psychic or bodily habits. Seeing is a property of the inner self ... and the more we see ourselves, the more we shall have the right state in front of children ... [and] evoke their confidence. (p. 164)

In my experience there is a subtle connection between our efforts, our general lack of presence (as described in the previous principle) and the availability of Help that is implied in the above material and captured in a quote from Gurdjieff (Bennett, 1974, p. 380): "Two things have no limit: the stupidity of man and the mercy of God." That is, if our efforts are genuine, despite the fact that our efforts may be completely "stupid" (in the sense implied by Gurdjieff's quote), Help may be available to provide us with what we need (perhaps not what we want!). This concept I believe is implied in the concept of a spiritual warrior (e.g., Trungpa, 1984 and Castaneda, 1974) who understands his/her nothingness, yet understands the need to impeccably make efforts (or live life), inviting Help and Spirit. I will cite one example from my life to hopefully clarify this process. When I was in the third month of the nine-month course at Claymont, I became impatient and wanted to be "enlightened" right then. I decided to make a super effort to "force" enlightenment. For example, I decided to stop eating and sleeping until I was transformed. In addition, I made other efforts such as trying to retrace at midnight without a flashlight an earlier guided walk in the woods of Claymont. In summary, I made what Gurdjieff termed as "stupid" efforts (in hindsight, it was hard for me to believe that I actually thought that this "plan" made sense!). The evening of the second day without sleep, I was peeling apples and, for the first and last time in my life, I was clearly hallucinating. At that point, I realized not only the futility of my efforts, but also the danger of those efforts. I gave up and went to bed. Amazingly, I woke up in time for the morning sitting and went to the sitting with the feeling of completely failing in my experiment. Suddenly, during the sitting, I "saw" what was needed for me to properly complete the course — that insight guided me for the remaining six months of the course. Although this is an extreme example (and not an approach I recommend), I believe it illustrates some of the characteristics of this type of interplay between our efforts and Help: (a) Although my efforts were clearly misplaced, they were genuine in the sense that I really did believe (before the experiment) the efforts made sense and I attempted to carry the plan out to the best of my ability. (b) The nature of my efforts somehow created a situation that allowed Help to enter. (c) Although that Help did not allow me to achieve what I sought, perhaps it allowed what was needed in that point in my life. (d) It was not until after Help that I realized the misconnection between what I perceived I needed and what was actually needed.

To clarify this process of the interplay of our efforts, our general lack of presence, and the availability of Help, I will cite some examples in the process of education identified by Bennett.

1. When Bennett (1995) was asked by someone on a Sherborne course how can a teacher see and understand the possibilities of a student, he commented,

> First of all, no one can see the possibilities of another. And we must know that, when we are in front of a child, we are in front of a being whom we cannot know. And if we try to begin knowing that being, already we are off on to personality [versus essence]. What I must remember — and that is itself a real discipline for me — is that this is an unknown being, and that it is the unknown possibilities of that being which matter — not the facts that I am inevitably putting into that child. I must bring that in

myself, by keeping present in me this memory that it is the invisible that matters far more than the visible one, and also accepting that I am not able to see that invisible child — any more than anyone else can — because invisible does not mean just around the corner; invisible means belonging to a different world. (p. 66)

Further, Bennett commented on how to work with this observation by advising the simple experiment of "not letting yourself, when in front of the child, think — what are the possibilities? What can the child become? — but simply to remember that this is a being who has possibilities that no one can know" (p. 66). Finally, Bennett explains somewhat the dynamics of what happens if we are able to work in this manner:

If you will keep that discipline with yourself, you will see that, so long as you keep it, something will be different in your relation with the child. Something will pass from you to the child which is more necessary to him than what you are able to give in the world of fact, and it will have the effect that the two [value and fact] will be able to be harmonized. (p. 66)

I would suggest that the dynamics of this approach are that we realize that we do not see the possibilities of the student, we make *attempts* to be present enough to keep this realization alive in us and Help transforms the situation, allowing something that is needed to enter.

2. Bennett was clear that the most important factor concerning meeting the spiritual needs of the student is the quality of our inner work, versus what we "teach" the student. He said "our task [as teachers] begins with ourselves; and there is much more benefit to be derived by children from what those in contact do to put their own house in order than what they attempt to do to put the child's house in order" (1984a, p. 82). Bennett (1984b) suggests,

it is not really necessary that we should have arrived at a state of freedom from psychic defects, but that we should have a genuine wish to be free. The genuine acceptance of the burden we place upon children by our own defects, and the wish to be free from them, is the secret of helping them. That in itself is enough to make a prodigious difference to the whole feeling of the child about life, to its confidence in this world, and also to its confidence that there is truly a meaning in its existence. (p. 157)

In summary, if we have a "genuine wish to be free" there is likely to be a quality to our efforts (despite, perhaps, the shortcomings of our actual efforts) that invites Help that transforms the situation.

In addition, it seems appropriate to identify some components of the educational process that seem essential to an effective school and *require* a combination of efforts (including struggling with our inability to be present) and receptivity to address effectively. For example, the faculty, individually and as a group, needs to recognize and address the fact we are not typically fully present and have tendencies to interfere with the student's natural tendency to develop spiritually. The first step in this process is a shared awareness of the reality of this difficulty and a shared commitment to address this issue, individually and as a group. Second, perhaps the most significant key to a successful school is the ability of the staff to collaborate to establish an effective learning community including students, staff, parents and both the local and larger community. This implies that staff development and community building should be an integral part of the school's life. The school needs to have a structure that allows faculty to determine what each student needs and the faculty needs the time to see the school as a whole. Thus, the school should provide time for the teachers to work together on their personal and spiritual growth. Finally, individually, teachers need to listen to the essence of what students are communicating, have a genuine respect for the students, and sensitivity to nonverbal aspects of communication.

Again, it is suggested that these are examples of issues that cannot be addressed effectively without a combination of receptivity and a quality of effort that includes a struggle with our inability to be consistently present.

## PRINCIPLE 5

There is a need for an approach in education in which the child's bodily, intellectual, emotional and spiritual needs are balanced.

Bennett supported the need for an approach to K - 12 education balancing the bodily, psychic and spiritual needs of the child, but emphasized the need for recognizing the spiritual needs of the child in this process. Bennett (1984b) stated that because the essence of the child is born into a human body there is a preparatory period prior to adulthood in which the primary need of the child is to learn to live successfully here on this earth, to cope with the physical and psychic needs of earthly life. But this should not be done in a way as to produce a complete forgetfulness of whence we came, and whither we shall return, and the reason for our presence here. (p. 148)

In terms of pedagogy, Bennett (1984d) saw spiritual needs connected with a reality that could not be reached through the senses or grasped by our minds. Also, he made it clear that the spiritual needs of children could seldom be addressed by direct instruction. Specifically, Bennett (1984a) states:

Gurdjieff advised us very strongly: Never attempt to teach children directly about high and deep spiritual questions, including questions of religion. If we did so, they would only be taken as a psychic, mental or emotional experience and would not penetrate into the deeper understanding of the child. One should always ... begin from afar in such a way that their own search would be encouraged. What we do with children should be a response to their search rather than an attempt to instill or teach them anything. (pp. 71-72)

In the rest of this section, I will identify some areas that Bennett suggested we could address in preparing students for a more direct spiritual quest as an adult.

1. Bennett (1984d) suggests that the environment that surrounds the student can be important in effecting certain spiritual needs of the student. He suggests that the environment should communicate qualities such as "trustworthiness, sincerity, and truthfulness that create the feeling that, 'I am in an environment that I can trust' " (pp. 11-12) versus an environment that focuses primarily on psychic stimulation. He asserts that such an environment can result in later years the student being able to trust in God (p. 12).

2. As previously mentioned, Bennett (1984b) considered it important for students to remember "whence we came, and whither we shall return, and the reason for our presence here" (p. 148). Bennett's advice to help the child preserve this spiritual recollection is that, "you should not attempt to teach your child anything about spiritual realities; but devote yourself, as far as possible, to the worship of God. From that worship of yours there will remain in the child a contact with Reality" (p. 158).

Bennett added that "worship of God" could be interpreted in many different ways by different religions or spiritual traditions, but what was essential is the adult's sincerity in the act of worship. He adds that for himself worship is, "the awareness, deep inside myself, that I am not here just to satisfy my own egoism, but that I belong to quite a different life, and that there is in that life ... a Source which gives a meaning to everything that exists, including my existence" (p. 159). Certainly, Bennett's definition of worship implies an inner state of the teacher that is "communicated" to the receptive student "indirectly" by the teacher's presence and actions rather than an outward form of worship that would be apparent to the student.

3. Educators should try to keep

> alive in children the sense of wonder, and the realization of how much there is that cannot be known and cannot be understood ... [versus] trying to impress upon them the extent of our own knowledge.... We should make it clear to them that all that we know is very little compared with the great wonder of the world in which we live, and that the great part of it is not to be explained by our scientific procedures (Bennett, 1984a, pp. 82-83).

Bennett (1984a) shared his observations of Gurdjieff: "I have seen him tell children things which were very surprising for children and have seen how this has left something behind which has been a preparation for an approach for the deeper and more spiritual problems of life" (p. 71). Bennett implied that this type of emphasis creates the conditions that will allow children to naturally ask questions that are connected with their spiritual needs.

## CONCLUSION

I have attempted to give the reader practical guidelines in applying the implications of the work of Bennett in education. As implied in the body of this text, there are serious limitations to this method of communicating matters concerning Spirit. My hope is that I have been at least somewhat successful, and that you, the reader, will experiment with some of the suggestions made in this chapter. In the final analysis, your experimentation with these ideas (perhaps in collaboration with others) is the only reliable way to make these suggestions meaningful.

## References

Bennett, J. G. (1961). *The Dramatic Universe*, Vol. 2. Sherborne, England: Coombe Springs Press.

Bennett, J. G. (1964). *Energies.* Sherborne, England: Coombe Springs Press.

Bennett, J. G. (1974). *Witness.* Tuscon, AZ: Omen Press.

Bennett, J. G. (1975). *The Sevenfold Work.* Sherborne, England: Coombe Springs Press.

Bennett, J. G. (1983). *Enneagram Studies.* York Beach, ME: Samuel Weiser.

Bennett, J. G. (1984a). Begin from afar — Gurdjieff's approach to the child. In *The Spiritual Hunger of the Modern Child: A Series of Ten Lectures* (pp. 44-65). Charles Town, WV: Claymont Communications.

Bennett, J. G. (1984b). The Subud approach. In *The Spiritual Hunger of the Modern Child: A Series of Ten Lectures* (pp. 146-168). Charles Town, WV: Claymont Communications.

Bennett, J. G. (1984c). A summing up and practical conclusions. In *The Spiritual Hunger of the Modern Child: A Series of Ten Lectures* (pp. 194-220). Charles Town, WV: Claymont Communications.

Bennett, J. G. (1984d). A survey of the problem. In *The Spiritual Hunger of the Modern Child: A Series of Ten Lectures* (pp. 1-21). Charles Town, WV: Claymont Communications.

Bennett, J. G. (1993). *Elementary Systematics.* Santa Fe, NM: Bennett.

Bennett, J. G. (1995). *Making A Soul.* Santa Fe, NM: Bennett Books.

Brown, R. (1998). The teacher as contemplative observer. *Educational Leadership* 56 (4), 70-73.

Castaneda, C. (1974). *Tales of Power.* New York: Simon and Schuster.

Flier, L. (1995). Demystifying mysticism: Finding a developmental relationship between different ways of knowing. *The Journal of Transpersonal Psychology* 27 (2), 131 - 152.

Gurdjieff, G I. (1969). *Meetings With Remarkable Men.* New York: Dutton.

Kessler, R. (2000). *The Soul of Education.* Alexandria, VA: Association for Supervision and Curriculum Development.

London, R. (1989). *Nonroutine Problems: Doing Mathematics.* Providence, RI: Janson Publications.

London, R. (1998, April). *A post-modern research model that takes into account the implications of spiritual psychology.* Paper presented at the American Educational Research Association National Convention, San Diego, CA.

Manheim, R. (1977). *Grimms' Tales For Young And Old: The Complete Stories.* Garden City/New York: Anchor Press/Doubleday.

Marshak, D. (1997). *The Common Vision: Parenting And Educating For Wholeness.* New York: Peter Lang.

Miller, J. (1994). *The Contemplative Practitioner.* Toronto: The Ontario Institute for Studies in Education.

Mitchell, S. (Trans., 1988). *Tao Te Ching.* New York: Harper and Row.

Montessori, M. (1966). *The Secret Of Childhood* (M. Costelloe, Trans.). New York: Ballantine Books.

Ouspensky, P. D. (1949). *In Search Of The Miraculous.* New York: Harcourt, Brace & World.

Steiner, R. (1995). *The Kingdom Of Childhood.* Hudson, NY: Anthroposophic Press.

Trungpa, C. (1984). *Shambhala: The Sacred Path Of The Warrior.* Boston: Shambhala Press.

Wilber, K. (1996). *A Brief History Of Everything.* Boston: Shambhala Press.

Wilber, K., Engler, J., & Brown, D. (1986). *Transformations Of Consciousness.* Boston: Shambhala Press.

Zimmerman, J. (1996). *The Way of Council.* Las Vegas: Bramble Books.

# CHAPTER 14

# Nourishing the Spiritual Embryo

## The Educational Vision of Maria Montessori

### Ron Miller

"We must take into consideration that from birth the child has a power in him. We must not just see the child, but God in him. We must respect the laws of creation in him."
Maria Montessori, 1935 (1989a, p. 98)

Maria Montessori pursued her educational work with a spiritual consciousness verging on mysticism. Although her ideas have been packaged and practiced for ninety years as a "method" replete with cleverly designed materials and recognizable classroom routines, Montessori's educational vision is far more profound than this, and essentially aims for a complete transformation of virtually all modern assumptions about teaching, learning, childhood, and the very purpose of human existence on this Earth. This was recognized as early as 1912 by one of the first Americans to visit Montessori's experiment in Rome, Dorothy Canfield Fisher, who reported that Montessori considered her "ideas, hopes and visions" to be "much more essential" than the techniques she had developed. Fisher continued,

> Contact with the new ideas is not doing for us what it ought, if it
> does not act as a powerful stimulant to the whole body of our
> thought about life. It should make us think, and think hard, not

only about how to teach our children the alphabet more easily,
but about such fundamental matters as what we actually mean
by moral life; whether we really honestly wish the spiritually
best for our children, or only the materially best; why we are really in the world at all. In many ways, this 'Montessori System' is
a new religion which we are called upon to help bring into the
world, and we cannot aid in so great an undertaking without
considerable spiritual as well as intellectual travail (Fisher,
1912, p. viii).

Much more recently, Aline Wolf, a Montessori educator for nearly
forty years, reaffirmed this position, arguing that it was time for her colleagues to make the spiritual vision at the heart of Montessori's work far
more visible and explicit (Wolf, 1996). This shall be the intent of my essay.

## An Educational Physician

Montessori was born in Chiaravalle, Italy in 1870 and grew up in
Rome. As she matured she became interested in mathematics and science, areas of study that attracted few women in her time or place. Overcoming prejudice and outright opposition, she became the first woman
to enroll in medical school in Italy, was an uncommonly diligent student,
and graduated with high honors in 1896. Immediately she embarked on
a successful career as a physician, scholar, research scientist, and internationally respected advocate of women's rights. Her practice and research
increasingly specialized in the problems of "mentally defective" children, and by 1900 she was involved in teacher training as well as direct
pedagogical work with children. She undertook extensive studies of
psychiatry, physical anthropology, and pedagogy, finding the pioneer-
ing work of Jean Itard and Edouard Seguin, earlier physicians who had
worked with deaf-mute and "idiot" children, to be most relevant to her
emerging understanding.

As I have pointed out elsewhere, this intellectual and professional
background is virtually unique among educational theorists, providing
Montessori with "an empirically disciplined approach to pedagogy and
a therapeutic interest in the individual child" (Miller, 1997, p. 158). Although she did hold strong views about women's rights and social reform, her educational approach was not the result of philosophical
speculation or a specific political agenda, as is the case for most educational theorists; she maintained throughout her long career that educa-

tion must follow the universal laws of human development as these are revealed in the lives of actual children, rather than seek to achieve social aims by imposing adult ideals on young people. We should keep in mind that any particular way of understanding or applying "universal laws" is affected by one's historical and cultural conditioning, thus no educational method is absolutely, universally superior. But it remains significant that Montessori's educational theory began with an unusually open minded experimental approach, which she enjoined her followers to emulate.[1]

Years later, Montessori's son Mario described her as a "positivist" and "disbeliever" during these formative years of her career, and her major biographer, Rita Kramer, called her a "freethinker" (i.e., essentially non-religious, skeptical). Yet Kramer also observed a "peculiar tension in Montessori between scientist and mystic, between reason and intuition," that showed itself as early as her years in medical school, when chance encounters with children inspired a sense that she had "a destiny to fulfill" (Kramer, 1976, pp. 91, 45). Her work with children, culminating in the founding of the first *casa dei bambini* (Children's Home) in 1907, seems to have touched a deep place in Montessori's soul. Kramer reports that during these years she began attending an annual two-week spiritual retreat at a convent, while Mario Montessori suggested that his mother's conversion was rather dramatic: thunderstruck by the transformations she observed in the children under her care, "she left her career, she left her brilliant position among the socialists and feminists, she left the university, she left even the family and followed Him [Christ]" (Mario Montessori, 1984, p. 51). For nearly half a century, until her death in 1952, Montessori was a tireless crusader for the spiritual renewal of humanity, which she believed could occur only by nourishing the divine creative power within the children of the world.

Outside the confines of academic discourse, she lectured around the world, held conferences, trained teachers, and wrote several books. Beyond propagating the "Montessori Method," this body of work represents a prophetic vision of human redemption. It rests on a foundation of medical/psychological/biological insight (Montessori's understanding of human development as well as her ecological conception of life were well ahead of her time), yet her work is laced with Biblical imagery and religious fervor. This respected physician/scientist would unflinchingly refer over and over again to God, Christ, Scripture and various saints.

Montessori had clearly become a devout Roman Catholic. By 1915 she was applying her educational insights to sectarian religious education and in 1929 published a book on *The Child in the Church*. Indeed, one extension of the Montessori movement, represented particularly by the work of Sofia Cavelletti and Gianna Gobbi, is an explicit Catholic approach to religious education in early childhood that nurtures the young child's personal relationship to God (Cavalletti, 1999; Lillig, 1999). Philosopher Robert G. Buckenmeyer asserts that Montessori's Catholic faith "is the basis for her educational philosophy, namely, that the child is created by God and merely loaned to parents and teachers whose job it is to respect the mysterious possibilities of each child. . . ." He argues that in contrast to the Calvinist Protestantism that has influenced American culture, the Latin faith underlying Montessori's vision emphasizes the essential goodness of creation and humanity (Buckenmeyer, 1997, pp. 232n, 203n). "It was Christ who showed us what the child really is," Montessori proclaimed—"the adult's guide to the Kingdom of Heaven" (Montessori, 1972a, p. 86).

Nevertheless, Montessori's faith was not merely sectarian—it was a transcendental, mystical spirituality, and as such it touched upon core religious teachings at the root of nearly all world traditions. Buckenmeyer himself found "oriental" elements in her thinking, and some commentators suggest that Montessori's seven-year stay in India during World War Two, as a guest of the Theosophical Society, influenced her worldview, particularly her notion of "cosmic" education which she expounded in the last years of her life. But I think Günter Schulz-Benesch (Montessori, 1989a, pp. 29-30) is correct in observing that Montessori's spirituality was universalist throughout most of her career and resonated with, rather than became substantially altered by, the "oriental" teachings of Theosophy. For her, the practice of Catholicism was an opening to a direct experience of divine presence, as it was for Meister Eckhart, Hildegard of Bingen, or her fellow Italian, St. Francis of Assisi. It is significant that her teachings have been respected and even revered by people of many cultures and faiths, including Jews, Hindus, Muslims, and Buddhists. It was during my own Montessori training that I first encountered Sikhs, and I was struck by their deep interest in her educational vision. Members of the Baha'i faith, too, have found this vision compelling.

## A Holistic Vision of the Universe

Kramer's biography showed remarkably little interest in the spiritual dimension of Montessori's life and work, and what she perceived as a "peculiar tension" between rationality and "intuition" was, in my view, neither peculiar nor tense. The blend of science and religion in Montessori's worldview forms the basis for a truly *holistic* conception of the universe. Similarly to fellow Catholic theologian/scientists Teilhard de Chardin and Thomas Berry (among others), and in a way not unlike the "spiritual science" of Rudolf Steiner, Montessori looked carefully and deeply into the world of nature and found, not isolated material entities interacting mechanically, but a living and purposeful Cosmos. "All things are part of the universe, and are connected with each other to form one whole unity" (Montessori, 1973, p. 8). She was deeply impressed by the *harmony* she discerned in the natural world, the ecology of existence that gives every living thing a meaningful function in the larger system. Every species, indeed every individual organism, contributes to the good of the whole by performing its inherent "cosmic" function. This harmony has not emerged randomly, but expresses "a pre-established plan" that is "of divine origin"; she was convinced that "the purpose of life is to obey the occult command which harmonizes all and creates an ever better world" (Montessori, 1989b). The Cosmos is engaged in a process of evolution toward ever greater harmony—toward the fulfillment of God's mysterious purpose.

The guiding belief of Montessori's educational philosophy, the fundamental point around which all her principles and techniques revolve, is her conviction that *humanity has its own special function to fulfill in this divine evolution.* The human species is "God's prime agent in creation" and it is our responsibility to "learn to do more effectively our share of work in the cosmic plan" (Montessori, 1973, pp. 26, 33). Evolution is not yet complete; God's purpose has not yet been achieved, and the mission of human life is to give expression to the formative forces within us that are yearning to complete the cosmic plan. We are called to work in partnership with the divine. This understanding of our existence places all our endeavors—our cultural, political, economic, and even our most personal strivings—in an entirely spiritual light: "The world was not created for us to enjoy," Montessori proclaims, "but we are created in order to evolve the cosmos" (Montessori 1989b, p. 22). In an earlier essay (Miller, 2000), I argued that this striking statement is consistent with the teachings of great moral sages such as Martin Luther King, Jr., Abraham Heschel, and Krishnamurti, who all similarly asserted that we are on this Earth to contribute to the unfolding of divine justice, harmony and wisdom, not merely to amuse ourselves or satisfy our many material and sensual desires. In this light, education is not to be seen merely as preparation for a successful career or any sort of social or intellectual distinction; rather, education is the process of awakening the divine formative forces within every person's soul that enable the individual to make his or her own unique contribution to the cosmic plan, to fulfill his or her own destiny.

Montessori wrote that humanity's role in evolution is to construct a "supra-nature"—a social, cultural and technological extension of nature that calls forth ever greater dimensions of human creativity and understanding—a notion very similar to Teilhard de Chardin's "noosphere." This is humanity's task because we, more than any other living species, "can receive the emanations of the Godhead" and transform divine plans into physical and cultural manifestations (Montessori, 1972a, p. 35). But she repeatedly observed that our material and technological progress had far outpaced our psychological, moral and spiritual development, and in the twentieth century it was imperative that we make a determined effort toward remedying this imbalance. Modern societies, due to their pervasive materialism, have neglected the spiritual forces that animate the human being, and our institutions, particularly schooling, have become repressive and damaging, turning people into "slaves" of the machine rather than cultivating their spiritual sensitivity, she wrote. Modern people are ill prepared to deal with the great moral challenges of our age, and are unable to resist the demons of nationalism and war that threaten to engulf the world.

To address this imbalance, Montessori envisioned a curriculum for elementary school students that she called "cosmic education." The purpose of this approach is to provide the young person with an expansive, inspiring vision of the grandeur of the universe and one's personal destiny within it. This is an education that gives life meaning because all aspects of creation are shown to fit into a complex, interconnected whole that is far larger than our customary limited worldview. Aline D. Wolf comments that

> The value of cosmic education, as I see it, is that it places the child's life in a spiritual perspective. No one can be confronted

with the cosmic miracle and not see that there is more to life than our everyday experiences. Fast foods, designer sneakers, video games and sports heroes all pale beside the wonder of the universe (Wolf, 1996, p. 97).

Cosmic education lifts the young person's consciousness out of the mundane, materialistic concerns of modern society and instills a sense of awe, touching a receptive and searching force within the soul.

This is exactly the sort of "spiritual reconstruction" that Montessori intended when she spoke at several international peace conferences in the 1930s, and asserted that only the spiritual renewal of humankind through education, not any superficial economic or political effort, could alter the violent course of human history: "The real danger threatening humanity is the emptiness in men's souls; all the rest is merely a consequence of this emptiness" (Montessori, 1972a, pp. 44, 53). In recognition of her efforts, Montessori was nominated for the Nobel Peace Prize in 1949, 1950 and 1951.

Consistent with her holistic understanding, Montessori saw all of humanity as one nation, even one organism—an "organic unity." She considered people as fundamentally being citizens of the Cosmos beyond their social or cultural conditioning. Given technological developments of the modern age, she argued, it was time to put partial identities and false distinctions aside, and work together globally to achieve our "collective mission" of furthering the evolution of consciousness. It is education's task to encourage peaceful cooperation "and readiness to shed prejudices in the interests of common work for the cosmic plan, which may also be called the Will of God, actively expressed in the whole of His creation" (Montessori, 1973, p. 74). Her views on peace, social justice and democracy flowed from this holistic religious conviction that human beings all share the task of building a divinely ordered world. Idealism born of economic analysis or ideological conviction alone would not be sufficient. A socialist early in her life, at one point later in her career she addressed a group of communists and bluntly informed them that their social revolution would fail unless people were uplifted "towards the laws that govern human nature, which are connected to the very laws of the universe" (Montessori, 1989a, p. 101). Democracy and justice *follow* from the unfolding of divine potentials, and social change is not authentic unless it springs from a genuine love of humanity, which is a spiritual, not simply an intellectual, commitment.

## THE CHILD AS SPIRITUAL EMBRYO

Montessori often compared the process of psychological and spiritual development to the physical unfolding of the human organism. Just as the material body first takes shape as a self-forming embryo, requiring during its formation the protection and nurturance of the womb that envelopes it, the human soul first appears in the newborn child in an embryonic form that requires nourishment from a psychic womb—the protective environment of loving, caring parents and a spiritually responsive education. Montessori's distinctive notion of the child as a "spiritual embryo" emphasized her key principle that the growing human being is not simply a biological or psychological entity, but a spiritual energy seeking expression in the form of a human body within the physical and cultural world. She compared the mysterious emergence of spiritual life in the child to the Incarnation of God in Christ described in the New Testament, "when the Word was made flesh and dwelt among us" (Montessori, 1972b, p. 29). For Montessori, the Word is made flesh in *every* child born in the world; each human being has his or her path of incarnation to follow, his or her destiny. Montessori, like Emerson, referred to the "secret" within the soul of every child—the personal spiritual imperative that transcends whatever social prejudices, ideologies, and mundane educational curricula that adults seek to overlay onto the child's personality.

Reflecting on the unusually lengthy period of physical dependence that human infants (compared to other species) experience, Montessori was convinced that early childhood is designed to be a time of intense psychic receptivity. The young child takes in the world through an "absorbent mind," literally incarnating (taking into its bodymind) the sensations, impressions, and feelings it receives from the surrounding environment. One of the guiding principles of Montessori pedagogy, the concept of "sensitive periods," expresses her observation that young children move through periods of development during which they are especially attuned to particular characteristics in the environment. When they are ready to acquire language they hungrily, effortlessly absorb it by hearing it spoken around them; when they are ready to develop fine motor skills they begin to act on their surroundings accordingly. It is the task of parents and educators to provide the stimulation and resources the developing child needs at these critical times. Keep in mind that for Montessori this is not simply a biological or pedagogical responsibility, but a profound spiritual task, because the child is being directed by its embryonic spiritual energies to reach out to the world to fashion a personality. Careless parenting or education, by stifling optimum development, frustrates the child's spiritual formation.

Montessori frequently commented that the child creates the adult—not, as our modern common sense has it, the other way around. The spiritual energy seeking expression through the child's encounters with the world is engaged in building a person in a way that no adult education or conscious effort can achieve. By adulthood an individual's psychological identity is deeply engrained, and learning no longer takes place through "incarnation" or absorption. Therefore it is crucial for parents and educators to allow the child's own inherent nature to emerge and act within the world. As Montessori put it in 1915,

> We must believe that all beings develop by themselves, of themselves, and that we cannot do better than not to interrupt that development. We must confess to ourselves that the psychic life of man is full of mysteries.... The preparation for the teacher is twofold: to be sensitive to the mystery and to be sensitive to the wonder of life revealing itself (in Buckenmeyer, 1997, p. 35).

Montessori called the spiritual embryo humanity's "most precious treasure" because it was only this divine formative power that could transform the world: "The child promises the redemption of humanity, and we might say that this truth is represented by the mystical symbol of the Nativity" (1972a, pp. 36, 104). By failing to appreciate the value of this treasure, and educating young people only to participate dutifully in a materialistic, mechanistic system of economic production, modern societies are diminishing the visionary creativity, the moral insight, and above all the loving compassion that divine energies promise to bring to bear on the problems of human life. Montessori was convinced that through the child, these energies could be released into the world as a powerful source of good. It is evident throughout her work that the heart of Montessori's educational mission was not to introduce special techniques or materials into pedagogical practice but to make a fervent plea to the modern world to become "sensitive to the wonder of life revealing itself" through the life of each child. That was the appeal she made for fifty years to audiences and readers throughout the world.

## THE CHILDREN'S HOME

If we perceive Montessori's message in this light, the *casa dei bambini* she established in Rome in 1907 cannot be viewed merely as a prototype for a child-centered preschool. The term is usually translated into English as "children's house," and even many Montessori schools are named with some variation of "Children's House" or "House of Children." But the learning environment Montessori sought to provide was not simply a house—a physical space with child-sized furniture and developmentally appropriate materials. The correct translation of *casa dei bambini*, as Dorothy Canfield Fisher insisted in 1912, is "children's home." Feminist philosopher Jane Roland Martin explicitly built on this understanding of Montessori's vision in her concept of the "schoolhome"—an educational setting that provides the love, caring and nurturance that young human beings vitally require for their healthy development (Martin, 1992). Martin observed that in the modern industrial age, as both men and women leave home to work, children are left without the strong "domestic context" that provides a nurturing womb for their psychological, emotional and moral unfolding. She argued that even though John Dewey, around the same time as Montessori, sought to address the problems industrialization posed to children's development, Montessori understood far better than Dewey the role of this "domestic," traditionally feminine, realm of nurturing. Montessori "had inserted family love into school," an endeavor Martin regarded as critically needed in our time (Martin, 1992, p. 14).

While this is not the place to discuss the details of classroom practice in Montessori schools, it is important to recognize that for Montessori and the movement she inspired, the design of a "home" for nurturing children's spiritual development suggests specific pedagogical requirements. First, it is necessary to understand the meaning of freedom in Montessori education. She often advocated the "liberty" of students in the learning environment, and emphasized the principle, quoted above, that "all beings develop by themselves" and adults "cannot do better than not to interrupt that development." However, she clearly did not mean to endorse the absolute trust in children's actions expressed by educators such as A. S. Neill or, later, John Holt. As long as a child is engaging in *constructive* activity, the adult must stay out of the way because divine forces are at work, but we need to be vigilant for lapses in concentration when a child's impulsive desires or negative reactions to earlier events start to dominate his or her activities. Montessori believed that the educator needs to be acutely sensitive to the meaning of children's behavior, and should distinguish between random, impulsive, destructive activity, and genuinely purposeful pursuits guided by "eternal laws" working within the child's soul.

Montessori sought, above all, to cultivate inner discipline through purposeful activity. In her view, the child becomes "normalized"—capable of acting responsibly, independently—through concentration. The educator's task is to assist the child in finding connections to the environment that call forth concentrated attention and effort.

It is the environment that educates, not the teacher directly; more precisely, it is the child's inherent formative energies, finding material in the environment to act upon purposefully, that calls or brings forth (the genuine meaning of the word "educate") the child's true nature. The educational process starts with the individual, with self-formation, and then extends out into the social life of the classroom. Progressive educators have always had misgivings about the Montessori approach because this emphasis on personal independence reverses Dewey's premise that all learning, and even the development of the individual personality, is grounded in social interaction. Montessori saw children growing from inside out, from a spiritual source, where Dewey saw the human being developed through dialogue and negotiation with the social environment. Montessori was not, however, advocating some sort of rugged individualism: She was convinced that a child allowed to develop "normally" would naturally forge a loving relationship with the larger world, starting in the classroom and radiating outward to all humanity.

Because Montessori emphasized the importance of the environment in learning, her theory has been criticized as being "empiricist" in a Lockean sense, meaning that she appeared to privilege sensory and intellectual content over imagination or the construction of meaning. The emphasis in her early childhood environment, in particular, is on "sensorial" materials, and she asserted that for the most part young children would gain more by being engaged in concrete activities (purposeful work) than in fantasy play. On this point, it is quite remarkable that even while Montessori's spiritual conception of the world paralleled that of Rudolf Steiner (Coulter, 1991), her educational approach is vastly different from Waldorf pedagogy's explicit and detailed cultivation of imagination, and it differs as well from "constructivist" educators' emphasis on free play.

In short, to create a proper home for the developing human soul, Montessori argued that educators must provide a "prepared environment" that would answer to specific patterns of development as she understood them. In assessing Montessori's vision, I think it is useful to separate the *principle* that the growing child requires a spiritual home that enables the true self to develop from the *prescription* of what that environment must entail. I believe that the principle is universal, and that Montessori deserves enormous credit for formulating it. Yet, it seems likely that Montessori's own understanding of learning and child development, despite her claim to scientific objectivity, was partially conditioned by her own historical, cultural and religious context, just as any theory of pedagogy is necessarily so conditioned. If we truly have faith in the dynamic, possibly divine creative energies seeking expression through us, then it seems to me that we must be willing to subject our assumptions, our methods and techniques to the test of ongoing experience. We will find, I believe, that various portions of the Montessori "method" will be more or less relevant to the needs of particular children in particular situations at particular times. I believe we can acknowledge this, even as we appreciate the genius of this brilliant woman's soaring, liberating vision.

This essay has provided only a brief overview of Maria Montessori's spiritual conception of education. Yet these reflections are enough to make us realize that current educational policies, with their single-minded emphasis on unforgiving standards, rigorous testing, and accountability to corporate and bureaucratic elites, are a sad perversion of education's possibilities. We have before us the living child, the incarnation of cosmic energies, the potential source of social renewal and harmony among humanity, and we treat this priceless treasure as "intellectual capital" to feed our voracious economic system. Montessori proclaimed an alternative to the deadening materialism of the twentieth century, but, except for her relatively small following of devotees, her vision has been ignored and bypassed in the march toward global technocracy. I suggest that it is time to rediscover her vision. It is time, as Fisher declared ninety years ago, to "think hard" about "whether we really honestly wish the spiritually best for our children, or only the materially best."

## NOTE

1. Readers familiar with my work will recognize the point I am making here. In all my writing on holistic education, I have insisted that we look beyond the differences in particular methods and techniques and consider the essence of holistic education to be an open minded, open hearted sensitivity to the actual life of the child and to the specific social and cultural context of that child's life. Montessori and Rudolf Steiner were ultimately exploring the same deep truths about human existence, but they formulated distinct methods in response to different cultural needs (see Coulter, 1991). John Holt, whom I mention later in this essay, derived his methodless educational approach (which finally evolved into what he called "unschooling") from an open minded sensitivity both to children and to the social and political milieu of his time and place that was every bit as acute as Montessori's to hers. To ask whose method (or nonmethod) is "correct" or even "universal" is the wrong question. What we need to know is whether our chosen pedagogical approach is truly nourishing the unfolding inner life of the young person standing before us. I believe this principle is reflected in the diversity of perspectives represented in this volume.

## REFERENCES

Buckenmeyer, Robert G. (ed). (1997). *The California Lectures of Maria Montessori, 1915: Collected Speeches and Writings*. Oxford, UK: ABC-Clio.

Cavalletti, Sofia (1999). "Discovering the Real Spiritual Child" *NAMTA Journal*, Vol. 24, No. 2 (Spring, 1999), pp. 7-16. (North American Montessori Teachers Association, 11424 Bellflower Rd., Cleveland, OH 44106.)

Coulter, Dee Joy (1991). "Montessori and Steiner: A Pattern of Reverse Symmetries" *Holistic Education Review*, Vol. 4, No. 2 (Summer, 1991), pp. 30-32.

Fisher, Dorothy Canfield (1912). *A Montessori Mother*. New York: Henry Holt.

Kramer, Rita (1976). *Maria Montessori: A Biography*. New York: Putman.

Lillig, Tina (1999). "The History of the Catechesis of the Good Shepherd" *NAMTA Journal* Vol. 24, No. 2 (Spring, 1999), pp. 29-38.

Martin, Jane Roland (1992). *The Schoolhome: Rethinking Schools for Changing Families*. Cambridge, MA: Harvard University Press.

Miller, Ron (1997). *What Are Schools For? Holistic Education in American Culture* (3rd edition) Brandon,VT: Holistic Education Press.

Miller, Ron (2000). "Education and the Evolution of the Cosmos" in *Caring for New Life: Essays on Holistic Education*. Brandon, VT: Foundation for Educational Renewal.

Montessori, Maria (1949/1972a). *Education and Peace*. Chicago: Henry Regnery.

Montessori, Maria (1936/1972b). *The Secret of Childhood*. New York: Ballantine.

Montessori, Maria (1948/1973). *To Educate the Human Potential*. Madras, India: Kalakshetra.

Montessori, Maria (1989a). *The Child, Society and the World: Unpublished Speeches and Writings*. Compiled and edited by Günter Schulz-Benesch; translated by Caroline Juler and Heather Yesson. Oxford, UK: Clio Press.

Montessori, Maria (1946/1989b). *Education for a New World*. Oxford, UK: Clio Press.

Montessori, Mario (1984). "Dr. Maria Montessori and the Child" in *The Spiritual Hunger of the Modern Child: A Series of Ten Lectures*. Charles Town, WV: Claymont. (The lectures published in this volume had been given in London in 1961.)

Wolf, Aline D. (1996). *Nurturing the Spirit in Non-sectarian Classrooms*. Hollidaysburg, PA: Parent Child Press.

# CHAPTER 15

# Waldorf Education

## Reflections on the Essentials

### Jeffrey Kane

I want to experience things not just learn about them.
(Emily Kane, 17)

## THE NEED FOR AN EXPERIENCE OF KNOWLEDGE

In early January 2001, after nearly two decades of a national obsession with educational reform, the polls indicated that Americans placed education as their number one national priority over tax cuts, issues of women's rights or the economy. Recognizing the importance of the issue, the newly inaugurated George W. Bush unveiled an education proposal as his first major policy initiative. On January 24, 2001, *The New York Times* carried a front page story on the Bush plan which began with the following sentence, "President Bush proposed a significant increase today in the federal role in public education, detailing an ambitious plan that includes requirements that states test all students in the third through eighth grades and report on their progress to the public, states and the federal government."

Clearly, the perceived problem in American education, a problem identified with the publication of *A Nation At Risk* in 1983, is that American students are not performing sufficiently well on standardized tests. With little analysis of the value of such standardized testing or the social, economic and political factors that make for dramatically different levels of educational achievement or of the merit of increasing test scores, a crisis has been defined and a solution proposed.

However, the plan for the future, and the path we have now being set for a national education reform effort, will likely only deepen an unnoticed crisis in American education: a spiritual crisis.

This spiritual crisis lies at the very heart of American educational policy and the daily experience of children in classrooms. This crisis is neither ephemeral or removed from the only partially perceived failure of our schools.

The problem is that children are given so little to enliven their thinking, engage their feelings or strengthen their character. There is so little to educate them, to draw them forth and guide them in their unfolding as people. They often leave school without a hint that the world may have a transcendent meaning, a meaning within which they participate and ultimately define themselves as human beings.

The process of educational reform over the past two decades has been driven by economic considerations where the global competitions of post-industrial markets have replaced concern for what children need to grow and learn. The principles guiding national educational policy in the United States and in countries, East and West, have nothing to do with children but with the expanding of global market share. Multinational corporations whose means and objectives are now virtually unmediated by national boundaries or loyalties, exert their influence in education, to sell their goods and services, to maximize (according to their perceptions) the supply of labor and to grow new consumers.

In terms of the need for labor in this "age of information," children amount to no more than "intellectual capital." The near universal corporate goal is to fill children's minds with information and to develop the skills necessary to process information. The primary methods used — increased intellectual standards and testing — reflect corporate operating procedures rather than insight into child development, learning theory or effective educational practice. The sole measure of educational quality is output, or as we say in education, "outcomes," outcomes governed by political and economic interests.

At the same time, the American public has viewed education as a means of continuous upward mobility for its children. Doubtless, few parents see their own children as "intellectual capital," but they do see them as future wage-earners and hope for their prosperity. The dramatic development of technology has created even greater urgency on the part of parents to see education as the only way of providing the new knowledge and skills that are perceived as necessary for the "information era."

At the same time, the clamor grows for character education. There is increased concern about violence in the schools, a lack of "family values" and the use of drugs (both prescribed and those popular on the streets) used to "cope" with life.

This second set of issues is not seen as related to the drive for the raising of test scores. The possibility does not seem to surface that the failure of reform and the troubling trends in children and adolescents stem from the same problem: a lack of inner experience, a vital experience of knowledge. Yet, with each passing year of failed reform, policy makers and the public reify their strategies rather than question their assumptions. All the while, schools become more shallow and lifeless. There is less and less to nourish children's souls.

Most children come to school with a natural curiosity, a love of the world and for discovering its secrets. This joy fades with the emphasis on intellectual study where detachment and analysis are the rule even as educators struggle to make their lessons interesting or simply "fun." The problem here is that we do little to promote children's inner activity — to give them a sense of belonging in this world in all its aspects, a sense of meaning, a sense of purpose. Our approach to knowledge is inwardly vacant and disenchanting, literally. We systematically diminish our children's natural sensibilities rather than bringing them to fruition as part of balanced human development.

Vaclav Havel, the Czech playwright, dissident, prisoner, and now president wrote,

> I think that the reasons for the crisis in which the world now finds itself are lodged in something deeper than a particular way of organizing the economy or a particular political system…. Where does the cause of this crisis lie?
>
> I'm persuaded that this [crisis] is directly related to the spiritual condition of modern civilization. This condition is characterized byloss: the loss of metaphysi cacertainties, of an experience of the transcendental …and any kind of higher horizon. (From *Disturbing the Peace*, quoted in Gardner 1992, p. 8)

The purpose of this chapter is not to analyze educational policy or to criticize the good intentions of people concerned about their children. My intention here is to suggest that the real crisis in education lies in our materialistic and mechanistic assumptions about the world, ourselves and in the interaction of the two in the process of education. The nature of this crisis requires more than innovations in curriculum, instructional methodologies and assessment. We need to examine not only our educational policies and practices but the assumptions they embody about what the world is, who we are and what we are doing here.

## WALDORF EDUCATION

In this context, the Waldorf School movement provides a substantial, well-developed approach to education that stands in stark contrast to contemporary educational theory. Waldorf Education is rooted in the spiritual scientific research of Rudolf Steiner (1861-1925), an Austrian philosopher and scientist. Steiner, a scholar with considerable formal training, had a remarkable capacity for spiritual insight. He combined these two in over 350 volumes of collected work on subjects as varied as agriculture, medicine, economics, social theory and, of course, education. His work attracted the attention of industrialist Emil Molt, the owner of the Waldorf Astoria cigarette factory in Stuttgart, Germany. He was asked to establish a school for the children of the factory workers. Steiner accepted the task and led in the creation of the first Waldorf School which opened its doors in 1919. Since that time students of Steiner's work have opened 750 schools in 44 nations.

The Waldorf Schools do not merely offer alternative "techniques" for motivating students, developing their thinking skills or making learning more interesting or entertaining. The pedagogy is rooted in a spiritual conception of the world and of the human being. For Steiner, the physical world is spiritual in nature, and we cannot separate out spiritual concepts or beliefs from our attempt to understand the world around us. Hence, spiritual concerns cannot be removed from the curriculum or made into a separate subject area for religion or moral values.

In Steiner's view, the spiritual world is fluid, dynamic, formative; it cannot be understood by concepts which are concrete, fixed or detached. Understanding the spiritual activity of the world requires inner activity within the human being; the creative in the world can only be understood through awakening the creative within us. Through this awakening, we can understand the forces operating in the physical world and tend to all manner and sort of practical issues. Steiner writes, "We want to use the subject matter in our Waldorf School in such a way that at each stage of instruction, it will improve the human development of the pupil regarding the formation of the will, feeling and intellect rather than serving to provide superficial knowledge" (Steiner, 1995b, p. 11).

A deeper kind of thinking is necessary than can be understood or recognized through our scientistic approach to cognition.

When we understand that the physical world is spiritually rooted, we can understand that each lesson we are taught not only provides information for our minds but is also an opportunity to draw forth and develop ourselves as full human beings. The task of the Waldorf educator, therefore, is not merely to develop in children the social and cognitive skills that may be required for adult life but,more importantly, the task of the Waldorf educator is to guide children to develop the depth of heart, capacities for the inner experience of thinking, and the strength of will in balance with one another so that they (the children) can do in the world what they have come to do.

It seems that in our attempts to make human beings effective processors of information in an age of information, we have diminished the capacity to see into and appreciate the world, ourselves and one another in such a way as to give us a sense of purpose, connection and commitment in our lives. Waldorf educator John Gardner explains that the aim of education is to ensure that *"knowledge shall grow out of a full human experience"* and that such experience shall be the foundation of whole human development.

> Ordinarily, the knowledge with which education confronts the child consists of facts that are to be observed and ideas that are to be thought. Such observations and thoughts certainly use a part of the human capacity for experience, but not the larger part. They leave out both the feeling and the active sides of a child's nature. Arithmetic, spelling, grammar, science, geography, and history, as these are generally taught in school, make little contribution to a student's desire to be humanly touched and moved. (Gardner, 1975, p. 8)

Gardner once said that, "the deep calls unto the deep." The deepest in us calls forth for the deepest in the world. Steiner writes, "Ordinary thinking is dead, a mere corpse of the soul, and one has to become aware of it as such through suffusing it with one's own soul life.... Then one realizes that [what] one possesses in ... living thinking has no connection whatsoever with the physical world but is none the less real" (1974, pp. 41-42). Steiner is not denying the reality of the physical world but explaining that it is governed by spiritual forces that are vital and creative, forces that can be known only as we become equally vital and creative within ourselves. In order to understand the experience of knowledge, it is necessary to develop a picture of the two poles of experience: the world and the child. It is, therefore, essential to look more closely at how Steiner understands the world and child development.

## THE WORLD WE KNOW

One way to understand the relationship between the spiritual and physical worlds is by way of a metaphor I developed in a previous book, *Education, Information and Transformation*. It goes as follows:

> Imagine there is a planet where the inhabitants have very refined skills equivalent to those we normally associate with inquiry in the physical sciences. They have the ability to observe with precision, identify discrete variables, and apply a calculus to describe the interactions of things they observe. The inhabitants have honed these skills but no other cognitive or expressive capacities. On their planet, the arts do not exist. There is no music.

> Now imagine that one of these extra-terrestrials visits our planet and finds him or herself outside a building listening to someone inside playing a violin. Using his or her skills, the visitor begins a study by listening carefully to each of the notes, identifying each of their characteristics and attempting to find explicit patterns in their relationships. Our visitor takes each note and defines it in terms of its duration, amplitude, and frequency. With this information, the visitor constructs a mathematical model to describe to colleagues "back home" exactly what was discovered.

> However, this would not be able to describe anything more than sound or vibrations in the air. He or she would not be able to observe or understand that each of the notes carries meaning. This exacting scientist would not be able to discern that each of the notes, each characteristic of each of the notes, and the configuration of all the notes together, including the intervals of silence between them, were governed by a meaning transcending physical characteristics.

Leaving our planet, this observent alien would not have a clue that there is music on our planet or that what he or she heard ultimately was more a creation of a musician's vision than simply the vibration of air. (Kane, 1998, p. 3)

This metaphor illustrates Steiner's view of the spiritual and physical worlds as well as the necessary limitations of the scientistic mode of thought undergirding Western thinking for the past 400 years. The music and, indeed, the musician, represent the spiritual dimensions of the world. The sound represents physical existence. Each chord, each note, each silence is governed by a spiritual meaning transcending the music itself. So it is with the physical world; all things and everything are imbued with a spiritual meaning transcending the world itself.

The largely reductionistic approach to understanding prevalent in the West (and now embodied in virtually all the modern world) is at once incapable of grasping the principles overarching the physical world and, at the same time, its own limitations. When listening to a piece of music, we know that it has meaning; it is not a matter of faith but of inner experience (even as our tastes are largely driven by culture). Depending upon the particular opus, it resonates within us. We are inwardly moved. Something experienced by the musician and composer is not only conveyed to us but becomes generative in us. We can be led to experience the sublimity or power of nature or an enormous range of human emotions from sheer joy to base disillusionment. The music quickens something of one sort or another in us or we soon lose aesthetic interest; we are not inwardly moved.

In our metaphor, the alien traveler begins his/her attempt at understanding by reducing all thinking to ideas that, for all their precision, do not allow for inner activity. In Western history this elimination of this personal dimension of thinking is most dramatically represented in Descartes' method of systematic doubt. His approach to thinking was to eliminate anything from his thinking that could be subject to doubt and in the process reduced the world to fragmented pieces which he then reconstructed using what he believed to be mathematical precision. The central problem here is that he removed all things from contexts and connections that could be understood through aesthetic or immediate intuition. He asserted that all things had to be related according to his concept of logic. In doing so, he precluded the possibility of principles and relationships beyond abstract reasoning. Descartes removed the knower from the known and consequently eliminated the possibility of apprehending the Creative in the Created.

When thinking is disconnected from feeling and will, it is dead. It severs the vital connections that animate and give form to things, including ourselves. The structure of our thinking, as Descartes' heirs, the implicit assumptions that play out in our explicit concepts, preclude the possibility of a higher awareness in us or higher meaning flowing through creation. Since the seventeenth century our methods of scientific inquiry have grown far more sophisticated than Descartes' speculations while sitting in his room. We have moved from "undoubtable" principles to publicly observable empirical phenomena. We do not apply logic as a method of constructing knowledge; we experiment through the manipulation of variables for the application of mathematical formulae. He developed a system of thinking. We have adapted and applied it to create a calculus of the empirical. Yet, the differences, as radical as they may be, have not changed the essential nature of the knower or the known. The modern paradigm has no place for the Creative in the world or the Creative in us. In this context, there is no possibility for meaning working through creation or quickening the Creative in us. We have inherited the habit of mind to segment, to fragment, phenomena in order to create a picture of the world. In doing so, we have amassed enormous power to control nature. However, we have diminished our capacity to see things in their relation beyond our limited focus. We have created a vision of the world and ourselves without meaning or purpose. Physicist Bohm explains that

> In essence, the process of division is a way of *thinking about things* that is convenient and useful mainly in the domains of practical, technical, and functional activities (e.g., to divide up an area of land into different fields where various crops are to be grown). However, when this mode of thought is applied more broadly to man's notion of himself and the whole world in which he lives (i.e., to his self-world view), then man ceases to regard the resulting divisions as merely useful or convenient and begins to see and experience himself and his world as actually constituted of separately existent fragments. (1980, p. 9)

A different kind of thinking is necessary to apprehend transcendent ideas active in creation, in the evolution of the world and in our unfolding as human beings.

While Descartes sought to ground his thinking in a detached objectification of the world, Steiner explains that "living" thinking requires that we be inwardly active, that we experience within ourselves the Creative ideas at work in all we perceive. There is a resonance where we engage the Creative in the world with the Creative within ourselves. Instead of standing back and reducing the world to abstract pieces, he encourages us to embrace the forces at work through imagination fired by both will and feeling.

American transcendentalist Ralph Waldo Emerson put it succinctly, "Every fact is a symbol of a spiritual fact. Every appearance in nature corresponds to some state of mind ..." (1965, p. 197). A spiritual fact is not isolated or complete unto itself; it is formative, enmeshed in the dynamic continuity of the Creative. As such, its apprehension requires that we respond with reciprocal inner activity. Emerson explains that

> Behind nature, throughout nature, spirit is present; one and not compound, it does not set upon us from without, that is, in space and time, but spiritually, or through ourselves; therefore, that spirit, that is the supreme Being, does not build up nature around us, but puts it forth through us, as the life of the tree puts forth new branches and leaves through the pores of the old" (p. 216).

Living knowledge is not simply information stored in our heads; it is not power over the environment. It is bound up in our very being and serves as a source of unity with all Being. Through encounter with the Creative, we are educated, drawn forth and become. Sometimes, when we see something new, unexpected or afresh from a new angle or in a new context, we can experience an inner resonance, a stirring of the Creative within us by the Creative within the world. By way of example, I recently went for a walk on a suburban university campus with a colleague from the city. As we walked, he noticed with absolute delight rabbits hopping from bush to bush. I could see that they struck a chord in him, and that he, in a very subtle way, experienced a bit of wonder in creation and expanded, ever so slightly, his own sense of appreciation for life. In a more universal illustration of our capacity to sense the transcendent quality of nature, Emerson writes, "If the stars should appear one night in a thousand years, how would men believe and adore; and preserve for many generations the remembrance of the city of God which had been shown!" (p. 188). What is true for the stars is true for all things. Coleridge declares, "Every object, rightly seen, unlocks a new faculty of the soul" (Emerson, p. 202).

## THE CHILD

Each fact, like a note in a symphony, is both physical and transcendent; it conveys meaning that we may or may not perceive depending on our own inner activity. Steiner explains that our inner resources, our capacities to experience meaning are not fully developed as we enter the world, but emerge in a metamorphic fashion over the course of our lives. As these capacities unfold, new possibilities emerge for the Creative in the world to awaken the Creative within us — to Become. The Waldorf curriculum is, therefore, centered on the development of the child; it is a correspondence between the emergent capacities of the child and the spiritual qualities that may be found in subject matter.

The focus of the curriculum is to "teach [children] only what the essence of humanity dictates" (1995b, p. 55). Steiner writes, "We want to learn from the very nature of the developing child how children want to develop themselves as human beings, that is, how their nature, their essence should develop to become truly human" (p. 55). This unlocking or unfolding is at the core of the Waldorf approach to education, and it requires that we respond to the potential for growth found at the various stages of childhood.

Steiner sees the child as descending from the spiritual into the physical world. This process of incarnation is metamorphic rather than linear. It is not a matter of the gradual accumulation of physical, social and cognitive skills. Rather, Steiner explains that childhood consists of a succession of stages each marked by the development of a predominant mode of experience. During the first seven years, until roughly the change of teeth, the central faculty is the will. The following stage, lasting until the onset of puberty is dominated by the image of feeling. The third stage, lasting approximately another seven years, is the time when the faculty of independent thinking matures. Given the importance of these stages in determining the Waldorf curriculum and instructional methods, let us look at each of them more closely.

Steiner observes that the first stage of childhood is dominated by the senses. Infants and young children are immersed in their immediate environments. Everything flows into them directly and without mediation. The environment is not limited to their physical surroundings but includes the behaviors, attitudes and dispositions of those around them.

These influences have profound importance in developing their physical bodies — the primary work at this stage of life. Waldorf educator Henry Barnes concludes,

> Everything — anger, love, joy, hate, intelligence, stupidity - speaks through the tone of voice, the physical touch, bodily gesture, light, darkness, color, harmony, and disharmony. These influences are absorbed by the still forming physical organism and affect it for a lifetime. (Fenner & Rivers, 1995, p. 9)

Children, at this age, are not passive observers. Steiner states that "the spiritual world is still fully active in a child in the first seven years of life" (1995a, p. 7). Children are active and their activity is shaped by their environment. In short, they imitate. The primary mode of learning at this stage is through imitation.

Imitation is not a simple mimicking, but, as Barnes notes, "the power to identify oneself with one's immediate environment through one's active will" (Fenner & Rivers, 1995, p. 9). The creative forces in the children resonate directly with the factors at play in the immediate surroundings. Children do not learn to understand the world through reflection or analysis. Rather, they imaginatively merge with their environment. They and the environment are one in a dance of activity. The children "indwell" in the world; they imagine into it through action. When young children play with dolls, they dwell in the world as another — as mother, father or family dog. They "try the world on" from multiple perspectives by imitating what they see. This recreation is the process by which children build their bodies and lay the cognitive foundations for the later development of the intellect. Writer M. C. Richards writes, "In early childhood, intelligence lives in the will. It metamorphoses then into intelligence of feeling, and again metamorphoses and awakes as the capacity for rational judgment" (1980, p. 52).

Given these considerations, Steiner stresses the importance of providing an environment worthy of imitation, an environment where children can imaginatively indwell in the world, identify themselves with it through activity as Barnes explains, and form the generative foundations for the next phases of human development. Waldorf preschool classes are filled with opportunities for imaginative play from a dress-up corner to little kitchens, to watertables and wooden blocks, trucks and tractors. The children paint in simple, bright watercolors, bake bread, sing songs, mold beeswax figures and play freely together. These are the active foundations for the later development of the intellect. The alphabet, readers, math materials and the like are nowhere to be found in Waldorf preschools. Such abstract objects do not provide for the immediate imaginative engagement of the will.

In the next phase of childhood, following the change of teeth, children begin to understand things more through their feelings than their wills alone. Certainly, infants and young children have feelings, but such feelings are not a primary mode of understanding. In this second phase of childhood, children sense their separateness from the larger environment and take a step back. They slowly shift from expressing in action what they see to mediating their activity with a sense of their own responses to the world. They begin to experience things through their own feelings. This experience is a stage between indwelling and intellectual distance. It is a precursor to the development of the intellect, but not yet the proper stage for intellectual study. Steiner explains, "it is no mere figure of speech to say that man can understand with his feeling, his sentiment, his inner disposition as well as his intellect" (1975, p. 37).

It is uncommon to assert that feeling has much to do with cognition in anything but a personal sense. We do not normally feel that we develop our understanding of the world through our feelings but rather through rational thought. These assumptions have been imbedded in our culture, as we have removed human experience from the development of understanding. However, Steiner maintained that human feeling is part of the awakening process of the creative within us to the creative within the world. Steiner explains,

> It is not easy, at first, to believe that feelings like reverence and respect have anything to do with cognition. This is due to the fact that we are inclined to set cognition aside as a faculty by itself — one that stands in no relation to what otherwise occurs in the soul. In so thinking we do not bear in mind that it is the soul which exercises the faculty of cognition; and feelings are for the soul what food is for the body.... Veneration, homage, devotion are like nutriment making it healthy and strong, especially strong for the activity of cognition. Disrespect, antipathy, underestimation of what deserves recognition, all exert a paralyzing and withering effect on this faculty of cognition." (1975, p. 23)

These feelings can be engendered through the experience of what Emerson calls "the miraculous and common." The "miraculous" refers to the spiritual forces that give all things their form and substance; the "common" refers to all things familiar or seemingly insignificant. The miraculous is the meaning running through all things. In an educational context, Steiner explains,

> As before the age of seven we have to give the child the actual physical pattern for him to copy, so between the time of the changing of teeth and puberty, we must bring into his environment things with the right inner meaning and value. For it is from the inner meaning and value of things that the growing child will now take guidance. Whatever is fraught with deep meaning that works through pictures and allegories, is the right thing for these years. (1975, p. 29)

These deeper meanings are found in the patterns and relationships that weave into and through things; as with experiencing a piece of music, a student requires an aesthetic imagination, an imagination through which we can perceive the Creative working through the created. Through this kind of perception we see things in their context, in their movement, in their relationship to one another, in their growth and metamorphosis. The creative forces that shape the world are fluid not static; ther apprehension requires fluid thinking, imagination.

At this stage of childhood, the imagination is nourished by images, pictures, parables and the like rather than fixed concepts. Concepts are abstract and do not generally spur the kind of inward movement necessary to experience the meaning in things beyond their immediate practical contexts. Through imagery and imaginative picture, through story and metaphor, children are spurred to inner movement, to create knowledge for themselves. Ideas, as such, are not abstractions but inward experiences mirroring the forces at work in the subjects they study. Steiner explains that

> The presentation of living pictures, or as we might say of symbols, to the mind, is important for the period between the change of teeth and puberty. It is essential that the secrets of Nature, the laws of life, be taught to the boy or girl, not in dry intellectual concepts, but as far as possible in symbols. Parables of the spiritual connections of things should be brought before the soul of the child in such a manner that behind the parables he divines and feels, rather than grasps intellectually, the underlying law in all existence. (1975, p. 33)

In the Waldorf Schools, reading and writing begin with a rich experience of language in fairy tales told by the teachers. Writing emerges from these stories, and the letters themselves are introduced through accompanying pictures which are gradually transformed into the symbols we know. Numbers are taught in such a way as to reveal their inner quality: the wholeness and unity of the number one, the polarities and symmetries evident in nature that arise with a division known as the number two. History is introduced through myth, legends and biography filled with colorful detail to awaken within children, as John Gardner points out, "… the kind of inner attitude, the psychological capacities that originally made each culture and civilization what it was" (Gardner, 1975, p. 16). In nature study, children are guided to look at the human characteristics in various animals and to see how each of them shares a common bond with the human being. In botany, children draw and paint the plants they observe in great detail focusing on the flowing patterns of leaf, stem and flower; they plant and learn to see the connections between the earth, soil and sky and the living plant. During this phase of childhood, the primary educational task is to draw forth and develop a child's sense of connection, belonging, appreciation and wonder through imaginative encounters with the world.

With puberty, the emphasis shifts to the child's capacity for thoughtful, independent judgment. Steiner writes,

> What the intellect has to say concerning any matter, should only be said when all the other faculties of the soul have spoken. Before that time the intellect has only an intermediary part to play: its business is to grasp what takes place and is experienced in feeling, to receive it exactly as it is, not letting the unripe judgment come in at once and take possession. (1975, p. 46)

This capacity for thought is not detached or abstract but an outgrowth of the capacities for will and feeling nurtured in the early years.

During this phase of development, students in the Waldorf School revisit many of the subject areas studies in the earlier grades. Their previous studies establish a ground of inner experience that now allows them to form their own judgments based upon their own observations, based upon their own sense of what is true. Whether studying the history of architecture, structure of revolutions, English literature or physics, students are encouraged to see the generative patterns and relations in and between things; they are encouraged to see creative ideas at work within the world by awakening these creative ideas within themselves. Such thinking is not sentimental but based on keen observation and penetrating imagination. In the process of thinking, students are encouraged to develop insight rather than power, a sense of intrinsic meaning rather than utility alone.

## PLAYING THE MUSIC

In all the phases of childhood, there is a third party engaged where the child is opened to the world and the world is opened to the child. There stands the teacher. In Waldorf schools, the teachers are given the primary responsibility for running the schools; they set the curriculum; they determine hiring and firing; they decide on the admission and educational program for the children. Steiner recognized that teachers, as examples of humanity, have to take responsibility for what and how they teach. If one would have children grow into free and responsible adults, so their teachers should be.

Steiner had remarkable trust in teachers and thus burdened them with profound responsibility. In the various stages of childhood, the teachers take on diverse responsibilities. At times, they must provide in every word and gesture an example worthy of imitation. At times, they must master themselves. Emerson said, "He who is more disciplined than I masters me." At times, their thinking and questions must be crisp and incisive. Yet, in all cases, the teacher must maintain a clear sense of who, directly, they are teaching. The teacher must interpret the curriculum in response to the children in the class. There are fundamental principles but no prescriptions. In all cases, the teacher must also intuitively understand the subject matter. He or she needs to awaken imaginatively. It is only when the teacher is inwardly alive that the subject matter can quicken the Creative within the children. In Waldorf Schools, there are no textbooks, until at least the middle grades; it is essential for the teachers themselves know the world well enough to teach about it creatively. There are helpful examples of methods in Waldorf literature but no techniques.

In this context, I'd like to give the reader a sense of what the "music" of Waldorf classrooms might sound like as one walks down a hall or visits a class. The examples illustrate a few of the principles at play in Waldorf lessons.

Several years ago, I taught a 7th grade class about acids and bases. At the close of school one day, I placed a spoon in a strong base and a second spoon in a strong acid. I did not tell the children anything about these substances but only that we would look at the spoons in the morning. The next day, the two spoons showed considerable erosion. I then asked the children to imagine what it would be like if we put these two powerful substances together. They agreed that we could expect some kind of explosion. I directed the children to the back of the room while I stood in front with heavy gloves, goggles, lab apron and tongs. Holding the acid beaker at a distance, I slowly poured it onto the base. Occasionally, I tested the ph of the solution (again without saying anything). I stopped adding the acid when the solution was of neutral ph. I then asked if there was a tough person who would step forward. One boy did, and I asked him to put his finger in the new solution. He thought I was crazy and refused. As he turned to go back to his classmates, I picked up the beaker and quickly drank it down. The children gasped. When the boy asked what happened, they shouted, "He drank it! He drank it!" I calmly asked the children to sit back down in their seats and started to teach them some math. I said nothing about what I had done. The next day, they came in with all kinds of theories about what happened, and we began a few experiments with acids and bases to test their theories.

I would not recommend this lesson to anyone unfamiliar with specific acids and bases. However, it does illustrate a few important Waldorf principles. One, the lesson attempted to demonstrate the miraculous quality of acids and bases. That is, part of my aim was to have the children experience, with some awe and wonder, this small aspect of the chemical properties of the world. Two, the lesson began with the phenomena; the phenomena were allowed to speak for themselves. The image of my drinking this witches' brew was left to play in the children's imaginations. Only after a night's sleep was there intellectual discussion. Three, the children were encouraged to theorize and experiment for themselves after the phenomena raised questions. The children did learn about the chemical properties of acids and bases, but they did so with a vivid feeling that they were studying something that, to a lesser or greater degree, was wondrous and meaningful.

In a fifth grade, a colleague of mine, George Benner, thought his children were ready to move from their studies in arithmetic to geometry. He wanted to do so in a context of the "connectedness of things." Benner writes, "I look at a snail shell or a leaf and am struck by the connectedness of these seemingly unrelated objects. I see the web of a spider and the structure of a honeycomb and the connectedness strikes me" (p. 120). George's educational aims are particularly important because he, as a Waldorf teacher, was setting out a problem for himself outside of the vast, specific pedagogical suggestions offered by Steiner. He used Steiner's remarkable insights and his own imagination to create a series of lessons bridging the order of mathematics with the patterns and symmetries of nature.

George introduced the children to a simple arithmetic progression first discovered by Leonardo of Pisa, better known today as Fibonacci. Fibonacci generated a pattern of numbers by beginning with one and adding successive addends to one another. Thus,

| | |
|---|---|
| 0+1=1 | 3+5=8 |
| 1+1=2 | 5+8=13 |
| 1+2=3 | 8+13=21 |
| 2+3=5 | 13+21=34 |

George then showed that this seemingly arbitrary number pattern is found in nature. Sunflowers and pine cones have interlocking spiraled seed formations, one spiral clockwise, the other counterclockwise. The seeds in each of the spirals are always found on the Fibonacci series. The two numbers will form a successive pair in the series. For example, pine cones might have 8 seeds running in one direction and 13 running in the other. In sunflowers, one will find larger numbers, perhaps 55 in one di-

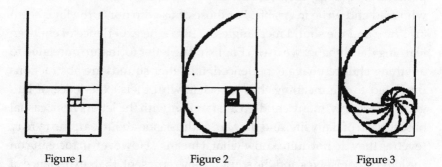

Figure 1                    Figure 2                    Figure 3

rection and 89 in the other. George went on to find the pattern in twigs of trees. The series occurs when you count the number of times you can go around a twig or leaf to leaf until you meet or come to a point directly in line with the one with which you began. "It is estimated that 90% of all plants exhibit the Fibonacci pattern of leaf placement and leaf number" (Knott, 2001).

The number series is also found in shells. One way to see the pattern emerge is to have the children cut two square inch squares. Then following the Fibonacci series, have them cut a two inch square, one three inch square and so on up to 13. Arrange the squares as in figure 1 below. Draw the arches as in figure 2 and compare with the chambered nautilus, figure 3.

In these lessons, children learn to see a mathematical order and harmony in nature. They begin to see common threads running through creation like the aesthetic streams that run through a piece of music. The children do not learn to abstract and analyze as the only way to understand nature but to observe things in their connections and to synthesize ideas. All this comes with a sense of one's own connectedness in the harmonies of the world — the experience of knowledge that transforms and nourishes the growing person.

The third, and last example for now, is one that Steiner provides himself. He had a great deal to say about the teaching of writing and reading, and I can only offer a minimal introduction to the way these basic skills are taught in the Waldorf Schools.

The key to understanding Steiner's approach to the teaching of writing and reading is to keep in mind what the child experiences. We, as adults, are so familiar with the letters of the alphabet and their role in the process of communicating ideas that we can forget how abstract they are to children. Imagine that you were told that every time you see a certain patterns of squiggly lines ش, say "sh." This is, indeed, the case of those who read and write in Arabic. For those of us who don't, the lines seem arbitrary and the sound meaningless. This is the experience of children learning the alphabet we use in English. The letter forms are unrelated to anything children have experienced; the letter sounds are abstractions unrelated to the meaning they associate with their experience of language. Certainly, many children are familiar with the letters from casual observation of daily life, and they are enthusiastic about learning to read (even as they do not quite know what it means). However, in focusing on the letters themselves and the sounds they represent, their experience of language becomes more abstract, more removed from the world they know both within and without. Writing and reading emerge as functional skills; they engender little enthusiasm except as a function of social approval. This is especially true of young children who struggle to refine the necessary perceptual and motor skills required. Given these factors in the larger context of child development as explained earlier, Waldorf educators do not stress early written literacy instruction and let children progress at their own rates through grade three.

Steiner suggests that we begin the teaching of reading and writing within in an imaginative framework of literature geared to the stage of development of a first grader. More specifically, he suggests the use of fairy tales. Fairy tales provide images that speak to the heart of children at this age about inner aspects of themselves and the world around them. Anthroposophic physician and philosopher, Franz Winkler explains that the fairy tales symbolize

> partly hidden realms of the human soul. In these realms, unselfish will and purified emotion must find their union as prince and prin-cess, to rule their domain with the help of reason grown into wis-

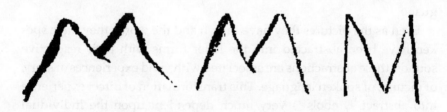

Figure 4

> dom. Such wisdom, according to the fairy tale, is to be found in nature. Her animals, forests, rivers, flowers, and stones can become man's teachers on his quest for inner kingship; and yet if his search for knowledge is selfish and overbearing, the power he acquires may become his undoing. For in the fairy tale, as in reality, every-one can grow up to be kind in his own soul only if he learns to re-spect the dignity and sacredness of his fellow creatures. (p. 206)

Waldorf teachers tell these stories to children. They do not read them. Each story is crafted in response to the mood in the classroom, the look in the eyes of individual children. After the children have had a full day to let these images enter their sleep, teachers may draw some simple pic-tures on the board from the story which the children may copy. In the

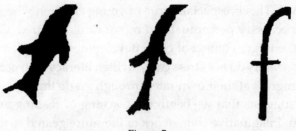

Figure 5

days following, the children, after being given many opportunities to re-tell the story, gradually follow the teacher in abstracting letter forms from the simple drawings they have made. For example, a picture of a mountain may be metamorphosed into the letter "m." A fish may be turned into the letter "f." (See figures 4 and 5.)

The words "mountain" and "fish" are then gradually abstracted to the sounds of the letter "m" and the letter "f." Waldorf teachers may lead children in tongue twisters using the letters they have just learned both to develop their elocution and to let children play with the sounds of language.

Even as the pictures they have drawn and the words they have spoken have been abstracted into the letter forms with their respective sounds, these abstractions are associated with vivid experiences of story, of picture, of spoken language. This transformation of direct experience into abstract symbols is very much dependent upon the individual imagination of the teacher in terms of the specific stories he or she tells and the drawings he or she makes.

However, this approach to the teaching of writing and reading is in fact a reflection of the way our alphabet developed over time. Steiner writes,

> When you start appealing to the nature of the child in this way you really transport him back to earlier cultural ages, for this is how writing originally arose. Later the process became a mere convention so that today we no longer recognize the connection between the abstract letter shapes and the pictures that arose purely out of seeing things and imitating what was seen in the form of drawings. All the letters have arisen out of such picture shapes. (1988, p. 12)

After children have had an initial introduction to letters, they may paint them, shape them with their bodies, or walk them in large forms out in the schoolyard. When children have learned a sufficient number of letters, the teacher guides them in writing their own first books which contain very simplified versions of the fairy tales they have heard. The children use these books as readers. It is important to note that writing is taught before reading. In practical terms, something may be read only after it is written, but in a broader sense Steiner maintains that it is important for children to understand that someone generates a written text to convey something of meaning to someone who will then read it. Soon, children learn to read other stories and move into more expanded reading with a sense of warm familiarity with their friends the letters.

These three diverse examples are intended to demonstrate how Waldorf educators attempt to provide children with the opportunities to experience knowledge inwardly. This inner experience does not merely make education entertaining or provide motivation; it is the very stuff out of which to actualize the will, deepen the heart and free thinking. It is this experience which educates and guides the child in healthy, whole development.

## CONCLUSION

There is a crisis in education. It is a spiritual crisis that pervades our society and culture. More than we need people of sharper intellect and greater facility in processing information, we need a transformation of consciousness. The narrow and economically oriented conception of knowledge that pervades our educational system provides little sustenance for the growth of individuals who will develop not only competence but compassion and commitment. Franz Winkler notes that "the problems of our time cannot be solved by political, economic or social reforms alone; they are deeply rooted in the unfulfilled and often hidden longings of the human soul" (1960, p. 32).

The gifted writer Parker Palmer stated,

> But the great insight of our spiritual traditions is that we — especially those of us who enjoy political freedom and relative affluence — are not victims of that society: we are its co-creators. We live in and through a complex interaction of spirit and matter, of the powers inside of us and the stuff "out there" in the world. External reality does not impinge upon us as an ultimate constraint: if we

who are privileged find ourselves confined, it is only because we have conspired in our own imprisonment. (1999, p. 89)

Steiner maintains that the fundamental problems of our time require individuals with a sense of purpose and meaning including but transcending their own interests, individuals who understand the invitation that all things and all moments offer to participate in the spiritual evolution of the world. In this context, Waldorf Education is not focused exclusively on the individual but on the larger need of modern civilization to respond to the social, political, economic and ecological problems of our time. Our response to these issues, as well as the responses of future generations, will very much depend upon our individual and collective capacities to develop what is most essential in each and all of us. In essence, it will depend upon the quality of education we provide for our children.

## REFERENCES

Benner, G. (1975). *Arithmetic.* Adelphi University, Garden City, NY: Unpublished Manuscript.

Bohm, D. (1980). *Wholeness and the Implicate Order.* London: Kegan Paul.

Emerson, R.W. (1965). Nature. *Selected Writings of Ralph Waldo Emerson.* New York: The New American Library, Inc.

Fenner, P.J. & Rivers, K.L. (1995). *Waldorf Education: A Family Guide.* Amesbury, MA: Michaelmas Press.

Gardner, J. (1975). *The Experience of Knowledge.* Garden City, NY: Waldorf Press, Adelphi University.

Kane, J. (ed.). (1999). *Education, Information, and Transformation: Essays on Learning and Thinking.* Upper Saddle River, NJ: Prentice-Hall.

Knott, R. "Fibonacci Numbers and the Golden Section," 2001, http://www.mcs.surrey.ac.uk/Personal/R.Knott/fibonacci/(17 April 2001).

National Commission on Excellence in Education. (1983). *A Nation at Risk: The Imperative for Educational Reform.* Washington, D.C.: Government Printing Office.

Palmer, P. J. (1999). *Let Your Life Speak: Listening for the Voice of Vocation.* San Francisco: Jossey-Bass.

Richards, M.C. (1980). *Toward Wholeness: Rudolf Steiner Education in America.* Middletown, CT: Wesleyan University Press.

Sanger, D. (2001). The new administration: The plan; Bush pushes ambitious education plan. *New York Times*, 24 January, sec A, p. 1.

Steiner, R. (1974). *Awakening to Community*. Hudson, NY: Anthroposophic Press.

Steiner, R. (1975). *Education of the Child in the Light of Anthroposophy*. London: Rudolf Steiner Press.

Steiner, R. (1995a). *The Kingdom of Childhood*. Hudson, NY: Anthroposophic Press.

Steiner, R. (1995b). *The Spirit of the Waldorf School*. Hudson, NY: Anthroposophic Press.

Steiner, R. (1988). *Practical Advice To Teachers*. London: Rudolf Steiner Press.

Winkler, F. (1960). *MAN: The Bridge Between Two Worlds*. N.Y.: Gilbert Church, Publisher.

# PRACTICES

# CHAPTER 16

# Eros and the Erotic Shadow in Teaching and Learning

## Rachael Kessler

> To call attention to the body is to betray the legacy of repression and denial that has been handed down to us by our professorial elders. Professors rarely speak of the place of eros or the erotic in our classrooms. Trained in the philosophical context of Western metaphysical dualism, many of us have accepted the notion that there is a split between the body and the mind. Believing this, individuals enter the classroom to teach as though only the mind is present, and not the body.... (hooks, 1994, 191)

Despite this conceptual split between mind and body, Eros finds its way into the classroom. It comes as an ally, or if we try too hard to keep it out, it catches us off guard and comes as an enemy. Eros enters the classroom because it is intricately intertwined with teaching and learning.

At the heart of good teaching is the ability to:

- care deeply for our students,
- be passionate about our subject,
- have full access to our senses to convey and elicit wisdom and meaning in a rich variety of modalities, and
- be receptive to new ideas, forms of expression and levels of synthesis.

Caring. Passion. Sensory aliveness. Connection. These are all expressions of an erotic impulse that infuses life with warmth, vitality and relatedness. Even the language of academic discourse reveals the presence of the erotic archetype: from the colloquial expression "to flirt with a new idea" to more erudite expressions such as a "seminal concept," teaching and learning are laced with Eros. In his article "Love and Despair in Teaching," Dan Liston (2000) captures the erotic energy inherent in good teaching:

> As teachers we share this love of learning with our students. To teach is to publicly share this love; it is to ask others to be drawn in by the same powers that lure and attract us; it is to try to get our students to see the grace and attraction that these 'great things' have for us. In teaching we reach out toward our students in an attempt to create connections among them and our subjects. We want them to love what we find so alluring. To love teaching is to be enamored of the attempt to share the attraction and hold the world has on us. To love teaching is to give of yourself in a way that can be so tenderly vulnerable. (p. 92)

Without access to Eros, our teaching becomes flat, mechanical, alienating. We are unable to engage or inspire our students; we are easy prey to burnout as our work becomes dry. But why would we teachers cut ourselves off from this vital stream?

We live in a culture which often reduces the erotic to sex and confuses sensuality with genitality. Sexuality — the broad range of needs and yearnings, the complex interweaving of the emotional, cognitive, physical, social and spiritual realms of our humanity — is reduced to "sex." Even our passion for our calling or our art has been reduced by some thinkers to a sublimated form of sex. Equating the erotic with sex, educators have often dismissed or ignored this vital force in teaching and learning. But this confusion is not simply conceptual — it can become emotional, and even physical.

When the profound energies of the erotic are awake and flowing in the classroom, when we allow ourselves to feel the depth of passion for our subject and the warmth of caring and connection with our students, it is possible for a dangerous side of Eros to be unleashed as well. Out of the Shadow come feelings that have been kept well-hidden by the force of cultural taboo, suppressed in our personal effort to maintain appropriate professional boundaries. We may feel romantic love, sexual attraction, even obsession about these young people in our charge.

These feelings have the power to sweep away our sense of responsibility and suspend our conscience. So closely tied to the beauty of our love, the feelings which erupt from the Shadow of Eros can obscure our ability to discern our motives, our rights, and our responsibilities. Is it any wonder we try to banish Eros from our work with the young?

But what happens when we try to suppress such a potent force? One danger is the Scylla of acting out feelings of attraction between teacher and student. The other is the Charybdis of repressing Eros, which can lead to stonewalling particular students or draining the warmth and life out of the classroom. This essay will examine these costs of forcing the erotic dimension of education into the realm of Shadow — the vast unconscious territory created by all those feelings we refuse to express and do not even want to know about ourselves. I will briefly explore the dynamics of Shadow and then focus on what I call the "Erotic Shadow" in education. Using my own stories, as well as those of teachers in my workshops on emotional intelligence, I will challenge this taboo which has kept hidden in shame information which is vital to the preparation and ongoing support for teachers at all levels.

## THE DYNAMICS OF SHADOW

Let us look at the basic theory of the creation of Shadow — how it is formed and how it functions in the personality. Originally introduced by C.G. Jung, the concept of Shadow presumes that we are all born whole, filled with expansive possibility and radiant energy. To ensure our survival in this world as fragile little ones, we seek to please. First we try to satisfy our parents, on whom we depend for our very lives. Then, we accommodate our teachers, whose power over us can determine much present and future well-being. Later, we can't alienate our peers because they are the gatekeepers to belonging. Children have extraordinary antennae for what pleases these arbiters of our physical and psychic survival. Based on their criteria, as well as more pervasive cultural criteria which the media infuse into the very air we breathe, we nip and tuck at our wholeness to make ourselves acceptable and lovable.

Those qualities which we attempt to discard do not really go away. They settle into the not-so-cold storage of the Shadow — a realm of unconsciousness which remains volatile and active as long as it is unknown. When I speak of Shadow here, I do not mean a synonym for our "evil" side or our "weaknesses." Our Shadows contain not only the negative "uncivilized" side of our nature, but also the positive — what has been called the "gold in the Shadow" (Johnson 1991, 5). Whatever we have disowned and hidden in our formative years will lurk in our shadows. Anger, aggressiveness, greed, or sexual hunger may sink into the Shadow because we felt shamed about them while we were growing up. But we also buried some of our gifts and aptitudes — the gold we have never claimed as our own. If our older sibling has been a star athlete, for example, we may disown our own athletic abilities and desires, focusing our development on intellectual or artistic pursuits. Or, we may disown our natural talent as a creative artist when it is mocked by a perfectionist teacher or provokes irritation in a parent who has little respect for art.

What we feel permitted to reveal are "the ordinary, mundane characteristics.... Anything less than this goes into the shadow," says Robert Johnson in his book *Owning Your Shadow*. "But anything better also goes into the shadow. Some of the pure gold of our personality is relegated to the shadow because it can find no place in that great leveling process that is culture" (Johnson, 1991, 8).

If, as teachers, we do not have the support or guidance to uncover what is in our own Shadow, we may hurt ourselves or our students. "Emotions that simmer beneath the threshold of awareness can have a powerful impact on how we perceive and react," writes Daniel Goleman in his groundbreaking book *Emotional Intelligence*. We begin to have the capacity to evaluate and choose our outlook and behavior only when "that reaction is brought into awareness — once it registers in the cortex"(Goleman 1997, p. 55).

Whatever our conscious agenda, our students perceive both what we put forward and what we are not yet ready to claim. Children and adolescents are particularly sensitive to the unconscious, unspoken psychological issues of the adults they count on for survival — parents and teachers. When we as teachers are unable to tolerate and understand certain feelings in ourselves, we risk either impulsive behaviors with our students and colleagues or a stonewalling stance that prevents students from receiving the knowledge, wisdom and support that we have to offer. Suppressing energies and capacities that are vital to our identity, teachers may feel unusually tired or become half-hearted about our work. The joy and playfulness we dare not express, the sorrow or vulnerability we are afraid to feel — these and other unclaimed dimensions of our wholeness become barriers which limit the freedom of discovery in both teacher and student.

## THE EROTIC SHADOW: THE COST OF SUPPRESSION

Now, let us look specifically at the Erotic Shadow in teaching. We have already seen that the expression of positive Eros in teaching — caring, passion, sensory intelligence and connection — can easily activate the more dangerous energies of the Erotic Shadow. We may feel attraction, longing, desire, even possession, love, affection, arousal, even sexual obsession.

For many teachers, this looming Shadow of the erotic is so threatening that they make an unconscious bargain which promises to banish Eros altogether from their teaching. But Shadow will not stay contained forever. As the poet Robert Bly says, "Every part of our personality that we do not love will become hostile to us. We could add that it may move to a distant place and begin a revolt against us as well" (Bly 1988, 20).

In recent years, the Erotic Shadow in the teaching archetype has certainly had its revolt:

- In Seattle, a thirty-five year old grade school teacher pleads guilty to child rape for having sex with her thirteen year old student. Released from jail after 100 days for good behavior, Marie LeTourneau is arrested again and sent back to jail for nearly 7 1/2 years after being caught again with the boy in an attempt to run away together.

- In Washington, D.C., fifty-year old President Bill Clinton finally admits to an adulterous affair with a young woman in her early twenties. While not technically "a teacher," Clinton was in the role of the teaching archetype because this young woman was a White House intern — relating to the President not as her "employer" but as a mentor and guide.

These "sex scandals" of the nineties shocked and fascinated the public not only because of the breach of marital fidelity, the evasions and cover-ups but also because of the abuse of power, the violation of the young and "innocent" by precisely those adults who are responsible for protecting them and shepherding their growth.

I did not need to read the national news to be reminded of how the fires of affection and positive identification between teacher and student can flame out of control into a sexual encounter. In my own home town, one of my son's favorite teachers was suspended pending an investigation into an alleged affair with a high school senior. From another state, a high school teacher writes to me about her colleague, whose husband has just been accused of engaging in sexual activity with a student while taking a group of students to Italy. "In its wake," she writes, "a wrecked marriage, he's been fired, and a ghastly time for this couple's two children." And in my own work as a teacher of adolescents, I wrestle with the very same forces inside myself.

Paradoxically, the more we try to keep Eros out of the classroom and out of our consciousness, the more likely it is to erupt into inappropriate, impulsive expression. The Seattle teacher who made national news was the daughter of a politician who "fiercely opposed sex education in public schools. His congressional career ended in 1993 after one term with the disclosure that he had two children with a mistress" (Klass, 1998, p. 46A). This biographical twist in the Le Tourneau story suggests the dynamic common to the Shadow of fierce repression turning into compulsive obsession. Many people speculate a similar dynamic at work in President Clinton's apparently compulsive behavior. Only a drive which has reached volcanic levels can account for the extreme levels of recklessness which brought down both these public figures.

The teachers and their students in these stories paid one kind of price for attempting to banish the Erotic Shadow — the violation that comes when a teacher impulsively acts out sexually because she or he is not *conscious* — and therefore not able to be *conscientious* — about erotic feelings in the classroom.

But there is another price for denying the Erotic Shadow of education. Stonewalling our students — rebuffing one or all of our students with cold professionalism — appears to be the opposite of affection run amok into inappropriate sexuality. Yet stonewalling is also damaging to students and grows out of the same impulse to suppress awareness of erotic feelings for our students at all costs. In her groundbreaking essay, "Eros, Eroticism, and the Pedagogical Process," bell hooks tells a story from her first semester of college teaching which illustrates this second price. "There was a male student in my class whom I always seemed to see and not see at the same time," writes hooks (1994):

> At one point in the middle of the semester, I received a call from a school therapist who wanted to speak with me about the way I treated this student in class. The students had said I was unusually gruff, rude, and downright mean when I related to him. I did not know exactly who the student was, could not put a face

or body with his name, but later when he identified himself in class, I realized that I was erotically drawn to this student (p. 192).

Once she saw that she was attracted to this young man, hooks realized that in an unconscious effort to avoid what most of us fear will lead to sexual transgression, she had closed her heart entirely to this student. "… My naive way of coping with feelings in the classroom that I had been taught never to have was to deflect (hence my harsh treatment of him), repress, and deny" (hooks, 1994, 192).

Between the the Scylla of acting out sexually and the Charybdis of stonewalling described by hooks, are other lesser but still damaging costs of going unconscious about our own erotic attraction to students. Sometimes we find ourselves giving undue attention, opportunity or even decision-making power to these students for whom we feel an almost numinous attraction. This "teacher's pet" is not beloved by the other students. Even when we strain to be temperate, suppressing our erotic feelings towards our students can distort our judgment in ways that undermine the quality of our teaching.

So how can teachers reclaim what has been lost to Shadow or heal what festers there? Only by embarking on the extremely uncomfortable journey of airing and examining these issues can we be spared the heavy price of remaining unconscious to the Erotic Shadow of our work. "Socrates' injunction 'Know thyself,'" writes Daniel Goleman (1997) in his chapter on the role of self-awareness, "speaks to this keystone of emotional intelligence: awareness of one's own feelings as they occur" (p. 46).

When we are dealing with the Shadow, self-awareness can be difficult. Our primary, presenting self has a great incentive to repress certain feelings, impulses and thoughts, which is how they moved into Shadow in the first place. But as Goleman points out, there can be no *control* of inappropriate feelings if we do not first become aware that those feelings are operating. "Self-awareness," says Goleman, "is the fundamental emotional competence on which others, such as emotional self-control, build" (p. 47).

In preparing teachers to work responsibly with the social, emotional and spiritual development of their students, I have found it essential to support them in finding ways to unearth what has been buried in Shadow so that such self-awareness becomes possible.

## BEGINNING THE JOURNEY

Because the Shadow of teachers and of teaching has been ignored, it continues to be taboo for many teachers — a forbidden, and consequently perilous realm. Naturally, we feel conflicted, because the feelings, beliefs and impulses in our Shadow are something we cannot know until they are drawn out by circumstance. We can't see them under normal light. That's why they are in Shadow.

Yet there are effective tools for discovering this hidden domain. To shed light on what wants to be unseen requires great delicacy. It reveals itself only when it feels safe, and then only indirectly. In my workshops with teachers, I find that symbolism and story are often the best language to speak in calling forth the Shadow. Once we have worked together carefully to build a safe container for authentic dialogue, I invite teachers to tell a story from their own childhood or youth about a teacher who inspired them, by positive or negative example, to be the kind of teacher they strive for today.

As the stories unfold from each teacher, we weave a tapestry of the best and worst in the teacher-student relationship. We meet the heroes and the demons who have shaped our own essence as a teacher.

> *Richard*: I was in first grade. I can see her face, but I can't seem to remember her name. My brother had just died before I started school. She had a rocking chair in the classroom and on the first day of school, she picked me up on her lap in the rocker and began to rock me. She rocked, and I sobbed. And sobbed and sobbed. It was something I couldn't do at home — not the way my family handled these things. And you know, she did that for months, every day for minutes or sometimes what seemed like hours. She took me into the chair and rocked me for about five months, when my crying was done.

> *Eduardo*: I came to this country in high school. I was sixteen and I knew only three words of English. We had no ESL in those days. I just had to struggle through my classes. I did pretty well in math — language was not such a block there. I had left all my family, my friends behind and was trying to make it in this new country. It's hard to convey my loneliness. One morning, I was coming into school and I happened to run into my math teacher, Mr. _____. He stopped me in the hall and then smiled. "Bue-

nos Días, Eduardo," he said. That was all. He moved on and so did I. I cannot tell you what that meant to me — that he would make the effort to greet me in my own language. I remember that moment always.

But there are also stories, which, like my own, recount a moment in time when some potential or voice or path was frozen in Shadow.

I was thirteen years old. I was so excited because my eighth grade teacher had recognized my love for writing and had recommended me for a free after school enrichment program in creative writing. I had been composing poetry and stories since I knew how to write. As a child of Holocaust survivors, I had spent much of my early childhood seeking comfort and joy in the sanctuary of my imagination. At twelve, I taught myself to type on my brother's little Royal, and started a novel.

It was the second week of class and our teacher, a big tall man with a blond crewcut (I forget his name) was reading back responses to the first assignment — describe a setting. I had described my own bedroom. Just that year, my parents had the money for the first time to buy me a bedroom set of my own — new furniture, curtains, bedspread, and even a dust ruffle. Proudly, I described every detail of the decor, which was dominated by the color pink.

My teacher began reading and with a quickened beat of my heart, I recognized my own words. As he first came to the word "pink," he emphasized the sound. As the word repeated, his tone became more mocking and each time he made the word sound more like "pig" or "oink." His sarcasm was thick as he finished the piece and barely needed to critique the repetition because his tone had so obviously demonstrated his disgust. I felt like a stone. And like a stone, my capacity to write fiction, to tell a story, to improvise, to even fabricate a lie became frozen for many years. I could write essays — sometimes even decent poems. But not until I was in my forties could I pry open the door in my mind that is marked "creative writing."

In Eduardo's and Richard's stories, we meet teachers who used Eros to inspire students with their capacities for courage, caring and wisdom. But there are many stories, which, like my own, recount a moment in time when some of our own gold — a potential talent, voice or path — was frozen in Shadow.

As Richard's story illustrates, overcoming the mind/body split creates opportunities in our teaching for wholeness and healing. Even at the college level, a professor may choose to respond with an appropriate, accepting hug to a student who feels tormented or ashamed, having learned her sister has just been jailed, or his brother has just committed suicide. But many teachers will not dare to reach out even though it comes from absolute integrity because of the current climate of mistrust and litigiousness in education:

> When I taught in Vermont, we had a union lawyer who in a strident, apocalyptic tone grimly warned us about laying hands on any student. "Don't touch a student ever. No hands on shoulders. No encouraging pats. No touching at all." We were told about teachers who had lost careers, families and reputations because of charges that were never substantiated. The price of indiscretion in these matters can be unthinkable. For me, these grim warnings, these tales of unimaginable shame were never far from my conscious behavior.

Professor Sam Intrator of Smith College, who shared this story with me, was expressing his concern that readers might take this essay as an encouragement to share their own erotic feelings for students with a colleague or mentor who would misunderstand and put them in grave danger. Indeed this danger is very real. In my own community last year, the high school brought the district lawyer in to warn teachers not only about their own behavior, but about liabilities of not disclosing any information or observation they might have about the indiscretions of their colleagues. Working in this climate, it is no wonder that teachers who actually feel attracted to their students have no safe place to air and reflect on their experience.

### Beyond the Taboo

The feelings and issues that arise from the Erotic Shadow for educators are charged with taboo. In over a decade of teacher training, in countless workshops where teachers courageously explored many aspects of their Shadows which had been frozen in shame, I have never once heard a teacher raise the spectre of the Erotic Shadow.

Over a decade ago, when I first worked with teenagers in a high school, I was shocked when I first felt attracted to one of my students. Fortunately, I had the guidance and support of colleagues, a mentor and a husband with whom I could talk about virtually every issue that arose. Because they helped me as I struggled in my early years of teaching to find a way of meeting this aspect of my Shadow with consciousness and integrity, I could and did learn to work with these feelings in ways that brought more responsibility and vitality to my teaching, instead of hurting my students and destroying my career. Eventually I discovered the blessings in this mysterious, almost numinous magnetism that arose with certain students.

But I was still unprepared to teach others about the Erotic Shadow of education. I feared I would be judged and condemned by the teachers I worked with if I shared the experiences that led to my insights. I thought they would be frightened and ashamed, as I had been, of the leaking of erotic feelings into life at school. So it never occurred to me to design this issue into my teacher development workshops.

It was the power of the unconscious which broke through my resistance. In my retreats with teachers I encourage my participants to pay attention to the dreams that come as we work together. "We can invite our unconscious to be an ally in this work," I suggest on the first evening. "And who knows? Once we become a close-knit, working group, sharing your dream might have as much or more relevance to someone else or for the group than it does for you personally."

My own Erotic Shadow broke through in a dream at one of my first workshops. I was extremely reluctant to tell this dream about a young colleague I had a crush on for years. How could I reveal such embarrassing material to these teachers that I wanted to respect me? But I had asked them to share *their* dreams. How could I have integrity if I didn't share mine?

Sharing this dream in a council with teachers, I was flooded with energy and feeling. I realized immediately that the dream was a catalyst: it was only there to provoke me to dive more boldly into the Erotic Shadow in education. For it was not just the "love" for a colleague that surfaced when I began to teach. More shocking to me was the erotic attraction I felt to my students. This was a topic that no one seemed to talk about in education. But for me, this dream made it inevitable.

Sometimes, we find ourselves attracted to an unsuspecting student. Other times, we feel the power of a student's crush on us. Here, I would like to share stories which illustrate both of these challenges.

I met Daniel in my first year of teaching. I felt so embarrassed, so ashamed, so strange to feel an erotic attraction to an eighteen year old boy. But that was not all. Daniel was perhaps the one student most disliked by the rest of the faculty — he was rude, completely self-absorbed, shamelessly materialistic, lazy about schoolwork, rich, spoiled, and disrespectful to women. Month after month, I asked myself — how can you feel intense affection for such a jerk? Yes, he was handsome; but in Los Angeles, there were scores of handsome men of all ages and no others stirred these feelings.

It was not hard for me to be honorable in my behavior — I was not only committed to my marriage but firmly rooted in the belief that in teacher-student relationships, the power imbalance could only produce damage to the younger person in a romantic relationship. But the feelings wouldn't stop. I began to wonder if there was some purpose for this uncomfortable, almost disgraceful yearning in my heart that stirred whenever I saw him.

Late in the year, clues emerged. On our senior retreat, we learned that Daniel had hurt one of my female students with his rude, distasteful, and chauvinistic behavior. My colleague and I were furious. Even though she was his primary teacher, I offered to speak to him.

I knew that Daniel had contempt for most of the faculty — as most of them did for him. No one could get through to him — he would not listen through his wall of defense and derision. But when I took him aside to talk with him, there was love in my heart. I saw his face soften in a way I had never seen. He looked thoughtful and curious as I spoke to him, telling him what it feels like as a woman to be treated that way. He got it. And later he apologized to the other student.

I began to feel that this bizarre episode in my life might be coming to an end. There seemed to be a sacred purpose in what had felt so long like a dangerous current. There was a gift that needed to be given — and only in the context of love could it be received. Daniel needed someone to wake him up, or at least to begin that process. There was some kind of guidance in the magnetism that pulled me to him and opened my heart, despite the harsh judgements of my mind.

But the exchange was not complete. On the bus going home from the five day retreat in the mountains with thirty students, I was exhausted.

As I drifted into the relaxed haze before sleep, I heard Daniel's voice. I cannot remember what he actually said — no doubt he was bragging about some famous movie stars he hung out with at his father's club. Instead of my usual disgust, I felt connected to him for a moment.

Listening to Daniel, I suddenly saw that I, like many, had a side of me that was utterly seduced by wealth and fame. Until I arrived in LA, this side had been locked tightly in my Shadow. My presenting self — which I had always believed to be all of me — was the anti-materialist, social activist, service-oriented woman my immigrant family had raised me to be. But surrounded by the glitz of LA, a glamour-lover was desperately trying to get out. As long as I tried to hide from her, she had the power to sneak up on me and run the show. I could not "handle" her until I accepted her — even loved her. And loving Daniel — who was the ultimate expression of this side of my own Shadow — was the way I could accept and bless this very real part of myself.

I received his gift, just as he had received mine. And when we returned to campus, the magnetism was gone. Like magic — it just disappeared. I would see him but the thrill in my heart would not come. I was relieved. I also felt the dissipation of my hankering for Hollywood parties; my screenwriter husband was relieved. But I would never again judge those glamorous folks with contempt now that I knew there was a little piece of them inside of me. And more than once, my ability to go beyond the glitzy exterior took me into some of the biggest, most generous and caring hearts I have ever known.

When I finished telling this story in a workshop, the teachers showered me with gratitude. "It's such a relief to know I'm normal when I feel attracted to a student." "And to know you can have these feelings without acting irresponsibly." "Thanks so much for telling us your story — we know how hard it is to talk about all this, believe me."

Each time I offer up one of my own stories in a workshop, I shoo away my anxiety and fear that one of my participants will judge me a pervert. Then I wait for their own stories to rush in. With other difficult subjects, I could almost count on it — when I introduced educators to the grieving process, I would begin by illustrating certain concepts with my own stories, but soon they would be adding their own.

With the Erotic Shadow of teaching, this has yet to happen. I look into their faces and see much emotion stirring there. Their pupils are dilated; the ice floes of memory have begun to thaw and move. It is a slow, almost imperceptible movement, but I can feel their deep reflection, their reconsiderations. They say nothing about themselves. Sometimes one teacher offers to write and send me his or her own story of encountering the Erotic Shadow of teaching; the stories never come. Even if we teachers successfully avoid having, or even *thinking* about having, "crushes" on students, we cannot prevent students from having crushes on us. So sometimes I tell the story of Pete.

With Pete, it was different. It was the student who had the crush — on me. He began to enchant me with his delightful charm, warmth and almost seductive attention. In each class, he revealed more of his depth, his fascinating mind, his playfulness. I don't think any man (except my husband) has ever bestowed on me the adoration I felt coming from Pete. Eventually, I was hooked. For the rest of the semester, it was a challenge to not play favorites with him in class.

One day, he dropped by my office. He shared his existential confusion and yearning for meaning, while lounging seductively on the couch. I felt my heart beating so hard — I thought this could get out of hand. He never dropped by again. But on graduation day, in the crowd of celebrating parents, teachers and students, Pete found me. "Hey, let's go out for breakfast to say good-bye." Excitement mixed with fear — excitement won and I said yes.

In the days before this meeting, I thought back to conversations I had had about the situation with Pete over the previous months with several colleagues. I talked with my husband about it and with a mentor as well. I knew that if I kept it all inside, the charge could get bigger and I would be in trouble. Many of the conversations were strengthening, urging me to feel whatever I was feeling and steer a steady course. Some of the conversations were quite troubling.

One young teacher in my department told me that she had had an affair with a middle-aged professor when she was just nineteen, a year older than Pete, already in college. "I've always regretted it. But you wouldn't believe how common it was," she said sadly. "There's nothing unusual about what you're dealing with; I just hope you can keep your wits about you and not do something stupid."

A colleague closer to my age shared matter-of-factly that she had had a two year affair with a student in the last high school she worked in as a teacher and coach. They had remained friends, she assured me with a smile on her face. I was shocked, appalled, confused. I felt forewarned not to be complacent about the energies I was dealing with.

The night before the breakfast with Pete, I awoke from a terrifying dream and clasped my husband close to me.

"What is it, honey?" he asked in a sleepy voice.

"I had a nightmare. I think it's because of this breakfast I have this morning." My husband had been a good sounding board as I wrestled with this and other conundrums in my teaching. His faith in my good intentions was perhaps the greatest anchor for me in those rough waters. "I dreamt about this huge monster — it was black like pitch, like tar, with lots of crags and layers coming out from everywhere. It seemed to rise up from inside me to devour whatever it wanted."

As I drove the half-hour to our meeting, I reflected on my nightmare. This enormous monster, I thought, must be the Shadow of my sexuality. Until that day in my early forties, I had a profound fear that if I ever really let myself actually feel my sexual appetite outside my marriage, it would devour and destroy everything in its path. In my thirties, I had dealt with this fear by unconsciously designing a life in which, except for my husband, all my relationships — both work and friendship — were with women. Now working in a large co-ed school, this was no longer an option. Somehow I had to confront this aspect of my Shadow; my relationship with Pete had clearly sprung the monster from its hidden depths.

The dream put me on notice that I must be absolutely clean and discerning in the way I related to Pete. I must be a strong and loving elder, committed to his growth — and not succumb to the least moment of girlish flirtation, no matter how he behaved. But the dream was so strong that I also felt that I had actually met this sexual Shadow head on and did not need to fear or suppress it any more. Pete and I had a lovely goodbye — he told me in great detail how much I reminded him of his mother. I described the gifts I saw in him that would take him into a strong future. In the final moment, we both hesitated, knowing that there are many kinds of hugs to say good-bye. Our embrace was warm, simple and extremely brief. Our relationship was complete and we never saw or spoke to each other again.

Why do I risk telling such personal and potentially embarrassing stories when I train teachers in social and emotional learning? I do so because I want them to understand the dangers and also the opportunities of the erotic in education. I hope they will see in my experience with both Daniel and Pete that it is often through the dynamic of *projection* that the shadow leaks out and wreaks havoc. What we will not tolerate or claim in ourselves, we often project onto others. Our shadow qualities for which we feel shame suddenly appear in other people who then disgust us. The golden shadow qualities we dare not claim show up in those we envy, and often in those for whom we feel an overwhelmingly magnetic, romantic attraction or even non-sexual infatuation. Sometimes, as in the case with Daniel, attraction and disgust become paradoxically mixed together.

If we stop to ask ourselves as teachers — "what is it that I love about this young person?" — we open the door to witnessing the projections from our own Shadow. And if we go further and ask — "do I have some of that quality unclaimed, unblessed inside of me as well?" — we can begin to let go of the shame and fear surrounding these erotic feelings and discover a map leading directly to the gold in our Shadow. Taking responsibility for our projections, we lift the burden off of our students and allow for a healthy exchange of gifts. "Perhaps all the dragons of our lives are princesses who are only waiting to see us once, beautiful and brave," writes Rilke. "Perhaps everything terrible in its deepest being is something that needs our love" (Rilke, 1986, p. 92). No longer suppressing the erotic, we can allow its energies of warmth, vitality and delight to stream into our classrooms for the benefit of all of our teaching.

In dealing with the Shadow, *consciousness* precedes the development and expression of true *conscience*. These two forces are so closely tied that one of the original, now obsolete meanings of the word conscience was actually consciousness. Genuine conscience is not simply about following rules; it is certainly not about denying the existence of our own potentially immoral impulses. Conscience arises when we can make ethical discernment and *choose* responsible behavior. We can do this only if we have first become conscious — aware of feelings which can lead to both healthy and dangerous consequences.

## CONCLUSION

What we do not acknowledge or tolerate in ourselves — the Shadow of educators — we are unlikely to appreciate or accept in our students, or in the colleagues and parents with whom we work to create a caring, learning community in which everyone can grow. If we deny the Shadow, it will surface in ways that are sneaky and often out of our control. It will catch us from behind, grab us by the tail, and swing us around until we lose our balance and our perspective. Teachers who refuse to look at the Shadow, in themselves or in students, cannot afford to open their hearts, cannot really afford to love, and cannot express the quality of power that ensures safety in a classroom.

If we want to be fully present for our students, if we want to invite the "whole child" into the classroom, we must find a way to attend to the "whole teacher." Acknowledging the Shadow, and discovering how to meet it with conscious awareness, containing it in our embrace without denying or repressing it — these are central challenges for those of us who teach and those of us who prepare and sustain others in their teaching.

Each encounter with the Shadow raises anew the question of how committed we are really to knowing ourselves. We can reach a point where we think we have processed, probed and healed our insecurity, anger or even grief and have them "under control." At such comfortable times, do we really want to know that we still have painful or shameful feelings which require attention so they can stop erupting in hurtful behavior towards ourselves or others? Only as we learn to be at home in these uneasy domains of our own unconscious do we become more capable of loving and actually seeing our students and our colleagues without the trickster of projection distorting our perception and stirring conflict.

"When we enlarge ourselves to touch the not-beautiful," says Clarissa Pinkola Estes, "we are rewarded. If we spurn the not-beautiful, we are severed from life and left out in the cold" (Pinkola Estes, p. 46). When we begin to handle with care and compassion the "not beautiful" traits that surface from our own Shadow, we also become capable of regarding the Shadow of our students with empathy and forgiveness.

"As the shadow is drawn up into consciousness, it becomes softer, more pliable, more gentle," says Robert Johnson (1991, p. 41) More gentle with our own Shadow, we become more gentle with the underbellies of all we meet.

There is an ominous aphorism making the rounds today: "If you don't feed the teachers, they will eat the children." Feeding the teachers means giving them the respect, nourishment and guidance that helps them grow and flourish. Part of this feeding, I believe, involves helping to discover and embrace their wholeness. The concept of the Shadow was introduced to our culture by psychologists and poets. But many teachers have neither the opportunity nor interest to seek this work in a therapeutic setting. Innocent of the Shadow, these teachers may court danger in the classroom without even knowing it.

Those of us who seek to prepare and sustain teachers in their work can provide teachers with an introduction to this potent domain. With care, caution and respect, we can use opportunities in professional development to guide teachers into beginning this lifelong journey.

In a teaching and learning process which thrives on deep caring and positive identification between student and teacher, I believe it is inevitable that erotic feelings will arise. But they do not need to rise up from the hidden depths of Shadow, threatening to flood all sound judgement and leave a trail of damage to students, families, the teacher and the teaching profession itself. Instead we can tend the fires of Eros with consciousness and care, bringing renewed warmth, vitality and compassion into our classrooms. If we ignore these fires, or try to smother them completely, they can engulf us in their flames or freeze our students.

## REFERENCES

Bly, R. (1988). *A Little Book on the Human Shadow*. San Francisco, CA: Harper & Row.

Estés, C.P. (1992). *Women Who Run With the Wolves: Myths and Stories of the Wild Woman Archetype*. New York: Ballantine Books.

Goleman, D. (1995). *Emotional Intelligence: Why it Can Matter More Than IQ*. New York: Bantam Books.

hooks, b. (1994). *Teaching to Transgress: Education as the Practice of Freedom*. New York: Routledge.

Johnson, R.A. (1991). Owning Your Own Shadow: Understanding the Dark Side of the Psyche. San Francisco: Harper.

Klass, T. (1998). Caught with Teen Lover, Ex-Teacher Sent to Prison. *Rocky Mountain News*, February 7, p 46A.

Liston, D. (2000). Love and Despair in Teaching. *Educational Theory*. Winter 50 (1), 81-102.

Rilke, R. A. (1986). *Letters to a Young Poet*. New York: Vintage.

# CHAPTER 17

# How Do We Live, Learn, and Die?

## A Teacher and Some of Her Students Meditate and Walk On an Engaged Buddhist Path

### Lourdes Argüelles

Every year, with a group of my students, I meditate on how we live, learn, and die. Based upon those meditations my students and I also begin to walk together on what we may call an engaged Buddhist path. The students, all of whom are teachers and many of whom have a long history of social activism, come from a variety of socio-spiritual backgrounds and age cohorts. Some were raised in poor and/or ethno-racial minority families while others, mostly Caucasians, remember growing up in an environment of privilege. Most have described themselves as non-practicing Christians. A few designate themselves as "pre-Buddhist" or come from Asian backgrounds in which Buddhism is the forgotten religion of their parents' homeland. Occasionally there is a student who is already deeply immersed in Buddhist practice or in a non-mainstream spirituality such as paganism. Their ages range from twenty-five to over fifty. These students, however, do share one thing in common. They are, as I am, searching for alternative ways of living and learning in an everyday life of growing social inequalities, brutal incarceration policies, rampant consumerism, environmental devastation, and destructive globalization processes. They struggle with a society

that spawns childhoods, family lives, and school environments of insta-
bility, violence, and despair. In the process of their search for alternatives, and faced with a generation of children and youth in their own
classrooms whose lives are often cut short by gang warfare, suicide, and
police brutality, they have also begun to interrogate and reflect upon
their students' and their own dying.

When I first meet new students in my office or in an initial class session I ask them what brings them to my particular classes. They often say
they are seeking a sanctuary in which to openly explore their ideas and
experiences, and they also seek tools to help them continue their search.
They come with the thought that Buddhism may have something to offer
them, though they are unsure just what that might be. At times I find
their eyes glued to the picture of my root guru, His Holiness, The Dalai
Lama, that hangs behind my desk or furtively glancing at the mala[1] that I
often wear around my wrist. I explain to them that I am not a scholar or
teacher of Buddhism, but merely a rather poor practitioner of an ancient
and powerful tradition of mind-training. I tell them that all I can do is to
share with them some Buddhist views and practices that have helped me
to deal with my own suffering as well as to engage with the suffering of
others. I also encourage them to meditate and walk with me and to begin
to wrestle with suffering inside and outside of themselves in different
ways than they have done before. I always try to arrange to introduce my
students to some of my Buddhist teachers and, whenever possible, we
attend teachings together.[2] Thus, this essay is the story of a teacher and
some of her students meditating and walking together on an engaged
Buddhist path in an advanced capitalist society.

## HOW DO WE LIVE?

My students and I must ponder the understanding that we live in a
world that is very similar and, at the same time, radically different from
any world that our fellow humans and other beings have shared in past
times and other places. Our world is the same one where the three omnipresent poisons of greed, hatred, and delusion have beset sentient beings since beginningless time as the cycle of birth, death, and rebirth
continues to revolve endlessly without regard to date or location (Dalai
Lama and Carriere, 1994). We also understand that our world is very different from other historical, and even some contemporary, worlds. It is a
world where the interrelated forces of capitalism, modernization, and
globalization have disconnected individuals from themselves, from one

another, and from the land in a way that has never been known before. This alienation has been accompanied by a severely reduced sense of social responsibility and accountability as well as by the emergence of new forms of individual and collective violence and alienation (Norberg-Hodge, 2000).

As my students and I consider these issues I remind them that, for those interested in walking the engaged Buddhist path, such meditations reinforce the importance of at least three familiar Buddhist practices. These three are: taking refuge; confessing negative or harmful thoughts, words, and deeds; and cultivating causes and conditions that will lead to the emergence of compassionate alternatives.

## REFUGE

In sharing the practice of taking refuge in the Buddha, the Dharma, and the Sangha[3] I like to frame this practice as a simple one that transcends sectarian and cultural values by interpreting it as finding a safe place where one can rely upon for support and guidance. This concept seems to resonate with, and provide the possibility of relief from, the typical mindset that my students bring with them. The words of one such student, a seasoned teacher-activist working in an inner city school, illustrate this sometimes desperate frame of mind. She told her classmates, "Sometimes I just want to give up! Everybody is so full of anger all the time that it is difficult to accomplish anything constructive. The moment we attain some desired goal everything seems to go up in flames. I no longer trust anything or anybody, including myself, to do what needs to be done to really help the children. I need to find time and space to think about what I am going to do with my life and with my teaching. This is why I came to this class."

During one session I related to my students how I had realized the tremendous power of refuge while participating in a Cuban exile delegation to Havana in 1979. The delegation was charged with negotiating the release of 3,500 political prisoners from Cuban jails.[4] I talked to them about the climate of mistrust among the delegates, some of whom had been prisoners themselves and were now having to negotiate with their former jailers in a location that brought to them so many painful memories. I shared with them how I had felt lost and with nothing to rely on while being intensely fearful that the other delegates and I would be unable to accomplish our very difficult task. One evening, I told the students, I went back to my room overlooking the Bay of Havana. From my room's window I could see my grandfather's home, now in ruins, and as tears flowed down my cheeks, I began to breathe slowly and consciously and to focus on taking refuge in the Buddha within myself, in the Dharma that is compassion, understanding, and love, and in the Sangha, that community of sentient beings, human and non-human, that walk with me and support me on the Buddhist path. When I awoke the following morning my fear had subsided considerably, and I went back to the meeting of the delegation with Fidel Castro and other Cuban government officials feeling settled and ready to face what needed to be faced. I was truly amazed at the power of such a simple practice. After relating this experience, I shared with my students some of the words of Vietnamese Zen teacher Nhat Hanh about refuge. He has written, "Whenever you feel confused, angry, or lost, if you practice mindful breathing and return to your island of self, you will be in a safe place, filled with warm sunlight, cool shade trees, and beautiful birds and flowers. Buddha is our mindfulness. Dharma is our conscious breathing. Sangha is our five aggregates[5] working together" (Nhat Hahn, 1998, p. 152).

After listening to my story some students seemed very skeptical, and one of them remarked, "That may have worked for you because you are a Buddhist, but I have no faith in the Buddha, the Dharma, or in the Sangha, so it will not work for me." I replied, paraphrasing to the best of my ability the words of Thich Nhat Hahn, that in Buddhism, faith does not mean accepting a practice or theory that we have not personally verified. Taking refuge is not blind faith but the fruit of practice. You can begin by breathing mindfully and taking refuge in the Buddha-nature of something familiar that gives you solace and feels particularly close and meaningful to you. You can take refuge in the Dharma of some encouraging words you have heard. You can seek refuge in a Sangha composed of trustworthy beings. As you continue to take refuge, the Buddha, the Dharma, and the Sangha will reveal themselves to you more fully. When I was finished with my mini-speech, skepticism had grown among some, as had the spirit of exploration among others. Several weeks later a few students reported that they had made a regular practice of taking refuge in their own way and that their experimentation had yielded interesting experiences. One student who worked as a teacher with homeless children in a shelter shared the following experience: "One night, when I was very depressed watching a little girl and her mother leave the shelter for a cold night in the streets, rather than becoming angry at the injustice of it all, as I often did, I began to breathe slowly and think of myself as taking refuge in a Jesus Christ dressed in rags, in his teachings of love, and in all the men and women who have worked with and for the poor and the dispossessed. Suddenly I felt an inner strength that I had not felt for years. I went out and looked for the little girl and her mother and took them home with me. When I went back to the shelter the next morning I knew that my life had begun to change. The work with the homeless is now longer a job or even a facet of my social justice activism. It has become my life. I do not know what the future holds, and in a way that seems less important than taking refuge every morning and every night. I am still active in fighting a system that condemns people to homelessness, but I feel I am now less angry. Most important, I am less paralyzed by it all. I seem to be more slowed down and that feels restful." Some of the students in the class nodded while other remained their skeptical selves.

## CONFESSION

My friend and Tibetan Buddhist scholar, José Ignacio Cabezón, in his reading of a UNESCO declaration on the role of religion in promoting a culture of peace, emphasized the importance, for Buddhists and for others, of drawing attention to the harm that we, as individuals and as a collective, have done and continue to do to others and to the world. He encouraged people to acknowledge and to take responsibility for such harm, to make it known publicly in what Tibetan Buddhists call "confession" (so sor bshags pa). Cabezón believes that this confessional practice can encourage us to seek to make restitution for the harm we have done as well as to seek forgiveness. In his opinion it is one way of renewing our commitment to the welfare of others (Cabezón, 1999).

Unlike the practice of taking refuge, confessional practice does not tend to resonate positively among the majority of my students. Some see it as a return to punitive patriarchal religious culture. Others see it as an inappropriate challenge to the conviction that it is "the system" that abuses, and that the majority of individuals are simply pawns (and victims) of this system. In addition, the idea that we have harmed, or continue to harm, other sentient beings and the world seems ridiculous to students who, though decrying many aspects of the Judeo-Christian tradition, adhere to the tenet that everything in the world is for the use of human beings. One student summed up this perspective by stating, "I am sure all of us are sorry for harmful things we may have done to others, but to dwell on it and make it public is a waste of time in an era where the system is abusing everyone. I also think that we can worry about trees and animals when we have taken care of human needs."

Finding the skillful means to work with those who conceptualize themselves as the abused, and never as abusers, and who remain unaware of non-human and ecological suffering, continues to be a challenge. Along with such a mind-set comes a strong tendency to reject any type of confessional practice. I have found that instead of focusing on the need for recognition and ownership of wrong-doing, it is sometimes more skillful to borrow from practices such as Naikan (Krech, 1999) with its emphasis on gratitude, or to encourage the expression of sadness for unthinking damage done to other beings. In this practice I suggest that a student recall all that a specific sentient being (human or non-human) or non-sentient entity (home, country, etc.) has done for him or her, and then what he or she has done for that sentient or non-sentient being. Only when the student seems ready (and this is a matter of intuition on my part) do I ask him or her to consider what troubles she or he has caused to the specific being under consideration. With the handful of students who are ready for a more confessional approach in their lives, I have held ceremonies in which they and I have quietly talked together about our common regrets and remorse. Through modeling I encourage their consideration of the suffering that we all may cause on an everyday basis in several realms of existence. I often focus, in the face of some of my students' snickering, on the suffering I have caused to animals by eating their flesh and using their skin as shoes. I speak also of the damage I do to the land and the planet through my consumerist lifestyle.

In contrast to my customary process in the past, in which the central focus of my courses was on moving directly to strategies for reducing collective suffering and resisting the lures of the aforementioned three poisons by fighting for social justice and for the restriction of consumption, I find that now my approach has become less hurried and, perhaps, more gentle. Meditating and walking with my students on an engaged Buddhist path, has meant that I only give attention to these action proposals after considerable work with the processes of taking refuge, gratitude, and confession. A former student who occasionally audits my courses described the difference between my current teaching approach and my previous one by saying, "Before there was such a sense of urgency, an urgency to act. The emphasis from the beginning was on individual and social change strategies and tactics. Now there is still a focus on resistance, reparation, and restitution, but there has been a shift to a consideration of our own role in our suffering and that of others and on finding a stable place within ourselves from which to act. I can't say that it is better or worse — just different, but I guess it makes sense to me."

## CULTIVATING CAUSES AND CONDITIONS

My students and I, embedded as we are in a society that promotes and nourishes delusion, hatred, and greed, are intent on finding other ways of living, learning, and dying within this lifetime. The philosophical school known as Madhyamika, referred to as "The Middle Way" within Mahayana Buddhism[6] gives us the understanding that being, non-being, doing, and all other phenomena have no inherent existence. They depend upon a complexity of causes and conditions for their emergence. Thus, simply wishing to live, learn, and die differently is not sufficient to bring about change. One must diligently cultivate the causes and conditions that will allow such alternatives to arise.

The means for beginning to cultivate the requisite causes and conditions for the development of alternatives to one's established habits of being and doing are complementary to the practices of refuge, gratitude, and confession. They also go hand-in-hand with the students' community work among oppressed people and communities. Because this approach shifts the focus from visible results to relatively invisible causes there is much less risk that emerging alternatives will be fetishized, commodified, and commercialized. Living, learning, and dying differently then can mean much deeper change than simply consuming "green" products, dressing more casually and adorning oneself with objects associated with a particular spiritual practice, or planning for a more "meaningful" death.

Cultivating the causes and conditions that can generate true alternatives is slow and difficult work in the context of late capitalism and accelerated globalization. It is a deep process of individual and group study accompanied by hands-on experimentation which may yield multiple and varied outcomes. For some individuals in this intensely materialistic society, the first counterhegemonic step may be a shift of focus from outward acquisition to inner cultivation. For others an initial step might be to look beyond their cocoons of privilege and face the suffering of proximate as well as distant others. For my students and myself, given our particular social locations of working directly with oppressed and exploited peoples and communities, the need to simultaneously cultivate both internal and external causes and conditions for the arising of alternatives seems necessary. Thus, together we have begun a search for like-minded people and alternative organizational forms from whom we can derive inspiration and/or with whom we can link in cultivating both the inner and the outer causes and conditions. One such organization is the Interfaith Order of Communion and Community[7] which provides common practices and precepts for several hundred participants around the globe, many of whom are incarcerated. The members, drawn from various religious groups but also including agnostics, take vows to abstain from killing, lying, stealing, sexual misconduct, and consumption of drugs or alcohol. They agree to engage in community service and social justice work and to meditate at pre-arranged times. The founders of the Order, social activist and ecumenical spiritual teacher Bo Lozoff and his wife Sita, live simply and communally as a personal response to planetary problems created by excess consumerism and debt. Lozoff realizes that all religions and wisdom traditions revolve around two primary spiritual principles, one dealing with inner cultivation and the other with the ethic of how we regard others. The organizational form that he has developed is anchored on the interrelation between the members' journeys of inner communion and their embarking on the outer path of community with others.

The exploration of the Interfaith Order and similar non-Buddhist as well as Buddhist organizations such as the Greyston Mandala[8] through the writings of their founders and members has helped in identifying vehicles and supports for cultivating causes and conditions for alternative modes of living, learning, and dying within our society. That exploration has also led to the surfacing of several fears among my students. One of the most salient of these fears concerns the feasibility and desirability of simple living and of communal living in particular. One of my younger students declared, "For me living simply or communally is old "hippie" stuff, and I see it as almost impossible in a capitalist society such as ours. I don't think we can have much of an impact on the society if we marginalize ourselves. I think living the way Lozoff lives is doing just that, marginalizing oneself."

Bo Lozoff, however, has written, "I am always struck by how strongly visitors seem to be affected by our simple daily practices — group meditation first thing each morning, then a brief spiritual reading led by one person; silence until breakfast; then a focused workday of joyful service, not chatting while we work or during meal preparation; little things like that. Small, enjoyable details to us who live here, but sometimes life-changing for the people who visit" (Lozoff, 2000). Distance and cost prevent me from organizing short visits to the home of the Lozoffs' Interfaith Order so that students can experience for themselves the joy of simple communal living informed by the practice of meditation and service. I believe that such visits, if they were possible, might serve to dispel some of my students' assumptions and fears. Instead, I encourage them to visit more local organizations which, though not imbued with a collective spiritual vision, are attempting to forge a new path in Southern California. One outstanding example is the Los Angeles EcoVillage,[9] whose members live simply, and in community, in several residential buildings north of the Koreatown area of Los Angeles. The organization is an ecologically sensitive association of culturally diverse individuals and families that, as a group, have had a tremendous positive impact in their own and surrounding neighborhoods, and have captured attention regionally and nationally. The group's practices of uncomplicated but mindful living have deeply affected some of my students, one of whom became a full-time resident shortly after her visit there.

## HOW DO WE LEARN?

Having studied for many years with Buddhist masters as well as with sages from other wisdom traditions, I have come to understand the importance of the energetic transactions between student and teacher and between these two and the communities in which both are embedded. The current which flows among these entities seems to be a critical element for learning. The current flows through and around structured, stable components of teacher/student/community relationships such as traditional monastic organization, standardized dharma instruction, and intense daily practice commitments, as well as more flexible, unpredictable elements of teaching-learning activities, such as a teaching being unexpectedly announced or cancelled, a ritual or ceremony scheduled without prior notice, or a retreat suddenly prescribed. The fluctuation of activity seems to parallel a fluctuation of potential or readiness for particular types of exchanges or interactions between student and teacher.

I have often experienced this current circulating between myself and students with whom I have been able to work closely. Together we have reflected upon the importance of recognizing and maintaining this principle of fluctuating learning potential within the contemporary academy. Practicing within this concept of fluctuation is often very difficult to accomplish with the emphasis in the university on strict temporal and spatial organization, fast thinking and disembodied learning. The standard academic environment requires that teaching and learning take place within rigid quarter or semester time frames and in the localized and constricted spaces of classrooms. The typical structures favor the sort of intelligence which involves explaining issues, constructing arguments, and solving problems in ways that keep learning separate from experiencing and doing.

For my students and I the maintenance of the principle of fluctuation of learning potentiality has brought about the need to challenge some of the above mentioned fundamental characteristics of the academy by experimenting with the development of non-mainstream forms of teaching-learning. These forms include such strategies as organizing teacher-student interaction in settings that are not normally recognized as "educational," allowing the cultivation of more relaxed attitudes, and recovering lost teaching and learning practices.

## GRASSROOTS SETTINGS

Whenever possible my students and I have organized our work together in settings that are not recognized as "educational" except in the context of narrow "service learning" agendas. These include settings populated by people who are, in a sense, counter-cultural in that they are place-bound, part of close-knit societies or sub-cultures, and not fully integrated into our industrial schooling complex. Some examples are enclaves within large urban areas of recent immigrants from mature cultures,[10] and ethnic minority communities whose values and everyday life practices are only partially anchored in the mainstream of the dominant population. Other such settings include contexts in which people have been voluntarily or involuntarily marginalized from the mainstream (e.g., "skid row", communes, gay, lesbian, and transgendered peoples' groups, etc.). It is in reference to these settings that the vernacular "grassroots" is often applied.

The reasoning behind the exploration of these different learning formats has two aspects. First, by involving ourselves as individuals and as a group in these "non-educational" or grassroots settings, we can develop intimate relationships with one another by engaging in diverse learning activities such as reflecting and contemplating on how to cease doing harm to others and to nature, sharing meals and casual conversation, and doing manual labor while awaiting the most propitious times to engage in other, perhaps more formal, teaching-learning processes. The words of an old student are instructive in explaining, "We came as a group with our teacher to spend some time among recent immigrants from Southern Mexico, and in the process we developed strong relations with each other. We learned some unexpected things including how to be of service to people, sometimes in surprising ways, while waiting for the right time to plunge into more formal academic work. At first it seemed strange to register for a class and then to be told to get out of the university and try to engage mindfully with people that I never dreamt had anything to teach me. I thought I already knew what I would see and hear from them. It is not like I had never before known people from indigenous areas of Mexico! In the first few weeks I often asked myself when the 'real learning' would start. It's been only recently that I've understood that there is no such thing as 'real learning'. There is only learning." Another student observed, "When I first met my teacher I was not as ready for sustained and formal interaction with her as I am now. My mind was too accelerated. The time I have taken just talking and being with people at a low-income housing project sort of settled me in, and I formed a bond with the other students and with the teacher in addition to the bonds with the people in the community. I also began to realize how some of the things that I do in my classroom and in my life can impact negatively on the lives of these people. That has made a real difference in my life and in my teaching."

Other students have been less enthralled with this particular approach to teaching and learning. One frustrated student protested, "I came here to get a Ph.D. behind my name, and if a teacher thinks I am not ready for formal work then they should not admit me into the program and take my money. Being among homeless people and having no research or intervention agenda, cleaning a bunch of alleys, planting a garden, and figuring out how "not to do evil" as a pre-requisite for getting on with my research is not my idea of graduate study." Another objected, "This is just one more way of delaying the social justice needed by oppressed people. We should do more strategic planning."

A second aspect in the reasoning for these different learning formats has been the need to alter somewhat the nature of my own and my students' already existing social activist agendas by emphasizing being with people in a relaxed, reciprocal manner without immediately trying to make them objects of our "service" or subjects for our research. This approach tends to bring about the discovery of other ways of knowing than the usual accelerated, focused, and goal-oriented style of cognition. These slower ways of knowing are essential in enabling us to recognize the gifts that others have to offer and the limits of our "expert" knowledge. That recognition is a necessary prerequisite to being able to craft a way of working with people that is not limited to the servicing of needs but which emphasizes the identification and mobilization of their capacities.

## SLOW MIND

Slow, non-deliberate, non-formal, and sporadic ways of knowing are more often than not devalued by students in their own lives and in their practices. As a colleague told me, "Our students are so busy trying to get ahead that telling them to relax the mind is like using a four letter word. They think only poets and saints can think and be that way. I also don't believe your friends in the faculty will be too happy to hear that you are in the business of slowing minds." Some students who are interested in the learning possibilities of "slow mind" approach it by expecting a cookbook of visualizations and meditative procedures through which they can immediately attain it. Though I do share with my students selected practices from my Buddhist training and encourage them to engage in other mindfulness exercises on their own, my teaching focus is on developing a different understanding of the mind and in creating learning environments in which the mind can become habituated to a slower more relaxed pace. Buddhist psychologist Guy Claxton has reminded us that "In order to rehabilitate slow ways of knowing, we need to adopt a different view of mind as a whole: one which embraces sources of knowledge that are less articulate, less conscious, and less predictable.... The crucial step in this recovery is not the acquisition of the psychological technology (brainstorming, visualization, mnemonics, and so on), but a revised understanding of the human mind, and the willingness to move into, and to enjoy, the life of the mind as it is lived in the shadowlands rather than under the bright lights of consciousness.... When the mind slows and relaxes, other ways of knowing automatically reappear" (Claxson, 1997, p. 13).

## RECOVERING OLD LEARNING PRACTICES

As we proceed in walking along an engaged Buddhist path some of my students realize the need, and demonstrate a willingness, to tackle some of the least recognized problems created by the schooling system in which we all participate. One such problem is the system's propensity to distance our bodies from our minds and to fragment our experiences. The students have identified pedagogies that contribute to this fragmentation by separating reading from talking, learning from doing, and knowledge from understanding, pedagogies that have been spawned by the ideology of literacy. Rather than merely resigning themselves to denouncing this ideology through articles, conference presentations, and other academic verbalizations likely to fall on deaf ears, the students have engaged in a series of "archaeological digs." These digs are intended to recover old learning practices from certain wisdom traditions and from the few remaining living mature cultures. What they have unearthed has caused them to question the universal worth of literacy itself and facilitated the rediscovery of the value and validity of orality as an educational process.

One discovery was that the advent of silent reading initiated the experience of learning about something without being in any way physically or experientially engaged with the object of learning. This represented a very significant change from learning by doing to learning by reading, in effect a separation of body from mind (Illich, 1992, pp. 113-114). As a small step toward the reintegration of mind and body the students have experimented with reading aloud both in class and when alone. Some, in spite of opposition, have been able to extend the experiment into their own classrooms and re-introduce reading aloud and reading while moving the lips as valuable practices. Those who have a bit older students have been able to have discussions with them about how and why silent reading practices have become so dominant and to question consequences such as the assumption that we act with our bodies but think with our minds. Some have also explored in their classes the processes of orality among members of mature cultures and how the last vestiges of oral traditions in those cultures is quickly being lost (Rasmussen, 2000). One student noted, "To inquire into the history and into the reasons given for the dominance of silent reading to the exclusion of other modes of reading in our society has been a formidable experience. To re-introduce in my high school class the value of reading aloud or of moving one's lips has been difficult but interesting in terms of the positive impact on my students' learning, their relations with each other, and the energy within the class. But the most amazing part of this experience is that I no longer make fun of my grandmother who comes from Oaxaca, Mexico, when she moves her lips while reading. I now know that for her reading always has been what it should be, a bodily as well as mental activity. Now I sort of envy rather than pity her."

The recovery of old learning practices which were integrative of body and mind has often led my students to further exploration of both ancient and contemporary ways of interacting with one another and with their students as fully integral beings. They have been able to experiment with some aspects of what Claudio Naranjo has called "integral education: an education of body, feelings, mind, and spirit" (Naranjo, 1994, p.67). Though not all reactions have been positive, some students have become enthusiastic about their experiments. One reports, "Reading aloud or silently moving my lips was for me the beginning of an interest in being more attuned to and working with my own body-mind as well as the body-minds of my students in a more sensitive way that I had done before. For the first time I have been able to identify and challenge some of the routine practices at my school that disciplined my students' bodies in ways that repress their minds. I have now begun to explore traditional models of energy work such as *Qi Gong* as well as some modern somatic education practices. I'm looking for possible applications in my own life as well as in my classroom work."

## HOW DO WE DIE?

Throughout our journey along a path that engages, with the transforming power of the Buddha's teachings, our own sufferings and those of countless other beings, my students and I carry a formidable walking stick, the walking stick of contemplations and reflections on death and dying. These contemplations and reflections take many forms such as the sharing of stories, critiques of academic and popular literature, mindfulness exercises, and working with those presently going through the dying process. These contemplations and reflections help us to familiarize ourselves with writings in the area of death and dying, to attend to issues of our own mortality, and to begin to engage in grief work. Reflecting in this way also helps us to discover the possibility and spiritual benefit of valuing *dukkha* (suffering, affliction) as true and noble, as the Buddha taught, particularly the affliction and suffering of the end of earthly life as we know it.

Recognizing the inescapable reality of death and of other unavoidable afflictions and sufferings tends to place our utopian idealisms, whereby we think we can attain happiness and well-being for ourselves and others through the implementation of our preferred reform or revolutionary projects, into a more realistic perspective. Ascertaining the nobility of affliction and suffering also transforms our view in several ways. Suffering, which so often brings about shame or judgement in some form, becomes worthy of respect as a simple and universal reality of life and a superb vehicle for spiritual practice. Suffering can then be understood a noble cause rather than something to be avoided at all costs. That certainly does not mean that one becomes fatalistic, hopeless, uncaring, or unfeeling. One is reminded of the Buddha's emphasis on compassion and the relief of suffering, but one then engages in that compassionate action with a more peaceful mind grounded in reality rather than from a grandiosity that is determined (usually with much anger) to "fix" society's problems. Looking deeply at the common experiences of suffering and affliction lets us observe the extremely powerful emotions that co-arise with negative conditions and situations, especially in the case of death and dying. The power of these emotions can be harnessed and transformed into positive efforts and compassionate action for the benefit of others.

History is replete with examples of people whose lives have been galvanized into compassionate action by unavoidable hardship or intolerable suffering. In a recent book Buddhist psychotherapist David Brazier highlights the life of Thich Nhat Hanh as an example of the power of redirecting the energy of suffering brought about by death. Brazier writes, "… after a particular awful day during the Vietnam War in which several of his friends had been killed he (Nhat Hanh) wrote, 'I hold my face in my two hands. No, I am not crying. I hold my face in my two hands, to keep the loneliness warm — two hands protecting, two hands nourishing, two hands preventing my soul from leaving me in anger.'" Brazier goes on to clarify that Master Nhat Hanh's words are not the words of one who is on the path of extinction. What is being illustrated is how the power of the emotions that co-arise with *dukkha* can be controlled and redirected to energize a vast amount of positive work. In this case it was Thich Nhat Hanh's work of helping refugees, boat people, orphans, and veterans, as well as whole villages and communities devastated by the Vietnam War. It was the use of the emotional energy surrounding the experience of death and dying to do something worthwhile while we are living for others who are still living (Brazier, 1998). Brazier also quotes the *Denkoroku* (Cleary, 1990), a Zen text of the early fourteenth century, and notes that many practitioners throughout the ages have used suffering, particularly the suffering of death and dying, as their driving force in walking the Buddhist path. Affliction and suffering, he says, provide the fuel that heats the fire without which spiritual life would remain feeble.

Coming to terms with and keeping mindfully conscious at all times of the very obvious fact that life naturally involves suffering and inevitably ends in death has not come easily to most inhabitants of the modern West and the modernizing East. Even less easy for us has been the task of sheltering the great energy that arises from affliction and suffering from the destructive winds of greed, hatred, anger, and delusion, winds which lead us to flee from afflictions and seek distractions, or worse, to lash out in rage. Such approaches not only ultimately fail, but also inevitably generate more suffering. Even the most affluent and powerful cannot buy or fight their way out of suffering. In a recent presentation at a conference held at the Drucker School of Management in Claremont, California, attended by corporate executives, business students, and managers of non-profit organizations, I departed from my prepared speech on asset-based community work and began to spontaneously share my understandings of the true and noble nature of affliction and suffering and of the energy that they can bring into our lives. My students watched with astonishment as conference participants who had pretty much ignored the earlier part of my talk and those of other speakers now began pay rapt attention to my remarks about suffering. They were rather amazed, as was I, at how my audience would not let go of the topic and proceeded to ask probing questions on how to develop the necessary character to welcome and value affliction and suffering. One student, a veteran of numerous radical struggles, commented, "For the first time I could see these privileged people as no different, at a fundamental level, from myself and from those with whom I work. Of course, at the relative level, I will continue fighting against them and what they stand for in this society. I realized in some deep way, though, that we all are in some form of the same predicament, and we are all trying to deal realistically with suffering. I guess I have to respect them for that."

Some of my students and I continue to try to humbly walk an engaged Buddhist path, patiently reflecting on how to live, learn, and die as we continue to experiment with multiple ways of doing so. As a source of inspiration through the sometimes difficult process of our journey, and in the hope that we might one day be able to truly incorporate its message into our hearts and deeds, we are guided by the prayer attributed to the Indian Buddhist sage Shantideva (1997, p. 169):

And now as long as space endures,
As long as there may be beings to be found,
May I continue likewise to remain,
To drive away the sorrow of the world.

## NOTES

1. Malas are necklace strings of 108 prayer beads used for Buddhist mantra recitation practice. When not being used to count mantras they are usually worn around the neck or wound around the wrist.

2. I am grateful to my teachers, the Venerables Geshe Lobsang Tsephel and Khenchen Thrangu Rinpoche for kindly agreeing to host and teach some of my students. I am also grateful to my teacher Master Si-Tu-jie, for instructing my students in the Fundamental Drill of the *Wei-Tuo Qi Gong* Buddhist lineage.

3. Fundamental to all schools of Buddhism is the practice of taking refuge in the Buddha, the Dharma (his teachings), and the Sangha (the ordained Buddhist community). These three entities are called the Three Precious Jewels or Gems because they are both rare and precious.

4. The first exile delegation to Cuba (1979) negotiated the release of 3,500 political prisoners and made possible the visits of exiles to the island for the first time in almost two decades. Two of the members of the delegation were executed upon their return to the United States by the extreme right wing of the Cuban community in exile. Many others, including the author, went into hiding for some time after being accused of communist collaboration and receiving death threats.

5. In Buddhism a human being is seen as composed of five aggregates or *skandhas*. These are: form, feeling, perceptions, mental formations, and consciousness.

6. Mahayana is a term used to describe a school of Buddhism based upon scriptures that appeared after the death of the historical Buddha Sakyamuni. It encourages practices based on compassion, emptiness, and interdependence. Madhyamika is one of the two main schools of the Mahayana tradition. The Madhyamika view was taught by the Buddha in the Perfection of Wisdom Sutra (texts).

7. The headquarters of the Interfaith Order of Communion and Community is at Kindness House, an interfaith community in North Carolina (USA).

8. The Greyston Mandala is the brainchild of Bernard Glassman, Roshi, and is located in Yonkers, New York (USA). It consists of a series

of self-sustaining social projects that assist homeless individuals and families, persons with AIDS and other people in need. The well-known Zen Peacemaker Order, which is committed to engaged Buddhism, was born within the Greyston Mandala.

9. Los Angeles Eco-Village, a member of a network of sustainable communities around the world, is coordinated by long-time ecological activist Lois Arkin.

10. Members of mature cultures do not grow up in a high-speed society experiencing placelessness and a mono-species and monogenerational existence. They are usually not plagued by feelings of pastlessness and by conflicts of identity. They tend to be fluent in conceptual pattern-languaged understandings.

## REFERENCES

Brazier, D (1998). *The Feeling Buddha: A Buddhist Psychology of Character, Adversity, and Passion*. New York: Fromm International.

Cabezón, J.I. (1999). The UNESCO Declaration: A Tibetan Buddhist perspective. In D.W. Chappell (Ed.) *Buddhist Peacework: Creating Cultures of Peace*. MA: Wisdom Publications, pp. 183-188.

Claxton, G. (1997). *Hare Brain/Tortoise Mind: How Intelligence Increases When You Think Less*. New Jersey: The Ecco Press.

Cleary, T. (1990). *Transmission of Light*. San Francisco: North Point Press.

Dalai Lama, H.H., and Carriere, J.C. (1994). *Violence and Compassion*. New York: Doubleday.

Illich, I. (1992). *Mirror of the Past: Lectures and Addresses*. New York: Marion Boyars.

Krech, G. (1999). *Naikan*. Vermont: To-Do Institute.

Lozoff, B. (2000). *It's a Meaningful Life — It Just Takes Practice*. New York: Viking Press.

Naranjo, C. (1994). *The End of Patriarchy and the Dawning of a Tri-Une Society*. Oakland: Amber Lotus.

Nhat Hanh, Thich (1998). *The Heart of Buddha's Teachings: Transforming Suffering into Peace, Joy, and Liberation*. Berkeley: Parallax Press.

Norberg-Hodge, H. (2000). Economics, Engagement, and Exploitation in Ladakh. *Tricycle: The Buddhist Review*, Winter 2000, pp. 77-79, 114-117.

Rasmussen, D. (2000). Dissolving Inuit Society Through Education and Money. *Interculture: International Journal of Intercultural and Transdisciplinary Research*, 139, 1-64.

Shantideva (1997). *The Way of the Bodhisattva*. Translated by the Padmakara Translation Group. Boston: Shambhala.

# CHAPTER 18

# Educating For a Deeper Sense of Self

## Understanding, Compassion, And Engaged Service

### John Donnelly

The whole idea of compassion is based on a keen awareness of the interdependence of all these living beings, which are all part of one another and all involved in one another.

(Thomas Merton)

One of the questions teachers are always asked is, "what is the purpose and meaning of education?" For me, it is relatively simple: *to make a difference*. How to achieve this goal begins with creating understanding.

#### UNDERSTANDING

Understanding does not mean formal literacy or separated disciplines, nor is its meaning related to standardized testing or national standards. Understanding unfolds in an appreciation of diversity and difference. It reveals its presence through imagination, creativity, and intuition. It flourishes through interrelationship and awareness, through harmony, tranquility, hope, and ultimately faith. Understanding reveals itself through a respect for the mosaic of all beings and all life, and it is through this understanding that we can begin to develop our own spiritual awareness.

… Spiritual experiences and development manifest as a deep connection to self and others, a sense of meaning and purpose in daily life, an experience of the wholeness and interdependence of life, a respite from the frenetic activity, pressure and over stimulation of contemporary life, the fullness of creative experience, and a profound respect for the numinous mystery of life. The most important, most valuable part of the person is his or her inner, subjective life — the self or the soul. (Gang, Lynn, and Maver, 1992: 114-115)

Education can be the vessel for this inner subjective life, for deep connection, for understanding. Education developed through a sense of understanding can lead to transformation that is both personal and universal in nature. This allows education to be a source of transformation. As Gatto stated (1992):

Whatever an education is, it should make you a unique individual, not a conformist; it should furnish you with an original spirit with which to tackle big challenges; it should allow you to find values which will be your roadmap to life; it should make you spiritually rich, a person who lives whatever you are doing, wherever you are. (75)

Through understanding we can also develop a sense of compassion.

## COMPASSION

Compassion is everywhere. Compassion is the world's richest energy source. Now that the world is a global village we need compassion more than ever — not for altruism's sake, nor for philosophy's sake or theology's sake, but for survival's sake. (Fox, 1979, p. i)

Compassion bases itself in caring and concern, and it deals with consequences and character. It is the thought and deed and direction from which purpose and meaning are generated. It is more than cognition. It is more than affect. It is a feeling that creates a sense of wholeness and integral understanding, and it is unconditional. Purpel (1989) goes on to state, when analyzing the works of Matthew Fox, that:

Compassion is feelings with moral meaning; its literal meaning of "suffering with" reveals profound understanding of the nature of being — that it is likely to involve pain and suffering, that the burdens are particularly severe when one is alone, and that it is part of the human nature to share burdens and efforts to ease them. It is the cluster of feelings that energizes our intellectual conceptions of justice as well as the statement of our deepest urges to love. Not to feel the connections with social and moral concerns is to locate the emotions we have in reacting to other people's woes in self-oriented, self-directed, ego-centered sentimentality. (pp. 42-43)

From an educational sense, compassion generates itself with the realization that one never acts alone and that suffering for one is suffering for all. It brings into question issues ranging from cooperation to competition and material acquisition. It is a sense, not a term. It is a feeling, not an intellectual concept. It is what we hope to generate from our students because they truly are the ones who have the ability to express "good" for all. The importance of compassion is the ability, as Daniel Quinn (1997) points out, to be a *"Leaver"* not a *"Taker"* (p. 52); to give from the heart and feel from the soul.

When there is inner understanding and compassion, one is moving from a deeper sense of self. It is this movement of self that seeks statement in engaged service.

## ENGAGED SERVICE

Engaged service emerges from the realization that one can create healing, allow for joy, participate in love, and radiate hope while developing from within and moving from without. Engaged service is more than just an act, it is a commitment. It is a commitment to life, to betterment, to self and other. It is a commitment to the realization that a singular act generated by a single individual is the pathway to heal the universe and that single steps are the root of all transformation. As Sandra Krystal (1999) points out:

The students do not have to learn about caring, compassion, and respect in contrived ways.... As a result of these real-life experiences that they reflect upon in the classroom, students develop compassion and respect both for themselves and for others. The programs in which they are involved connect them with their communities so they feel needed, contribute something to the adult world, and earn respect.... How is the spirit nurtured? From the feeling of accomplishment; from the knowing they have achieved goals; from the rewards of giving and realizing how much they have received; from knowing they have made a difference in someone's life or in the community; from discovering their special talents; from having fun and learning at the same time; from the tears shed at the end of the service experience; from knowing they are part of their community and will perform service in some form for the rest of their lives. (p. 61)

Engaged service is many things: It is a curriculum in which all may participate without the fear of separation, segregation, or evaluation. It is an action that can take place every moment of one's life. It is a dynamic force that connects education with living in a positive, palpable way. It comes from the soul and radiates outward in directions that can benefit all.

## Teaching for Understanding, Compassion, and Engaged Service

Gaining a deeper sense of self through understanding, compassion and engaged service is the most important principle that guides my life and allows me to have hope for all the lives that I have encountered.

My passion is working with children in the less advantaged countries where a knowing smile, an intuitive suggestion based on experience, a heart-felt presence can positively influence their education and their lives. The gift that I have received from them is the knowingness that there is hope for all and a way by which every child can be reached. This way is very simple: it is honoring the abilities that a child has and the space that the child is in at the moment. There is no such thing as a "high risk" student; there are only high risk institutions.

Children learn in a variety of manners and styles. Their intelligence is shown in many ways that go unmeasured simply for the sake of formal literacy requirements. When I think of successfully meeting a set of objectives, I don't think of grade point averages, or test scores. I think of children writing poetry, helping those who are less fortunate, and interacting with Nature. But I have to do more than think, I need to go deep within myself to know right action. I witness students' joy and satisfaction in their unique and creative statements; I hear their laughter and song and honor their ability to achieve peaceful resolution among themselves; and, I observe the wonder on their faces as they explore the unknown and make new discoveries in their own way, in their own time. I never know when a student will have these experiences, but I do know that in the right, supportive educational environment their dreams can become their reality and their accomplishments can spread hope to those who feel hopeless.

From my work with children with special needs, I have found that change is not gained through conventional educational or authority-based consciousness, but by cultivating imagination and creativity within each student; by encouraging their sense of moral and ethical judgment, empathy, individual thought, and societal concern; and by the teacher's own willingness to change and grow. Teaching like healing, goes both ways.

Many times, my students work best when taught the least. This sim-ply means that one should allow for individual attainment through self-actualization and individualized instruction. The elements of freedom, dignity and respect should be the overriding concerns of curriculum de-velopment. When I look through my students' folders, I realize that there can be a sense of attainment achieved that far surpasses the intellectual ability gained through an atomistic approach to individual develop-ment.

Students must be given their own source of knowledge through an ar-ray of varied experiences. This is consistent with a broader vision of ho-listic education. As Jack Miller (1988) points out:

> The focus of holistic education is on relationships — the rela-tionships between linear thinking and intuition, the relation-ship between mind and body, the relationship between the individual and the community, and the relationship between self and Self. In the holistic curriculum the student examines these relationships so that he/she gains both an awareness of them and the skills necessary to transform the relationships where it is appropriate. (p. 3)

As part of these varied experiences, students should be encouraged to develop a sense of ritual and celebration. This can be as simple as mark-ing the passing of time, the stages of life, or the accomplishment of goals. An example of a simple ritual comes from the different seasons. I like to take students to different places in nature. In the fall we go to a bird estu-ary and discuss migration and interrelationships of all species. During the winter, we go to local, snow covered mountains and do projects con-nected with the winter season, such as hibernation and the various shapes of snowflakes. In the spring, we go on a whale watching trip.

Finally, during the beginning of summer, we go to the tidal areas and view sea life and many of the migrating bird species that utilize the area during the summer months. Each student chooses a differing exhibit and the end of each season culminates with a change of classroom display and a discussion of nature's changes.

From these rituals and celebrations, children can get in touch with their own sense of the sacred, gain a feeling of communion and connectedness with others, and reach a state of contemplative knowing.

For all the practitioners who question the present educational system; you are not alone. It is very easy when questioning the present system to feel frustration rather than hope. When one stays in a state of frustration and anger, this process becomes counterproductive. It is helpful to take the broader view as outlined by David Purpel (1992):

> Those who willingly engage in a struggle for a better world do not, alas, constitute a majority, albeit they are a forceful and influential group. This group is highly diverse, critical, imaginative, skeptical, and creative — not the characteristics of homogeneity. Their vitality and idiosyncrasies are essential elements in the struggle for a world of freedom and justice for all people.... (25)

In our daily struggles and work, it is important for us to take a few moments to find that peaceful space within which we can quiet our mental activities and hear our intuitive voice, where we can contemplate and reflect, where we can pursue our deeper sense of self. We should move not only from our heads, but from our hearts, converting the wealth of our experiences into wisdom. Everyone does this in his or her own way. Some follow a deep meditation practice, others embrace differing belief systems that integrate body, mind and soul. For others including myself, "My work is my prayer."

## THE IMPORTANCE OF ENGAGED SERVICE

Why then engaged service? What purpose does it serve in education, and how does it help children? From my point of view, nothing replaces the application of human contact and intervention. I believe that students in secondary schools could benefit from two hours spent each day in engaged service.

What I have personally observed is the incredible turnaround that can occur when you allow individuals to work with others. Those with serious antisocial behavior find the empowerment and empathetic understanding they have been lacking when placed in a position of responsibility. I have seen children benefit from activities that range from peer tutoring, to landscaping, to caring for the elderly.

The opportunity to participate in engaged service can occur at any time. It is more a state of awareness than a structured activity. On one occasion during a field trip, ten of my students helped one student who was confined to a wheelchair gain mobility around a mountain camp that had not been adapted for children with specific physical needs. They assisted him off the bus, folded his wheelchair, set out his silverware at the table, and by splitting into three different teams, helped him hike on trails that were inaccessible to children with special needs. They then finished a full day of these activities by helping him get ready and go to bed. These students came together and worked together as a team, initiating the activities and taking full responsibility for the results. I doubt if any more love or concern could be shown by a group of students, and I am thankful to have been a part of this wonderful experience.

As a practitioner, I think the most difficult thing to realize is that no matter how hard you strive, no matter how many times you intervene, no matter how much you care, there will be students who will not reach all of the life-long goals you wish for them. It is emotionally challenging to see them writing poetry, having hands-on experiences at an aquarium, and feeling the awe of a museum one day, only to deal with the violence of the street, the dysfunction of families, and the anguish that can push them to acts of rage and self-destruction. I had one student, "Angel," who one day was writing poems about family, love, and relationships, and that afternoon was shot multiple times for standing on a street corner and claiming eight blocks of a neighborhood for his gang's territory. I had another student who empathetically helped challenged students within the community and after an evening's family discussion went out into the community and randomly fired on any individual that happened to be on the streets. One of the most tragic events for myself, is having to cope with one of my former students, some months after dropping out of school, taking his own life. It is painful to accept that some children have given up on life before they have had a childhood. This always causes one to speculate, "What could I have done differently?" or "How could I have intervened?" All one can ever do is to not give up hope.

Children around the world have a common bond: a thirst for understanding and knowledge. I have seen children in Thailand walk ten miles each way without shoes to get to a one room hut so they could practice their writing and gain communication skills. I have seen children in Indonesia rotate a textbook between fifteen individuals on a twenty-four hour basis so they could obtain a basic understanding of elementary mathematical principles. I know of teachers in Africa, who during war, drought, famine and other disasters, have stayed in their classrooms because they believed that the next day would be better as a result of this action, even at the ultimate cost of their lives.

## MAKING A DIFFERENCE

Education, to me, is not theory. It is not requirements. It is not lesson plans. Education is felt. It is shared. It is a commitment to all the children of the earth and to all the flora and fauna of the planet. It is the realization that holistic learning, spiritual practices, and sacred space are not elements to shy away from or fear, but instead are the bonds that hold all of us together. Education includes the understanding that the search for a deeper sense of self is not a passive activity. We know that curing the ills of the world may not come overnight. It may not come in a generation, or even in a century or a millennium. But I believe it will come, and it starts with each one of us: one teacher providing understanding to one student; one practitioner creating a compassionate act; one facilitator creating the opportunity for engaged service. Simply put: it is making the world better, one step at a time. As Gill (1989) stated:

> As long as there is strife and human suffering in the global village, there will be a need for educational reform. As long as there is a need for human rights and for an informed society, there will be a need to consider morality and literacy. Until all the world's citizens can function effectively in their native lands and be their "brother's keeper," there will be a need for educational change. The highest reward for a man's toil is not what he gets for it, but what he becomes by it. (p. 20-22)

There lives within each human spirit a sense of doing what is right. There is something that creates feelings of helpfulness, caring and giving. To this end every educator in every classroom throughout the world should strive to bring this sense of potential to each child they meet. As Purpel (1992) states:

> I believe that in order for individuals to be compassionate, they must be open to feel the inner impulse to feel connected to all people; people need to have a sense of freedom, agency, and hope. I further believe that those capacities are very much connected to living in a secure, nourishing, and joyful community.... The voice of the spirit that urges us to care for one another is more likely to be heard when we have enough to eat and drink, and a decent place to live, and when we are in good health. We are more likely to have enough to eat, have good health care, have peace, justice, equality when we are in touch with those powerful and mysterious impulses to dedicate ourselves to the creation of a world that is true, good, and beautiful. (p. 25)

Throughout our careers as teachers, it is important both to teach with conviction and to strive to be exemplary in our actions toward students. Whether we are teaching the multiplication tables or discussing the ethical implications of political interactions, we should promote an understanding that crosses socio-economic barriers. We should act in a compassionate manner that recognizes there is a standard by which we can interact, by which we can observe, and by which we can transform. For ourselves and for our students let us see, let us feel, let us *make a difference*.

A deeper sense of self is the feeling that I bring back from overseas and which I try convey to my students. No one, I believe, can remain untouched by the experience of going to a rural village in Cambodia and seeing children helping other children whose legs have been blown off by a land mine get to their classroom. No one can remain untouched by the experience of going to Nigeria or Uganda or the Central African Republic and passing frail children begging for water; or going to Brazil or Peru and watching children die from dysentery or other common diseases for the lack of a dollar's worth of medicine. These images go beyond all borders and take away all boundaries, leaving you with the realization that we are truly one people who suffer or grow as one entity, uplifted by compassion and understanding. If I can convey these feelings, thoughts, deeds and events to the children in my classroom, and have them act upon them, then I won't simply be replicating a standardized citizenship, but instead will be helping nurture the human spirit. I do not have to strive to create this, I just have to allow the spirit which we all possess to emerge — the same spirit that lights the morning, creates the tides, and enables us to be benefactors of our universe, the same spirit that moves us from deep inside to engage in service to humankind. Engaged Service *is* Compassion. As Ram Dass (1992) stated:

> Compassion in action is paradoxical and mysterious. It is absolute, yet continually changing. It accepts that everything is happening exactly as it should, and it works with a full-hearted commitment to change. It sets goals but knows that the process is all there is. It is joyful in the midst of suffering and hopeful in the face of overwhelming odds. It is simple in a world of complexity and confusion. It is done for others but nurtures the self.... Compassion is bringing our deepest truth into our actions, no matter how much the world seems to resist, because that is ultimately what we have to give this world and one another. (pp. 3-5)

These principles are brightening cities once blighted by squalor. Hands are reaching out to others who lack the sense of movement, smiles are creating kindness in turmoil and abuse. Envision a situation where children can be children again. I see the restoration of wilderness areas because humanity realizes at last that all ecology is one and that posterity resides within our children. I see children helping the elderly and those with Alzheimer's, as they make paper figures together, assist them with moving, read them stories, and bring them hot meals. Even very young children can help in hospitals, hospices, and other care facilities. They can help by simply by being themselves, sharing their innocence and faith that "life" can be better simply by trying. As the Dalai Lama (1999) reflected in prayer:

> May I become at all times, both now and forever
> A protector of those without protection
> A guide for those who have lost their way
> A ship for those with oceans to cross
> A bridge for those with rivers to cross
> A sanctuary for those in danger
> A lamp for those without light
> A place of refuge for those who lack shelter
> And a servant to all in need. (p. 237)

We can build houses and shelters for those who have none. We can create homes for the homeless, protection from the storm, and personal space for those who have only known the streets as the beast of chaos. If children can selflessly help other children on and off buses, to touch the sand, feel the water, or honor the wind and breeze as it caresses their face, then we will have created a curriculum that is dedicated, not to rudimentary knowledge, but to the creative force within each one of us. When we accomplish these things, then we truly have an educational system dedicated to learning and the realization of a higher calling.

If you want to stimulate a deeper sense of self within your students, look to the pockets of poverty, look to the have-nots. Guide your children in the exploration of these areas through field trips, the internet, school partnership programs, international counterparts, and the inspiration of their own hearts. By doing so, you affirm what I feel is most important for children: creating a sense of connection. With this, they have the opportunity to shift their perception of life from one of survival or mere existence to one of hope and regeneration. They find the tools to improve their lives by broadening and reframing their experiences. As Devall and Sessions (1985) point out:

> Spiritual growth, or unfolding, begins when we cease to understand or see ourselves as isolated and narrow competing egos and begin to identify with other humans, from our family and friends to, eventually, our species. A nurturing non-dominating society can help in the "real work" of becoming a whole person. The "real work" can be summarized symbolically as the realization of "self-in-Self," where "Self" stands for organic wholeness…. Biocentric equality is intimately related to the all-inclusive Self-realization in the sense that if we harm the rest of Nature then we are harming ourselves. There are no boundaries and everything is interrelated. (pp. 66-67)

## LOOK TO THE CHILDREN

Look to the children and they will show us the way. Ask them what they need, do not explain to them what they want. Ask them how they can help, do not tell them what is required. Make the subject of the day a life that can be enhanced. Allow children to dream, allow children to run free, allow children to have their own answers to complex questions. Approach learning in an interdisciplinary manner that links body, mind, heart and soul. As Michael Murphy (1992) states:

We need to develop integral practices, which I define as transformative practices that address the somatic, affective, cognitive, volitional and transpersonal dimensions of human nature in a comprehensive way.... If we focus on our inter-development and bring forth our extraordinary capacities, we can learn to live more lightly on the earth, conserve the World's precious resources, and find meaning and delight through an inner-directed, more compassionate approach to life. (pp. 171-173)

This can be done through a multitude of activities. We must look to the children for our answers. We must integrate their voices into our process of education. We must teach that violence is not a solution as much as we teach the history of the Civil War. The understanding of sentence structure should be no more important than the realization that peace and prosperity on Earth are our consummate goals. If we understand the functions of the physical body, we must be able to understand that starvation in Rwanda, the Balkans, or India is abhorrent and unacceptable. If we understand that a grade point average is important to get into a chosen institution of higher learning, we must be able to understand that compassionate reasoning, integral learning, spiritual quests, and a sense of the sacred create what truly is the essence of the human spirit.

Throughout my life, my love of education has joined with my love of people to teach me that there are abundant opportunities for learning and growth. I find the beauty and depth of indigenous cultures around the world as fulfilling and exciting as the most celebrated museums, the most diverse art galleries, and the latest technological advancements. I feel as much joy in seeing children with limited means rolling in the grass, swimming in ponds, or hugging one another as I do with well-dressed children playing in the park. I believe that we are all conceived as a vehicle of beauty and a conveyance of good. Transformation happens every day, in every moment, whether or not we are conscious of it. It can start with ourselves and continue with our students, or it can start with our students and continue with ourselves. It is something we can work on every day, starting with ourselves, and continuing with our students. A solitary act of kindness can lead to outcomes beyond our greatest expectation. We must hold the intent to be the best practitioners that we can be. By being ourselves and living in integrity and truth, we can positively influence all whom we touch.

In conclusion, we need to create new patterns in education: patterns that convey and encourage the good of all people; patterns that make learning something students want to participate in; patterns based on a philosophy of hope rather than fear, on initiative rather than force, on love rather than hate. In order to do this, we must look to ourselves. Then we must look to each other and to the children. As Stephanie Chase (1998) foresaw:

> Children of the earth, come out of the darkness — light your candles from the stars.... Keep vigil for all the world. Let no heart deny the other ... let your love be the sign of peace made visible. (p. 183)

We must look to the heavens. We must look to the earth. We must look within. The answer is in us. The answer is us. We are the solution. I pray that we may all be an active force for educational change, and find that deeper sense of self from which all is possible.

## REFERENCES

Chase, S. in Crowell, S., Renate N. Caine, and Geoffrey Caine. (1998) *The Re-Enchantment of Learning*. Tucson, AZ: Zephyr Press.

Dalai Lama (1999) *Ethics for the New Millennium*. New York: Penguin Putnam.

Dass, R. and Mirabia Bush (1992) *Compassion in Action: Setting Out on the Path of Service*. NY, NY: Bell Tower.

Deval, B. and G. Sessions. (1985). *Deep Ecology: Living as if Nature Mattered*. Layton, Utah: Gibbs Smith.

Fox, M. (1979). *A Spirituality Named Compassion and the Healing of the Global Village*. Minneapolis: Winston Press.

Gang, P., Lynn, N., and Maver, D. (1992). *Conscious Education: the Bridge to Freedom*. Atlanta: Dagaz Press.

Gatto, J. (1992). *Dumbing Us Down : The Hidden Curriculum of Compulsory Schooling*. Gabriola Island, B.C. Canada: New Society Publishers.

Gill, W. (1989). Proper Behavior for the 21st Century in Our Global Village. *MiddleSchool Journal*. (21).

Krystal, S. (1998/1999). The Nurturing Potential of Service Learning. *Educational Leadership*. Vol 56, (4),

Miller, J. (1988). *The Holistic Curriculum*. Toronto: OISE Press.

Murphy, M. (1993). "Integral Practices: Body, Heart, and Mind" in Roger Walsh and Frances Vaughn (Eds.) *Paths Beyond Ego: The Transpersonal Vision*. Los Angeles, CA: Putnam Publishing group.

Purpel, D.E. (1989). *The Moral and Spiritual Crisis in Education: A Curriculum For justice and Compassion in Education*. Granby, MA: Bergin & Garvey.

Purpel, D.E. (1992). Bridges Across Muddy Waters: A Heuristic Approach to Consensus. *Holistic Education Review*. Vol. 5(1).

Quinn, D. (1997.) *My Ishmael*. New York: Bantam.

# Conclusion

## Yoshiharu Nakagawa

> The ignorant man is not the unlearned, but he who does not know himself, and the learned man is stupid when he relies on books, on knowledge and on authority to give him understanding. Understanding comes only through self-knowledge, which is awareness of one's total psychological process. Thus education, in the true sense, is the understanding of oneself, for it is within each one of us that the whole of existence is gathered.
> (J. Krishnamurti)

Growing discussions about "spirituality in education" have gradually made us recognize that the exclusion of spirituality from education may have caused some of the suffering we face today. Introducing spirituality into education could resolve some of the difficulties we face in our educational practices. Spiritual hunger is one of the deepest needs to be met in our life, and to gratify this spiritual need would provide a basis upon which we could live more completely. In this sense, spirituality is at the core of our existence. Education that tries to actualize our wholeness needs to involve spirituality as its essential component.

As a crucial problem, modern education has been based on a narrow vision of the human being. Infused with an overwhelming worldview of materialism, it fails to see the spiritual aspects of the human being, reducing us to the level of material existence. Also, a large part of mainstream pedagogy has been inclined to identify the human being within a solely socio-cultural context which also has contributed to narrowing human potentialities. Therefore, educational practices have stressed developing the materialistic and socio-cultural aspects of being a human. The narrow framework of modern education cannot meet spiritual needs that arise from our deepest heart, causing a variety of spiritual sufferings including meaninglessness, anxiety, and malaise.

Discussions about spirituality in education could lead to a radical transformation of our vision of education to encompass the wholeness of our life. Given today's situation in which we have few studies in this relevant field, the publication of this book, *Nurturing Our Wholeness: Perspectives on Spirituality in Education*, could be a significant contribution to increasing our knowledge and understanding about spirituality in education. Drawing upon various traditions, great teachers, and personal experiences, the authors respectively explore what is meant by "spirituality" and the practical implication for education. Thanks to the efforts of the authors who are committed to spiritual cultivation for themselves and their students, this book describes a wide variety of spiritually-oriented philosophies and practices in education. It is true that this volume is not comprehensive enough to include every possible approach, but it can serve as a steppingstone to further studies.

Here I am tempted to introduce a term "pedagogy of spirituality" to address this growing discipline which acknowledges the importance of spiritual cultivation in the whole enterprise of education.

The pedagogy of spirituality can explore the nature of spirituality in relation to education as a whole and examine what kinds of practices are useful for spiritual cultivation. Spirituality is a complex subject that involves attitudes toward spiritual development, experiential processes during spiritual cultivation, transformative moments called "enlightenment" and "awakening," and expressive actions flowing from the awakening process. The pedagogy of spirituality can see the importance of spiritual development under the perspective of lifelong education. It can design curricula for spiritual development with connection to other educational practices. It can also show the need for spiritual cultivation in teacher training programs. In this way, the pedagogy of spirituality can develop theoretical models and practical ways of a spiritually-oriented education.

To fulfill these tasks, the pedagogy of spirituality needs to learn from various sources. Among them, this book refers to traditions and teachers from East and West as well as personal experiences of the authors.

It is important to acknowledge here that the Western tradition of pedagogy gives a rich source for the pedagogy of spirituality. For example, Socrates and Plato laid a foundation of spiritually-oriented education in their educational activities and philosophies. Johann Amos Comenius (1592-1670), the great founder of didactics, developed a philosophical and pedagogical system of what he called "pansophia," a holistic system inspired by Christian mysticism. Friedrich Froebel (1782-1852), the originator of the kindergarten, conceived a mystical philosophy of child education. The "cosmic education" addressed by Maria Montessori involved ideas put forth in the circle of Theosophy. The pedagogy of spirituality needs to examine the history of pedagogy in a new light of spirituality.

The pedagogy of spirituality can learn best from those authentic thinkers and mystics who realized spiritual qualities within themselves and also engaged in education. This book includes some of them – Aurobindo, Tagore, Krishnamurti, Emerson, Thoreau, Alcott, Steiner, Merton, Buber, Huxley, Bennett, and Montessori. Unfortunately, mainstream pedagogy has so far largely ignored their work on education and paid no serious attention to the gifts they have given us. It is time for mainstream pedagogy to include these important thinkers.

The pedagogy of spirituality can also learn from the wisdom traditions around the world, including Hinduism, Buddhism, Zen, Taoism, Sufism, Tantra, Gnosticism, Jewish mysticism, Christian mysticism, and others (e.g., Nakagawa, 2000). This book discusses some of them along with Tibetan Buddhism, the Quakers, and the Hebrew Prophets. Indigenous teachings of living and learning are also a great source for developing the pedagogy of spirituality, for they provide balanced visions between community, spirituality, and nature. The wisdom traditions are storehouses that accumulated numerous methods of contemplation as well as comprehensive philosophies. In this respect, the pedagogy of spirituality can walk hand in hand with transpersonal psychology, for it has explored the wisdom traditions with new perspectives accessible to our contemporary mind. History shows that "transpersonal education" did not develop adequately but a pedagogy of spirituality could develop the educational part of transpersonal psychology.

The pedagogy of spirituality can provide useful maps for spiritually-oriented education. We definitely need a map to start an inner journey; however, it must be remembered that we often confuse the map with the terrain. A map is like a finger pointing to the moon, while what we need to see is the moon itself. The pedagogy of spirituality has to be aware of the paradox that personal experiences of spirituality ultimately go beyond any definitions, patterns, or theories that can be written in a book, for the human being is infinitely open in the deepest level of being. Spirituality seems to imply this infinite openness disclosed directly in our deepest existence.

## REFERENCES

ASCD. (December 1998/ January 1999). *Educational Leadership.* Issue: The Spirit of Education. Vol. 56, (4).

Bennet, J. G., et al. (1984). *The Spiritual Hunger of the Modern Child.* Charles Town, WV: Claymont Communications.

Glazer, S. (Ed.). (1999). *The Heart of Learning: Spirituality in Education.* New York: Jeremy P. Tarcher/Putnam, Penguin Putnam Inc.

Hendricks, G., & Fadiman, J. (Ed.). (1976). *Transpersonal Education: A Curriculum for Feeling and Being.* Englewood Cliffs, NJ: Prentice-Hall.

Kane, J., & Snauwaert, D. (2000). Editorial: Defining the "spiritual" in spirituality and education: Critical realism, religious pluralism, and Self-realization. *Encounter, 13*(4), 2-3.

Krishnamurti, J. (1953). *Education and the Significance of Life.* New York: Harper & Row.

Lerner, M. (2000). *Spirit Matters.* Charlottesville, VA: Hampton Roads.

Nakagawa, Y. (2000). *Education for Awakening: An Eastern Approach to Holistic Education.* Brandon, VT: Foundation for Educational Renewal.

Teasdale, W. (1999). *The Mystic Heart: Discovering A Universal Spirituality in the World's Religions.* Novato, CA: New World Library.

Walsh, R. (1999). *Essential Spirituality: The 7 Central Practices to Awaken Heart and Mind.* New York: John Wiley & Sons.

Wilber, K. (1997). *The Eye of Spirit: An Integral Vision for a World Gone Slightly Mad.* Boston: Shambhala.

# Biographies of Contributors

## LOURDES ARGÜELLES

Lourdes Arguelles (Ph.D., New York University) is Professor of Education, Claremont Graduate University. She is also a psychotherapist and community organizer working to enable individual and collective resistance to globalization and industrial ways of living, learning, and dying. Arguelles is a Buddhist practitioner in the Tibetan tradition. A former member of the Board of Directors of the Buddhist Peace Fellowship and a founding member of the Spirituality in Education Network, her work has appeared in academic and popular journals around the world. She lives with her life companion, Anne Rivero, in the San Jacinto Mountains of Southern California. She can be reached at idyllcuban@aol.com.

## RICHARD C. BROWN

A practicing Buddhist since 1978, Richard integrates Tibetan contemplative principles and practices into contemporary teaching and learning. Richard has been an educational therapist, a public elementary teacher, and a contemplative K-8 teacher. He led in establishing the contemplative Shotoku School at Rocky Mountain Shambhala Center. In 1990 he founded the Department of Education at Naropa University, including an undergraduate degree in Early Childhood Education and a Masters in Contemplative Education. He has been actively involved in holistic and spirituality in education movements since 1990.

## SAM CROWELL

Sam Crowell is a professor at California State University and a member of the Spirituality and Education Network. He founded and coordinated a Master's degree program in Integrative Studies. He is a poet, writer, naturalist, and consultant. His latest book is *The Reenchantment of Learning*.

## THOMAS DEL PRETE

Thomas Del Prete is past president of the International Thomas Merton Society and author of several articles on Merton and education, as well as *Thomas Merton and the Education of the Whole Person*, for which he was recognized with the Society's award for "scholarship and fresh insight into Merton studies." A former secondary school teacher, he currently serves as Director of the Hiatt Center for Urban Education and Chair of the Education Department at Clark University in Worcester, Massachusetts. In these roles he has sought to form learning communities among diverse groups within and across traditional institutional borders. He coordinates a school-community-university partnership focused on urban teacher education and education reform. He is recipient of Clark University's "John W. Lund Community Achievement Award."

## JOHN DONNELLY

John Donnelly is a Special Needs teacher in Anaheim, California. He is also Director of the International Foundation for Social and Educational Dimensions which works with schools in Europe and Asia.

## SCOTT H. FORBES

Scott H. Forbes taught at Brockwood Park, the Krishnamurti School in England for 10 years. He was also Principal at the school for 10 years. He recently completed a doctorate at Oxford and is now working at EnCompass in California.

## JEFFREY KANE

Jeffrey Kane is the Dean of the C. W. Post School of Education. He has written essays and articles on existential issues in teaching and on educational policy. Most recently, he edited and contributed to the book, *Education, Information and Transformation: Essays on Learning and Thinking*, published by Merrill/Prentice Hall. Dr. Kane also serves as Editor of the journal, *Encounter: Education for Meaning and Social Justice*. Earlier in his career, he was a classroom teacher in the Rudolf Steiner School in New York City. He lives on Long Island with his wife, Janet, and three children.

## Takuya Kaneda

Takuya Kaneda, Associate Professor of Art Education, at Otsuma Women's University in Tokyo, spent a number of years in India and Nepal doing research as well as visiting Tagore's school at Santiniketan. He was a visiting teacher at J. Krishnamurti's Rishi Valley School in India in 1999. He has written many articles on art and education.

## Rachael Kessler

Rachael Kessler, whom Daniel Goleman called a "leader in a new movement for emotional literacy," is Director of the Institute for Social and Emotional Learning in Boulder, Colorado, and consults on curriculum, staff training, and organizational development for schools and communities. Kessler is a co-author of *Promoting Social and Emotional Learning: Guidelines for Educators* (ASCD, 1997) and author of *The Soul of Education: Helping Students Find Connection, Compassion, and Character at School* (ASCD 2000). Her work has been supported and endorsed by educators and civic leaders from across the spectrum of belief. She lives in Boulder with her husband, Mark Gerzon, and three sons.

## Kathleen Kesson

Kathleen Kesson is Director of Teacher Education at Goddard College, an historic progressive college in Plainfield, Vermont. She also holds an appointment as Research Associate Professor at the University of Vermont, where she directs the John Dewey Project on Progressive Education. She has written extensively on the topics of spirituality, holistic education, and democracy for academic journals and edited books, and is the author (with Jim Henderson) of the book *Understanding Democratic Curriculum Leadership* (Teachers College Press, 1999).

## Karen Litfin

Karen Litfin is an associate professor of political science at the University of Washington where she teaches and writes about global environmental issues. She has a strong interest in the social and political dimensions of Sri Aurobindo's approach to spiritual life.

## Bob London

Bob London is a professor of education at California State University, San Bernardino. For over 25 years he has been a student and teacher of the process of spiritual transformation, primarily in the tradition of G. I.

Gurdjieff and John Bennett. Professionally, his interests include the process of problem solving from a spiritual perspective, strengthening our connection with nature, and identifying principles of education consistent with a variety of spiritual traditions. He is the founder and chair of both the Spirituality and Education Network, an international collaborative group studying the implications of a spiritual perspective in education, and the AERA Spirituality and Education SIG.

### DAVID MARSHAK

David Marshak is an associate professor in the School of Education at Seattle University. He is the author of *The Common Vision: Parenting and Educating for Wholeness* (Peter Lang Publishing, 1997), an exploration of the teachings of Sri Aurobindo, Rudolf Steiner, and Hazrat Inayat Khan about human nature and human unfoldment — and an explication of the "common vision" of these three teachers.

### JOHN (JACK) P. MILLER

John (Jack) P. Miller has worked in the area of humanistic/holistic education for 30 years. Currently he is Professor and Coordinator of the Holistic and Aesthetic Education Focus at the Ontario Institute for Studies in Education at the University of Toronto. He is author of ten books including *Education and the Soul* and *The Holistic Curriculum*. The latter book has been translated into Japanese and Korean and Jack has traveled frequently to Asia to work with holistic educators there.

### RON MILLER

Ron Miller is currently the Executive Editor of *Paths of Learning* magazine and President of the Foundation for Educational Renewal. Previously he was founding editor of *Holistic Education Review* (now called *Encounter*). He is a historian of alternative and progressive educational movements and has written or edited six books, including *What Are Schools For? Holistic Education in American Culture* and *Caring For New Life: Essays on Holistic Education*. He is also a co-founder of the Bellwether School near Burlington, Vermont.

### YOSHIHARU NAKAGAWA

Yoshiharu Nakagawa is an associate professor at Ritsumeikan University in Kyoto, Japan. He holds a Ph.D. from the Ontario Institute for Studies in Education of the University of Toronto. His current concerns involve holistic education, spirituality, and Eastern philosophy. He is also the vice-president of the Japan Holistic Education Society. He is the author of *Education for Awakening: An Eastern Approach to Holistic Education* (The Foundation for Educational Renewal, 2000).

## DAVID E. PURPEL

David Purpel is Professor of Education at the University of North Carolina, Greensboro, and author of several books including *The Moral and Spiritual Crisis in Education*.

## ATSUHIKO YOSHIDA

Atsuhiko Yoshida is a professor at Osaka Women's University in Japan. He is the author and co-author of several books, including *The Holistic Education: Philosophy and Movement, Waldorf inspired Education in Japan, Inquiries into the Psychology of Religion, Cosmology of the Child, Introduction to Holistic Education*. He is the President of the Japan Holistic Education Society.